DANIEL W. FOSTER, M.D.

A Layman's Guide to

Modern Medicine

SIMON AND SCHUSTER · NEW YORK

PUBLISHED BY SIMON AND SCHUSTER
A DIVISION OF GULF & WESTERN CORPORATION
SIMON & SCHUSTER BUILDING
ROCKEFELLER CENTER
1230 AVENUE OF THE AMERICAS
NEW YORK, NEW YORK 10020
SIMON AND SCHUSTER AND COLOPHON ARE
TRADEMARKS OF SIMON & SCHUSTER

DESIGNED BY EVE METZ
MANUFACTURED IN THE UNITED STATES OF AMERICA

1   2   3   4   5   6   7   8   9   10

LIBRARY OF CONGRESS CATALOGING IN PUBLICATION DATA

FOSTER, DANIEL W.
A LAYMAN'S GUIDE TO MODERN MEDICINE
INCLUDES INDEX.
1. MEDICINE, POPULAR.   I. TITLE.   [DNLM:
1. MEDICINE—POPULAR WORKS.   WB130.3 F754M]
RC81.F782   610   79-28399
ISBN 0-671-24366-7

*For Dorothy, Danny, Mike and Chris, wife and sons
who have given me continual joy.*

Contents

Preface

ON THE FACE it might seem strange for a professor of medicine and working scientist to attempt a book on medicine for non-physicians. I would like to explain its genesis. In 1973, in response to the request of KERA-TV, the Public Broadcasting channel for Dallas-Ft. Worth, and Dr. Charles C. Sprague, President of the University of Texas Health Science Center at Dallas, I became host of a weekly television series on medicine. On each program a guest authority and I discussed a major medical topic in serious fashion—the content was not much different from a presentation for physicians, but a major effort was made to avoid scientific jargon. Put simply, we tried to communicate top-grade information in understandable language. Subsequently the program was carried nationally on the Public Broadcasting System. Shortly after the first episode was aired in New York City, I was contacted by Bill Adler, a literary agent in Manhattan, who said very simply, "I think you ought to write a book." Because of time constraints (I had not given up any of my teaching, research, editorial or government advisory duties despite the demands of the television program), I was hesitant. Yet I knew from innumerable personal conversations and letters that there was a widespread interest in obtaining sound medical information. The quest for facts becomes particularly urgent if one is himself ill or if there is disease in a significant other. Endless questions arise: "What did he mean by heart failure?" "What is an arteriogram?" "What does BUN

9

mean?" "How does chemotherapy work?" Answers to such questions can and should be provided by the personal physician. But the physician is busy. Moreover, he or she is available only to the sick while one may wish to learn about medicine out of intrinsic interest.

Perusal of currently available books on medicine indicated that an adequate, up-to-date reference source was not available. Almost all published material dealt with narrow subjects or fad topics, and essentially none was written by an author with scientific credentials. On the basis of these considerations, I fairly early on became convinced that a broader book on medicine containing reliable information might be helpful to a significant number of people. I was less sure that I wanted to be the one to attempt it. In the end, however, I decided to give it a try. My academic background had equipped me to know good medicine from bad and scientific fact from fantasy. In addition I had been moderately successful doing the same thing on television. I finally told Bill Adler I would write it if he could find a publisher. Simon and Schuster said yes and so the book was started.

A word about intent. It was not my aim to produce a comprehensive medical encyclopedia. Rather, I wanted to give a summary view of modern medicine that concentrated on the description of normal physiology and explained the nature of the common diseases of Western man. In this sense what is presented is the central core of medicine rather than the far perimeters occupied by rare afflictions. Much that constitutes the disciplines of pediatrics, obstetrics and gynecology, surgery, psychiatry and a variety of subspecialties has been omitted because of problems of space and limitations in my own experience in these areas.

When one writes in the scientific literature, all statements are buttressed by presentation of data or reference to published work. I have chosen not to do so here since the necessary bibliography would be nearly as long as the book. However, I have tried to make no statement that is not consistent with available experimental evidence and have attempted to identify those areas where speculation exceeds the bounds warranted by current research.

It is my hope that the book will be considered balanced by my peers and both useful and interesting to the reader who is not a physician. Having spent my entire professional life in teaching, research and care of the sick, I would be disappointed if the lessons learned were not worth sharing.

It has been an honor for me to work the last 17 years in what I consider to be one of the great departments of Medicine in the world. Much of what I know was taught me by my distinguished colleagues in that department. I also wish to express gratitude to my scientific collaborator and friend, Dr. J. Denis McGarry. Over the past few years he has carried (always cheerfully) a vastly disproportionate load in our own research activities. Finally, Ms. Rita Koger was entirely responsible, from first draft to last, for the preparation of the manuscript. I deeply appreciate her care and concern.

DANIEL W. FOSTER, M.D.

1

Modern Medicine:
Achievements and Problems

THE ACHIEVEMENTS

The accomplishments of biomedical research and their clinical application in the past five decades can only be described as dazzling. The roots of medicine can be traced to the time of the New Stone Age (perhaps as early as 9000 B.C.) when trephination—the cutting of a hole in the skull—was carried out, presumably to allow demons (schizophrenia? epilepsy?) to escape. Yet the explosive age of scientific medicine did not begin until the third decade of the 20th century with the discovery of insulin for the treatment of diabetes mellitus. It is almost incredible that so much happened in a period of 50 years. Antibiotics were discovered and now almost every infectious disease of man can be specifically treated. The disciplines of microbiology and immunology eliminated the threat of poliomyelitis and provided the means to protect against an increasingly larger number of serious infectious diseases. Even now new vaccines against certain forms of meningitis and pneumonia are being prepared. Surgical techniques of astonishing complexity have been developed, and essentially no area of the body is currently beyond the surgeon's reach. Even the tiniest infant can be successfully operated upon. The genetic code was broken and the science of molecular biology, with all its promises, was born. Organ transplantation became a reality and dozens of hormones were identified and synthesized. Psychotropic drugs were discovered and revolutionized the treatment of mental illness. Even unsolved problems such as cancer and heart disease have been restricted in their scope. One-third to one-half of patients with acute lymphocytic leukemia can now be cured, and chemotherapeutic procedures have drastically prolonged life in patients with cancer of the breast and other tumors. The rampant increase in coronary artery disease has been slowed through widespread adoption of low-fat diets and education regarding the hazards of smoking, high blood pressure and stress. Diagnostic procedures have become increasingly specific. At the turn of the century, illness was recognized only through the physician's use of his five senses and the memory of previous experience. Now precise laboratory tests are available for almost every disease. The development of radioimmunoassay techniques has allowed accurate measurement of hormones and other important constituents of blood and tissue in quantities as low as one trillionth of a gram. Technological applications of electronics and physics have produced sophisticated instrumentation such as the computerized axial tomographic (CAT) scanner, which transforms X-rays of the head and body cavities into photographlike projections of their constituent parts. Hundreds of other examples could be given. In short every area of medicine has seen tremendous advances and the end is not in sight.

THE ROLE OF RESEARCH

The accomplishments just described and the evolution of medicine from an empiric discipline (with little to offer except kindness and comfort) into a powerful semi-science can, without argument, be attributed exclusively to the biomedical research apparatus of the Western world. While not widely recognized outside the scientific community, most of the major *clinical* advances have flowed from the observations of the *basic* scientist. To cite just one example: penicillin, which doubtless has saved more lives than any other single agent in history, owes its discovery to a soil microbiologist, Sir Alexander Fleming, who in 1928 noted that a contaminating mold had gained access to one of his bacterial culture plates and dissolved adjacent bacterial colonies. The thing that is noteworthy about the discovery is that Dr. Fleming was not searching for an antibiotic or a cure for human disease. Indeed, the observation was made by chance. Similar experiences have repeatedly occurred. The lesson to be learned is twofold: first, basic research must be supported at all costs and second, it cannot be programmed. The solution to cancer will not likely come from a "war on cancer" but from some critical observation made by a biologist studying the mechanisms of cell differentiation and its control. Atherosclerosis will not be defeated by a task force assigned to examine clinical manifestations of the disease but more likely from study of how the cholesterol-carrying lipoproteins of the blood regulate cholesterol synthesis and disposal.

It should be noted that the United States, in one of the great success stories of any government at any time, early recognized the importance of biomedical research and through the National Institutes of Health provided the financial resources without which the advances just described could not have happened. With unbelievable farsightedness, the leaders of the NIH understood that basic research could lead to clinical answers. Currently the crush of inflation and the limitation of federal dollars have produced strong pressure to cut back funding for research. An informed public should demand that this not be allowed to happen. It has been repeatedly pointed out that the money required to develop, test, synthesize and commercially produce the polio vaccine was a tiny fraction of what it would cost to maintain even a relatively small number of paralyzed patients in iron lungs. The same will hold for cancer, heart disease, diabetes, the neurological illnesses and all remaining unsolved problems in human disease. Research, by and large, is cost effective.

The success of biomedical research has had one other important effect on Western medicine. Its success has trained the physician to demand experimental data rather than unsupported opinion when he reads the medical literature. Rational inquiry, the heart of the scientific method, has also directly affected patient care. In a high percentage of cases, the physician consciously or unconsciously demands evidence before he makes a diagnosis and some proof of efficacy before a given treatment is used. The importance of such a mind set cannot be overemphasized. Unfortunately, there is now a powerful movement in some academic and clinical circles to de-emphasize the "science" of medicine. Proponents of this view believe that too much time is spent in the foundation disciplines (such as biochemistry and physiology) during medical school and too little time in training the student to treat the whole man. As discussed in the following section, there *is* a trend to depersonalization in medicine that needs to be remedied. But a solution to this problem does not require the medical schools, as is usually recommended, to weaken or abandon the scientific foundation of medicine which has made it great. It is this foundation, and this alone, that has allowed transformation of the physician from a kind and gentle (but helpless) comforter into the questioning, probing, rational, modern practitioner who can do something about human disease in real and measureable ways. Preservation of the research apparatus and protection of its progeny, the modern physician, should be a high priority item for society and its government.

THE PROBLEMS

Despite the monumental achievements mentioned before, there are problems associated with medicine which, paradoxically, are at least in part related to its successes. Four deserve comment.

Depersonalization–Specialization. The technological advances of medicine have had two effects. First, the physician's reliance on laboratory tests and special procedures has tended to decrease the amount of time spent in eliciting the history of the patient and talking to him or her. This is understandable when one considers that an inexpensive, highly accurate screening test for 18 or more blood chemicals can rapidly provide accurate information about liver and kidney function, the state of nutrition, the presence or absence of diabetes and the presence of disease in a number of other systems while questioning the patient about possible dysfunction in these areas may take up to 30 minutes and even then be of only suggestive diagnostic help. There is little doubt that the availability of these tests and a myriad of other diagnostic procedures has enhanced the quality of medical care, and a great deal of pathology that would otherwise have been overlooked or incorrectly diagnosed has been properly defined as a consequence of their use. On the other hand, the person who is rushed from test to test with little chance to explain his or her symptoms or, sometimes more important, the emotional feelings about these symptoms, may rightly feel depersonalized by the process. Further, there may be the suspicion that more diagnostic procedures have been ordered than would have been needed if the doctor had narrowed the focus of investigation by careful and sympathetic interrogation. Doctors do order too much laboratory work and do overutilize procedures not only to save time but because of the fear that they might miss something of importance to the patient. (Unfortunately also, some procedures are done in the hope of avoiding a malpractice challenge.) It is probably better to err on the side of too much rather than too little laboratory work, but academic faculties are increasingly concerned with teaching the judicious use of procedures to medical students and house staff. The aphorism is simple: every test is not needed in every patient. In addition, the teachers of medicine need to re-emphasize to students what some have called the "priestly function" of the physician. We do not do it well now. When a person is ill, a wide spectrum of emotions are produced. These vary from simple irritation over a cold or earache to feelings of fear, depression, anger and isolation as the illness becomes more serious or is perceived to be more serious. Anxiety about what lies ahead—fear of the unknown—is particularly devastating and almost universal with life-threatening disease. At the very simplest level, the priestly function means communication by the physician that he cares for a patient at the level of personhood, not simply at the level of a case to be solved. Physicians who do it best are characterized by a willingness to listen. They are prepared to indicate sympathetically but honestly the patient's current status and future prognosis. They are free enough (secure enough) to say "I don't know." And they convey the assurance that whatever experience the illness might bring (up to and including death), they will be present to help and comfort even if they cannot cure. The cynic will say such physicians do not exist. But there are many of them. The hope is that somehow their numbers will increase, that such behavior will become ordinary, not extraordinary. Incidentally it is my observation that the priestly attitude is good for physician as well as patient. Those who have it seem to be at lesser risk for boredom and fatigue in later years than those who do not.

The second consequence of the technological age of medicine is the emphasis on specialization and subspecialization. Changes in clinical medicine have come extremely rapidly, and knowledge has expanded to the extent that no one physician can encompass it. Many diagnostic and therapeutic techniques (both medical and surgical) are so sophisticated as to require extended training in order that they may be used. The stimulus for specialization arises in these facts. It is likely that most persons do not object to specialization per se. After all, if I have to have replacement of a heart valve, microsurgery of the ear to restore hearing, or a transsphenoidal hypophysectomy to remove a pituitary tumor, I do not want a family practitioner or even a general surgeon to do the work. I want experience and specialized skill. The same can be said for complicated diagnostic radiology or difficult problems in medicine such as cancer chemotherapy or the management of bizarre cardiac arrhythmias. Yet, there are valid objections to a specialist-oriented medical care system. First, many common medical problems do not require the competence of a physician who limits his practice to a narrow field; yet, frequently the patient is shunted from specialist to specialist as though each symptom demanded such expertise. Second, in a multispecialist system, the patient as a human being is sometimes lost; no one physician directs overall care, explains the nature of the illness or speaks to the fears and emotions that are generated therefrom. An even more serious problem is that medical care may suffer. Thus the specialist, seeing the patient through the narrow lens of his own interest, may focus on one symptom complex (because it is in his specialty area) when in reality the major problem is something else. For example, patients with overactivity of the thyroid gland may develop an abnormal heart rhythm called atrial fibrillation. It is not impossible that a busy cardiologist might treat the atrial fibrillation and overlook the presence of an enlarged thyroid gland and other signs of the thyrotoxicosis that caused it in the first place. Third, there is the continual danger that specialized knowledge or specialized procedures will become self-directing, particularly if the monetary yield is high. To illustrate, gastroenterologists are now incredibly skilled in the procedure called endoscopy where flexible fiberoptic probes can be used to visualize directly the entire gastrointestinal tract from mouth to anus. In many instances the technique is invaluable in locating a bleeding site or identifying a malignant lesion. However, in many hospitals endoscopy has become routine in every case of bleeding from the upper gastrointestinal tract even though senior academic gastroenterologists feel that it is not especially helpful in routine situations. The underlying reasons for this practice are complicated. Many times the physician does the procedure, recognizing that the yield will be small, to reassure himself or the patient that nothing has been missed. Frequently the referring physician will demand that endoscopy be done. And finally, because insurance plans pay more for procedures than for judgment, there is an economic drive to do the test.

Solutions to the problems of specialization are not easy. Abolition of the system would almost certainly be detrimental, though this has been recommended. It has been my observation that those who urge return to the days of the general practitioner usually mean for someone else; when they develop a complicated illness themselves, they want consultation by the most highly trained individual available. Ideally the delivery of medical care should be vested in the hands of a primary physician, probably a well-trained family practitioner or general internist, who would handle routine problems and coordinate the use of consultants when needed. Establishment of such a system nationwide (in the absence of a federal health service where doctors would be assigned to training and service regardless of their own wishes) would require limiting the number of training programs available for each specialty and restructuring the reward system to increase income potential for the primary physician compared to the specialist. There is little doubt that a career in primary medicine would become much more attractive if the economic penalty for not specializing were removed.

False Expectations and Inappropriate Anxieties. The second major contemporary problem—a two-headed monster of unwarranted hope and unreasonable fear—is a direct result of the successes of medicine coupled with widespread publicity regarding diseases yet to be solved. Because medicine has done so much, many have assumed that everything is in its power.

Such is not the case. Physicians not only cannot eradicate many cancers, they cannot even cure the common cold. Granting that there are unsolved problems, the physician has done pretty well when the arena of activity is the fight against human disease. Most of us readily accept that our role is to prevent premature death, to palliate symptoms where cure is not possible and to comfort (always) the afflicted. But recently more has been asked. Because the doctor has been frequently successful in the battle against disease, now it has been assumed that he can also provide "health." The World Health Organization has defined health as "a state of complete physical, mental and social well-being, and not merely the absence of disease or infirmity." In short, the physician is to be the provider of happiness for all mankind. This is nonsense and yet many have bought the dream. So, the doctor's office is crowded with people complaining of minor aches and pains, of boils and colds and constipation, of wrinkled faces and drooping bosoms, of minor cuts and simple sprains, of anxieties and unhappiness in all its myriad forms. A decade or so ago these complaints would have been considered trivial annoyances at best—a simple part of living. Now they are the doctor's problem. Little wonder that the single most prescribed drug in America is the tranquilizer, Valium. The cost in dollars and time of the myth that medicine can solve all problems is enormous; the surrender of inner toughness and self-reliance may, in the end, cost even more. When one is sick, particularly when one of the principal manifestations of disease is present (see chapter 3), the physician should be consulted and probably can help. For happiness, someone or something else is required.

The second aspect of the desire for health which deserves comment is the unreasonable fear and inappropriate anxiety that has been provoked by consumer groups, by federal regulatory agencies and by extensively publicized animal experiments of dubious import for man. Enormous good has come from the recognition of such high-risk environmental hazards as toxic chemicals, carcinogenic dyes, inhaled silica or asbestos fibers and contaminated water. Such hazards need to be exposed and regulated. Publicity regarding the dangers of smoking or alcohol abuse or of too much fat in the diet is useful. But the pendulum has swung too far and a fear complex has been the result. Food does not have to be grown in organic fertilizer to be safe or nutritious. Sugar is not dangerous in moderation except for diabetics, or in excess as a cause of dental caries. Salt does not harm one if there is no heart failure or high blood pressure. It is possible that a rare human being might develop cancer from using saccharin (though the evidence based on massive intakes in rodents does not persuade me) or that one might be protected from cancer by eating food with high fiber content. The point is that even if true, the risks and benefits, respectively, are so small as not to warrant a change in behavior. Sensible judgment is required. Where risk is high and proven (as in smoking), on rational grounds it might be considered foolish not to alter the life-style (stop smoking). When the risk is low or unproven (as with saccharin), one might rationally decide to continue its use, particularly if sweetness of food is an important need but sugar is proscribed, as in obesity or diabetes. It is not my purpose to argue the merits or demerits of individual potential hazards. The message is more simple: relax. Common sense indicates that the world is not filled with powerful and invisible agents all of which are risks to life. Be skeptical of media reports that make wild and fearful claims. If they are true, the reports will be confirmed by reliable scientists and action will be taken. If they are not, why worry?

Maldistribution. Current studies indicate that sufficient numbers of doctors exist to care for the population. Because of the large increase in the number of medical schools in the United States and in the size of entering classes in most schools, it is entirely possible that within 10 years there will be a surplus of physicians. Yet, large segments of the population do not have access to a doctor. These segments are located in two areas: rural communities and inner cities. The reasons for the absence of doctors differ in each. Physicians generally do not locate in small towns because no other doctors are there. It is not simply a matter of fearing the work load of a solo practice. It is because the complicated advances in medicine require the availability of specialized facilities and consultants to practice at a modern level. It is perfectly possible, doing things alone, to provide care equivalent to that available 20–30 years ago (which was not bad). But it is not possible in isolation to practice in conformity with the best contemporary standards. A young physician who has had a CAT scanner routinely available during training is not likely to be comfortable practicing in a village where there is no radiologist for 50 miles. The identical problem plagues Third World physicians who train in the West and then must return home where equivalent facilities are a rarity. Medicine is difficult and it helps to have someone to talk to about complicated issues. Even in the most advanced medical center, such informal consultation goes on regularly among persons who may be leaders in their fields. The situation is not made easier by the fact that most medical schools are located in cities where the future practitioner (and spouse) is exposed for 6–8 years to the convenience and attractions of a metropolitan area. Rightly or wrongly (and many would argue, wrongly) young physicians feel that living in a village or small town requires sacrifice because of small school systems, lack of orchestras and museums, minimal opportunities for eating out and entertainment and an inability to maintain a private life.

The problems of the inner city are much easier to understand. Most physicians will not practice in a ghetto because they are afraid of robbery and physical violence, because poverty limits the ability of the patient to pay for diagnostic and therapeutic procedures and because hospital facilities are limited. Even if a municipal hospital is provided by the city, the forbidding environment turns away most who have a choice. A few, for reasons of personal dedication, will come. Most will not.

Several solutions have been proposed. The first would accept the fact that physicians will not voluntarily go to places they find unattractive for medical or personal reasons. The alternative would be to provide a network of paramedical personnel (often called physician associates) as a first line of medical care. Such a system has already been started in North Carolina. Minor illnesses and routine preventive medicine such as immunizations would be managed by the physician associate. Serious illness would then be handled by transfer of the patient to a regional medical center where modern equipment and multiple physicians are present. This is the model adopted by the armed forces during the Korean and Vietnam conflicts. The old idea of care for the injured in field hospitals was abandoned, and seriously wounded personnel were rapidly evacuated to specialized centers. In the Vietnam conflict, for example, burn victims were immediately flown to San Antonio for treatment at the Army's burn center. Center-oriented medical care is extremely effective but requires an efficient transportation system to work. Its disadvantages are primarily those of dislocation (one is sick away from home and friends) and impersonality (one may not know the doctor as a person).

Alternatively, the reward system could be restructured to favor voluntary relocation to less desirable areas: physicians who choose to practice in the inner city or a rural area would be paid sufficiently more than their more pleasantly situated counterparts to make it attractive. Once several physicians are attracted to a deprived community, the major objections mentioned disappear. Consultation becomes available and the critical mass required to justify specialized equipment is achieved.

The third solution would involve direct federal intervention with sufficient expansion of the Public Health Service to allow direct assignment of doctors to duty where needed in the same way that the Indian reservations are now staffed. How to get doctors to serve in such a corps is a difficult problem. Presumably significant economic reward for young physicians immediately after they finish training, establishment of a two-year mandatory tour of duty in exchange for financial support during medical school and house staff training, or a coercive measure like the military draft would be required.

Costs. The cost of medical care is enormous and increasing steadily. In 1978 the overall figure for health-related expenditures was about $200 billion or close to 1/10th of the nation's total output of goods and services. The largest component of this increase has been hospitalization costs which have risen far out of proportion to inflation. The national average charge for a semiprivate room in 1978 was $105, up from $33.50 in 1967. Hospital care in some major centers is greater than $300 per day. The genesis of these costs is complicated and beyond the scope of this discussion. It should be noted, however, that hospitals are labor-intensive institutions and that pay for hospital workers, until recently among the lowest in the labor force, has increased significantly. A second cause is the drive to stay up with technological advances. Sophisticated medical instrumentation is incredibly expensive. The previously mentioned CAT scanners, to cite one example, cost $500,000 to $700,000. Regardless of cause, expenditures cannot be allowed to increase at the present rate without bankrupting the nation. Society cannot afford unlimited medical care for every citizen. The problem can be illustrated by a brief look at the renal dialysis program. It is now possible to keep patients with kidney failure alive for many years using dialysis procedures. With this technique each such patient spends several hours thrice weekly attached to a machine that removes waste products ordinarily handled by the kidney. In 1972 the Congress passed legislation that put the costs for chronic dialysis under the federal budget. By 1974, 15,400 patients were on chronic dialysis at a cost of $200 million per year. In 1980 the number of patients will increase to 47,000 at a cost of $1.3 billion per year. The program will presumably level out in the mid-1980s, with 75,000 patients under treatment annually at a yearly cost of between 2 and 6 billion dollars. And this is just one category of disease. Strong pressure exists (understandably) from victims of hemophilia, diabetes, cancer, stroke and multiple sclerosis, to name a few, to have their medical costs paid as well. Why, they ask, is the patient with kidney failure more valuable to society than one with hemophilia or another disease? In Britain the Directors of the National Health Service have decided to invest no more funds in dialysis equipment and by that decision have doomed 3,000 persons a year to death. Despite the wrenching emotional impact of the ruling, they judge that with limited funds for medical care the money could save more lives if used elsewhere. To the present, monetary considerations have never entered the equation in this country. The philosophy has been simple: if life can be prolonged, no matter the cost, prolong it. It is highly unlikely that the philosophy of unlimited support can be continued indefinitely, and costs will almost certainly have to be considered in the future. The sort of calculus that may be required can be illustrated by the following comparison. It has been estimated that the cost of saving one life from cancer of the cervix in women is a little more than $3000 (calculated by dividing the total cost of yearly Pap smears for all women by the number of cancers discovered). If the mean life subsequent to successful treatment is arbitrarily taken to be 30 years, the cost per year of life saved in cervical cancer is $100. This can be compared to the $30,000 per year required to keep a patient with renal failure alive. In terms of cost:benefit ratios, obviously the screening program for cervical cancer, given a limited number of dollars, is a better buy than an unrestricted renal dialysis program. I feel strongly that physicians cannot and should not decide how much medical care the country can afford. That is a societal decision which must be made legislatively with input from multiple sources. There is even an outside possibility that regardless of cost society will decide there should be no limit on medical care because no one wishes to make the decision that some should live and some should die. In the more likely event that the general principle of limitation is accepted, the level of support will be hotly argued. Whatever its upper limit, the minimal requirements seem clear to me:

1. All persons should have prompt access to competent medical care for serious, acute, potentially reversible illness regardless of cost.
2. All persons should be provided with that level of ordinary care necessary to prolong life and relieve symptoms throughout the course of chronic disease and for the duration of terminal illness.
3. All persons economically above the poverty level should pay something for medical care, but no person should be economically devastated by any illness.

Some comments about these three principles are in order. Item (1) emphasizes the words serious, acute and potentially reversible. Society should not be expected to pay for nonserious illnesses even if they are important to the patient. For example, the common cold, cosmetic surgery (such as face lifts, breast enlargement) and mild anxiety would not be covered. Acute and potentially reversible indicate that the change in health is something new and there is a chance that the illness is reversible. By way of illustration, a young person in an automobile accident with multiple life-threatening injuries but measurable neurological function would be treated by all ordinary and extraordinary means including respiratory support regardless of cost, while a similar patient with brain death evident by electroencephalography would receive only ordinary supportive care.

Item (2) means that patients with chronic, nonreversible or terminal illness would receive excellent medical care of the ordinary type, but extraordinary measures would not be taken. Thus a patient with malignant disease throughout the body would be kept pain free until death but would not have life prolonged through use of artificial support systems. The difficulty here is defining ordinary and extraordinary care. Is chronic dialysis for renal failure ordinary or extraordinary? Is lifetime provision of antihemophiliac globulin for hemophiliacs ordinary or extraordinary?

The (3)rd item indicates the need for a deductible insurance plan (whether private, federal or a combination of the two) for all except those citizens in the poverty level of the economy. The latter would receive medical care absolutely free. The purpose of a cash outlay in every illness is to avoid abuse of the system. The actual amount of the deductible should be graduated and can be set only after careful study; one possibility would be a maximum of 5 percent of the annual taxable income on the lower side of the scale, increasing to 20 or 25 percent for the wealthy. Such a system, in effect a universal major medical insurance plan, should protect both the system and the citizen from economic catastrophe.

Obviously many other things are needed to control costs. Wasteful duplication of facilities should be eliminated (every hospital in the city does not need a cancer center or a cardiac catheterization lab); hospital construction and the provision of new beds should be tightly regulated (beds, once available, have to be filled for economic reasons); health insurance plans should be rewritten to cover outpatient diagnosis and therapy (many coverages now pay only for hospitalization); the rise in physicians' fees should be limited to reasonable levels. Many persons concerned with these problems, including a number in the Congress, believe that these goals can be attained only if the federal government takes full responsibility for the medical care delivery system in this country. Any such proposal should be looked at with great caution if the aim is cost control. The chances are overwhelming (based on experience in other countries of the world) that a federal system, particularly a national health service, would cost more, not less. Some form of federal participation is obviously required, but ideally it should formulate priorities and regulations and directly participate only as a co-insurer with the private sector.

THE PHYSICIAN AND THE QUEST FOR HEALTH

As noted earlier medicine has, against its will, become the hope for health and happiness in the world. When health and happiness have not been forthcoming, the blame is often laid at the feet of the doctors. It is widely believed that the technological achievements of medicine have done very little for health. It is further stated repeatedly that if doctors were interested in the problem—if they cared about nutrition and preventive medicine—health would improve. I do not wish to be defensive and protective of physicians. I know firsthand their faults. But it is a myth that doctors can do anything about health or infant mortality or life expectancy in society as a whole. The physician can often restore health to an individual who is ill. He may advise patients about the values of a wholesome diet, exercise and immunizations. But he cannot heal the diseases of society. The most common causes of premature death are not illnesses but accidents, murders and suicide. Huge losses come from drug usage and alcohol. Thousands die because they continue to smoke. Within the last few years epidemics of diphtheria have returned to the United States because parents neglect to have children immunized. In some areas of the country, up to 30 percent of children are not protected by polio vaccine. Malnutrition exists not because doctors are negligent but because of slums and poverty. How can the physician force people to wear seat belts while driving cars or to quit smoking? By what means can medicine ban hand guns or block illicit drugs? What is the role of the physician in replacing slums? All of these are social, cultural and political, not medical, problems. We can do our part. We can try to teach good habits and we will continue the best we can to repair the damages of the bad. But no discovery of medicine—no new drug or surgical procedure —will have the slightest influence on these tragic social events themselves. As Dr. Donald W. Seldin, a careful medical scholar, has said:

Medicine is a discipline which subserves a narrow but vital arena. It cannot bring happiness, prescribe the good life or legislate morality. But it can bring to bear an increasingly powerful conceptual framework for the mitigation of that type of human suffering rooted in biomedical derangements.

That is what this book is about: the physician and his struggle to prevent premature death, to relieve suffering and to provide comfort for the individual patient who is ill.

2

Nutrition

The subject of nutrition is widely discussed in contemporary Western society. Interest in how much and what kinds of food we eat has been generated from many different directions. Since obesity is a common problem, literally millions of people worry about the caloric content of their diet. At the opposite end of the spectrum, concerned persons are haunted by the fact that children and adults are starving to death in the famine belts of the world and in those Third World countries where population growth is uncontrolled. The medical profession itself has contributed to the everyday awareness of nutrition by implicating diet in the pathogenesis of some of the most serious diseases afflicting humans and by recommending alterations in eating patterns as a prophylactic measure for the prolongation of life and maintenance of health. Even the United States Senate has become involved and through its Select Committee on Nutrition and Human Needs has issued a set of dietary goals for the nation. Finally, capitalizing on this interest, nutritional entrepreneurs have entered prominently on the scene urging the adoption of one diet or another, ostensibly to benefit the health of the nation but in reality to make money.

The emotions generated by nutrition are quite remarkable. Many times I have encountered patients who defended certain fad diets with a zeal that one would ordinarily expect to be reserved for an attack on motherhood or one's belief in the Deity. The variety of diets recommended and attested to by their followers is almost infinite. Some believe that even a spoonful of salt is life-threatening; others feel that meat is poison. High fiber intake is in, but refined sugar is out. Interestingly many of the diets are based on valid scientific observations that are taken out of context. There are a number of clinical situations where salt restriction is mandatory, but it does not follow from this that the general public should be on a salt-free diet. Similarly, a recommendation for rigid restriction of refined sugars is appropriate for diabetic patients but is inappropriate for the average healthy person. Some diets, of course, have no scientific basis whatever but are simply the result of eccentricity. I once was asked to see a woman who had turned yellow. The yellow pigmentation (which was truly astonishing) turned out not to be jaundice but *carotenemia,* the presence of high levels of a vegetable pigment called carotene in the blood. She had eaten nothing but carrots for months. An obsession with vitamins is part of the nutritional mania that has grasped large segments of the American population. *Megavitamin therapy* refers to the ingestion of quantities of vitamins that are orders of magnitude greater than the maximum known requirements for the human. Megavitamin intake may be with a single vitamin (such as vitamin C taken to prevent colds) or mixtures of vitamins. It is not uncommon for athletes and other health conscious persons to gulp dozens of multivitamin capsules every day in the belief that vitamins increase strength or protect against disease. The view seems to be that if a little is good, a lot is better. It is one of the great myths of our time.[1]

If addiction to fad diets and nutritional obsession represents one extreme of the population spectrum, unconcern with nutrition represents the other. Large numbers of people completely ignore the detrimental effects of inappropriate diets on their health. The stereotypic pictures of the obese subject who continues to overeat, the diabetic who will not restrict sweets, the patient with heart failure who refuses to limit salt, and the teenager who lives on soft drinks, chips and hot dogs are extremely

---

[1] The intake of vitamins or any drug may make the patient "feel better." So may a sugar pill. This is called the *placebo effect.* Put simply, if a patient expects something to make him better, it usually will—by the power of suggestion. That is why all new drugs are tested in *double blind* fashion; i.e., the real drug and an inactive lookalike (placebo) are given under circumstances where neither doctor nor patient knows what is being taken. At the end of the experiment a code held by a third party is broken, and the effects of the drug under test are compared to those produced by the placebo.

familiar to every physician. In addition there is a problem of true undernutrition and malnutrition which continues to exist even in the affluent societies of the Western world. While the classical nutritional diseases (pellagra, scurvy and rickets) have been largely eliminated and true starvation almost never occurs in the United States, subclinical malnutrition is common and overt malnutrition is not rare. This is surprising in view of the fact that personal income is at an all-time high, that public assistance programs are almost universally available and that a great many foods are fortified with vitamins and minerals. In fact malnutrition is not a problem for the average person eating a normal diet; its appearance is limited to certain high-risk segments of the population who for economic, social or cultural reasons are peculiarly vulnerable. These include the very poor, the elderly, the chronically ill, alcoholics, food faddists and pregnant women.

In this chapter I propose to review current concepts of good nutrition and cover briefly the syndromes of malnutrition. I will also say a word about the relatively new technique of total parenteral nutrition. I hope the reader will learn that the principles of good nutrition are quite simple and based on common sense. I trust also that the sensational claims of the food faddists and the slick advertisements of the nonessential food industries (candies, chips, soft drinks) will come to be seen for what they are: skillful propaganda designed to facilitate the transfer of money from buyer to seller under the guise of health or pleasure.

THE NUTRITIONAL PROCESS

Food is the source of the energy necessary to sustain life. All foods contain one or more of three basic components: carbohydrate, fat and protein. The initial step in the formation of all the food in the universe is the conversion of atmospheric carbon dioxide to simple sugars by plants under the influence of energy derived from the sun (a process called *photosynthesis*). These sugars, the primordial form of carbohydrate, are then used for the synthesis of more complex carbohydrates, fat and protein. Plants may be eaten by man directly or may be ingested first by animals or fish which can be considered intermediaries in the energy transfer process. When food derived from meat or plants is eaten, it has to be broken down to release the energy originally stored from the sun and to provide the building blocks (sugars, fatty acids, amino acids) necessary for the formation and maintenance of the body tissues.[2] For this process to occur, *enzymes, hormones, vitamins* and *minerals* are required. *Enzymes* are specialized proteins which serve as biological catalysts: they cause chemical reactions to occur in the cell with great rapidity and against unfavorable energy barriers. In their absence food could not be broken down, converted to free energy or utilized for synthesis of new tissues. Every cell in the body contains hundreds of enzymes, each designed to carry out one specific biochemical reaction. *Hormones* are small molecules that have the capacity to regulate the rate (velocity) of a wide variety of biochemical reactions. They do not themselves catalyze chemical transformations but stimulate or inhibit the enzymatic reactions under their control. They may act directly or through other chemicals called *second messengers. Vitamins* are chemical substances contained in the diet which are required in trace amounts for normal growth, development and maintenance of the organism. Commonly vitamins serve as *coenzymes,* meaning that the vitamin combines with the protein portion of an enzyme that is inactive in its absence, to form an active complex. In other cases vitamins appear to act directly (not as coenzymes). *Minerals* function in the body in a variety of ways. First, many enzymes require a

[2] For those who are chemically inclined, the life cycle of the universe can be summarized as follows:

$$In\ plants:\quad 6CO_2 + 6H_2O \xrightarrow{\text{sun's energy}} C_6H_{12}O_6 + 6O_2$$

$$In\ man\ and\ animals:\quad C_6H_{12}O_6 + 6O_2 \xrightarrow{\text{energy}} 6CO_2 + 6H_2O$$

This says that in plants one *mole* (the molecular weight in grams) of glucose (sugar) is made from 6 moles of carbon dioxide and 6 moles of water with the release of 6 moles of oxygen under the driving force of the sun's energy. (Fat and carbohydrate are subsequently formed from glucose.) In animal tissues one mole of glucose is oxidized by 6 moles of oxygen to yield 6 moles of carbon dioxide and 6 moles of water with release of the energy that was originally stored from the sun. (Energy is also released by oxidation of fat and protein derived from glucose.) Both sets of reactions require the activity of multiple enzymes acting in sequence.

mineral cofactor to be active. Second, they are important in tissue structure. For example, bone is made up almost completely of calcium salts and soft tissue cannot be formed in the absence of phosphorus. Finally, minerals are functional units of some important molecules in the body; e.g., iron is the oxygen-binding component of hemoglobin, the oxygen-transport chemical of blood.

Against this background we can now define good nutrition. It is the intake of sufficient food to provide for the energy and structural needs of the body together with adequate amounts of vitamins and minerals to assure efficient function of the enzymes and hormones required for proper utilization of that food. Three categories of poor nutrition are commonly recognized. *Undernutrition* means a deficiency of calories and in the extreme is synonymous with starvation. *Malnutrition* means an imbalance in food intake such that one or more essential elements is missing or inadequate. Undernutrition and malnutrition frequently occur together. *Overnutrition* means excessive caloric intake.

NORMAL NUTRITIONAL REQUIREMENTS

It has been pointed out that although the human body contains thousands of different chemicals, only 21 organic and 15 inorganic compounds are required for health,[3] apart from the calories necessary to meet body energy demands. These 36 compounds are defined as *essential* nutrient requirements, meaning that they cannot be synthesized in the body and their deletion from the diet produces disease. All other nutrients are *nonessential;* either they can be synthesized from other compounds within the body or their absence from the diet does not produce disease. The *essential organic compounds* include water, one unsaturated fatty acid, 8 amino acids[4] and 11 vitamins. The *essential inorganic compounds* include: calcium,

---

[3] Organic, in the chemical sense, means any compound containing carbon atoms. Synthesis by living organisms (plant, microbial or animal) is also implied. Most organic molecules contain hydrogen and oxygen as well as carbon. Nitrogen is also a common constituent. Inorganic compounds are generally derived from minerals. With rare exception they do not contain carbon.

[4] In children two additional amino acids, arginine and histidine, are required, bringing the number of essential molecules to 38.

chloride, chromium, cobalt, copper, iodine, iron, magnesium, manganese, molybdenum, phosphorus, potassium, selenium, sodium and zinc. The simplicity of these requirements attests to the incredible sophistication of the biochemical machinery of the human organism which can synthesize on demand all of the vast array of chemicals needed to sustain life, provided the 36 building blocks are available in adequate amounts. It also marks as foolishness any claim that the body can remain healthy only if it is supplied with special foods and excessive supplements of vitamins and minerals.

Two terms need to be defined in discussing normal nutritional needs. *Minimal daily requirement* refers to that amount of an essential nutrient that has been determined to be necessary to maintain normal structure and function of the body, including growth in children. The *recommended daily allowance* is an amount of nutrient 2 to 10 times the minimal daily requirement. It is designed to provide a margin of safety such that even individuals with greater than normal demands will be protected. While emphasis in nutritional discussions is usually placed on *deficiencies* of essential nutrients, *excesses* can also cause disease. Examples of the latter will be given below.

Calories. The calorie is the unit of energy commonly used by nutritionists, although in some scientific journals the *joule* is now preferred (1 calorie equals 4.184 joules). A calorie is the amount of heat needed to raise the temperature of 1 gram of water from 15° to 16° C.[5] Confusion sometimes arises from the fact that the calorie used in calculating diets (and the one with which the public is familiar) contains 1000 times the energy of the scientific calorie defined above (technically it is called a *kilocalorie*). Throughout this book the term calorie will refer to the familiar dietary unit. When we say that a certain food contains so many calories, we mean that it contains energy sufficient to provide that amount of heat if all of the energy could be released. The three major food types, whatever their source, have standard caloric values; thus a gram of carbohydrate and a gram of protein are both equivalent to 4 calories while a gram

[5] Scientists and most of the world apart from the United States use the centigrade (°C) rather than the Fahrenheit (°F) scale for temperature measurement. The temperature in degrees centigrade can be converted to degrees Fahrenheit by multiplying the former by 1.8 and adding 32. The reverse conversion requires subtraction of 32 and multiplication by .556.

of fat contains 9 calories.[6] In considering changes in body weight, the rule of thumb is that 3500 calories is equivalent to 1 pound; thus a cumulative excess of 3500 calories above body needs will result in a weight gain of 1 pound. The converse is true for negative caloric balance, a deficit of 3500 calories producing a 1-pound weight loss.[7]

No universal figure for caloric requirements can be given since even individuals of the same weight will have different energy needs. Ordinarily about half the calories ingested during a day are utilized for what is called the *basal metabolic rate* (BMR). Theoretically this value is equal to the energy required to sustain body structure and function in the total absence of activity (suspended motionless by a cushion of air). The larger the individual, the higher the basal metabolic rate since the total number of active cells increases with increasing size. The BMR is usually determined by measuring oxygen uptake in the individual over a given interval of time and relating it to body surface area. In the absence of disease the basal metabolic rate does not vary much from day to day. The range of normal values from individual to individual is also fairly narrow. The second large category of caloric demand is the *activity component,* and this obviously varies tremendously from person to person. A professional tennis player will require far more calories to sustain his weight (or can eat more calories without becoming obese) than a business executive who is seated behind a desk throughout the day. The third component of caloric demand is called *specific dynamic action,* a peculiar phrase which means the number of calories that must be expended to absorb food after a meal. Ordinarily this amounts to about 6–10 percent of the total daily caloric intake. It is higher for protein (about 30 percent of the ingested load) than for carbohydrate (6 percent) or fat (4 percent). This partially accounts for the fact that protein, gram for gram, is less fattening than carbohydrate.

While it is not possible to know *a priori* the number of calories required to maintain weight in a given individual, a rough rule is that 10 calories per pound of ideal body weight will suffice for basal metabolism. For a sedentary person about 30

---

[6] One pound equals 454 grams (.454 kilograms). Other helpful equivalents are as follows: 1 liter (1000 milliliters) equals 1.06 quarts; 1 liquid ounce equals 30 milliliters; 1 inch equals 2.54 centimeters.

[7] The 3500 calorie rule is useful but should not be considered precise. It will vary somewhat from individual to individual.

percent of the basal calories are added for exercise, while 50 percent or 100 percent are added for moderate or heavy activity respectively.

Water. It might be considered strange that water is listed as a nutrient. Water is formed in all tissues of the body as food is oxidized but not in amounts sufficient to sustain life. Thus it has to be considered a dietary nutrient in the essential category. Water is the largest single component of the body, constituting 60–70 percent of the total body weight. It is necessary for the absorption of food, for the circulation of blood and for the excretion of waste products in urine and stool. It also plays a key role in a number of biochemical reactions. Under normal circumstances water loss in a 24-hour period includes about 1500 milliliters in the urine, 400–600 milliliters via respiration and evaporation from the skin (these are called *insensible losses,* indicating that they are not visible) and 50–100 milliliters in the stool. From these figures it is clear that the average person must drink around 2 liters (about 2 quarts) of water a day to avoid dehydration. Insensible losses increase during exercise, in high environmental temperatures and with fever (about 200 milliliters per day per degree centigrade). Illness may dramatically increase water requirements. Diarrhea and vomiting, for example, may cause fluid deficits of several liters in a day's time if severe and protracted. Water loss in the urine can also become very large under two circumstances. The first is *diabetes mellitus* where the markedly elevated plasma glucose levels result in high urinary glucose concentrations which require large volumes of urine for excretion. The second is a condition called *diabetes insipidus* in which there is a deficiency of anti-diuretic hormone. This hormone is secreted by the pituitary gland and controls water reabsorption in the kidney. In its absence urine flows of 6–10 liters per 24 hours are not uncommon and on occasion may reach 20 liters. Patients with either condition must drink inordinately large amounts of water to stay in fluid balance.

Protein. Dietary protein is important because it is the source of the amino acids required for the synthesis of enzymes and other critical proteins of the body.[8] There are 20 common amino

[8] Proteins are not absorbed into the body as such. Ingested proteins are broken down in the gastrointestinal tract to their constituent amino acids which are then absorbed. Totally new proteins are synthesized in the body from these amino acids. Fats and carbohydrates are also broken down in the absorptive process and resynthesized in the body.

acids found in food proteins, but only 8 cannot be synthesized in the body. They are: isoleucine, leucine, lysine, methionine, phenylalanine, threonine, tryptophan and valine. In their absence new protein cannot be made. The distribution of amino acids in proteins varies widely. Those containing high concentrations of essential amino acids are described as having *high biologic value*. Eggs and milk have the highest biologic value of the common foods, and animal proteins in general have higher biologic value than those of plants. Plant proteins tend to be limited in one or more essential amino acids, and for this reason it may be difficult to meet amino acid requirements on a vegetarian diet. This difficulty can be partially overcome by eating complementary mixtures of vegetables so that deficiencies in one are supplied by another.

The recommended daily allowance for protein varies with age and a number of other factors. For the first half-year of life, it is 1 gram per pound body weight, gradually decreasing to about 0.7 gram per pound at 6 years of age.[9] In the adult about 0.5 gram per pound is required daily. Pregnant women and nursing mothers need an additional 20–30 grams of protein per day to supply the growing fetus and to provide for milk production. Protein requirements increase significantly with fever, infection and injury.

Fat. It is quite remarkable that while most Americans eat 80–120 grams of fat a day (about 40 percent of their calories) only 3 grams of one fatty acid (linoleic acid) are required to maintain health. Humans and other mammals cannot synthesize linoleic, linolenic or arachidonic acids, the three important *polyunsaturated fatty acids* of the body.[10] However, if linoleic acid is

---

[9] I am aware of the incongruity of using grams and pounds together (mixed measurement systems). The requirements should be given as grams per kilogram body weight. The reason for using pounds is that most Americans do not yet think in terms of kilograms.

[10] The term *saturated* means that no double bonds are present between carbon atoms and that each carbon bears two hydrogen atoms ($-\overset{\text{H}}{\underset{\text{H}}{\text{C}}}-\overset{\text{H}}{\underset{\text{H}}{\text{C}}}-\overset{\text{H}}{\underset{\text{H}}{\text{C}}}-\overset{\text{H}}{\underset{\text{H}}{\text{C}}}-$). *Unsaturated* indicates the presence of one or more double bonds. The carbons on each side of the double bond contain only one hydrogen ($-\overset{\text{H}}{\underset{\text{H}}{\text{C}}}-\overset{\text{H}}{\text{C}}=\overset{\text{H}}{\text{C}}-\overset{\text{H}}{\underset{\text{H}}{\text{C}}}-$) and thus are unsaturated (each could hold one more hydrogen). Fats containing high concentrations of unsaturated fatty acids are called *polyunsaturated* and have the capacity to lower the blood cholesterol. Linoleic acid contains two double bonds, linolenic three and arachidonic four.

provided in the diet, the body can use it as a precursor for synthesis of the other two. Unsaturated fatty acids are necessary for the synthesis of *phospholipids,* which in turn are critical for the formation of cell membranes, for normal nerve function, for expansion of the lungs at birth and for a variety of secretory processes in the body. Arachidonic acid is also now recognized to be the immediate precursor for the synthesis of *prostaglandins.* The prostaglandins are involved in the regulation of numerous important physiological processes, including the initiation of labor during pregnancy, the secretion of insulin, the regulation of water reabsorption in the kidney, the control of blood pressure and the aggregation of platelets during clot formation.

In the past it was thought that essential fatty acid deficiency was rare in man. It is now recognized that under certain circumstances, particularly total parenteral alimentation (see page 44), it can develop rapidly.

Vitamins and Minerals. The recommended daily allowances for vitamins and minerals vary widely from gram quantities (sodium, potassium, chloride, calcium and phosphorus) to amounts in the millionths of a gram (vitamin B_{12}). Individual values can be obtained from the authoritative monograph on the subject published by the National Academy of Sciences (Food and Nutrition Board: *Recommended Dietary Allowances.* Washington, D.C. National Academy of Sciences, 1974). This volume should be available in most libraries.

FOODS AND HEALTH

The Normal Diet. If one eats a typical American diet utilizing a mixture of foods, it is impossible to become malnourished. In this sense good nutrition is both simple and easily attained despite widespread allegations to the contrary. Surprisingly, one can even get a balanced diet eating in franchised food restaurants provided one chooses carefully. A hamburger with lettuce and tomatoes and a glass of milk, prepared under sanitary conditions in a reputable franchise, represents a good meal in the sense that it is not deficient in the essential nutrients (including vitamins and minerals, since milk and bread are artificially fortified). An important question is whether the typical

American diet, even if it meets minimal nutritional requirements, is the healthiest that could be devised, particularly in
regard to the prevention or amelioration of the chronic diseases
that cause the majority of deaths in this country: atherosclerosis
and its complications (heart attacks, strokes, peripheral vascular
disease), diabetes, high blood pressure and cancer. Many think
not. The aforementioned Senate Select Committee on Nutrition
and Human Needs, for example, has suggested fairly drastic
modification of the typical American diet.[11] At the present time
the average person in the United States eats a diet consisting of
40 percent fat, 12 percent protein and 48 percent carbohydrate.
Currently about 16 percent of the total calories is taken in as
saturated fat and 24 percent as refined sugar. If the dietary goals
recommended by the Senate Select Committee were completely achieved, the caloric breakdown would be 30 percent
fat, 12 percent protein and 58 percent carbohydrate, with a significant decrease in saturated fat, salt and refined sugars. To
obtain these goals the American people would have to increase
their consumption of fruits, vegetables and whole grains; decrease consumption of meat and increase the intake of poultry
and fish; decrease the intake of butter, fat, eggs and other high
cholesterol sources; substitute nonfat milk for whole milk; decrease the consumption of refined sugar and foods containing
high concentrations of processed carbohydrate; and sharply
curtail the use of table salt. Proponents of the modified diet
suggest that the decreased sugar intake would lower the incidence of dental caries while increased use of fruits, vegetables
and grains would result in a substantial increase in the fiber
content of the diet, at the same time providing needed carbohydrate. *Fiber*, the nonabsorbable carbohydrate residue of
foods (previously called *roughage*), has been claimed (without
any proof) to reduce the incidence of appendicitis, cancer of the
colon, constipation, diverticulosis, hiatal hernia, and possibly
diabetes and ischemic heart disease. Limitation of dietary fat
and an increase in the polyunsaturated fat component are considered the best dietary prophylaxis for atherosclerotic heart
disease; limitation of cholesterol plays a secondary role. Decreased intake of salt is recommended in the hope of preventing
high blood pressure in those prone to develop this disease.

[11] A list of the goals and a discussion of the issues can be found in *Nutrition Reviews*
36:161, 1978.

These recommendations have stirred enormous controversy among physicians and nutritionists. I have no idea whether they will prove to be beneficial if widely adopted by the populace. Given the current state of knowledge regarding the relation of diet to disease, they appear to me to be reasonable although I feel the sugar and salt restrictions are too severe.

Health Foods. A word should probably be said about the so-called health foods since the commercial sale of these items has mushroomed over the past several years. Every major city has multiple health food stores and it is not rare to find them now even in small communities. Several categories of food are sold. "Organic" foods represent plant products grown in soil enriched with humus and compost. No commercial (chemical) fertilizers are used and herbicides or pesticides have not been applied. "Natural" food means no synthetic or artificial additives are present and that processing has been minimal; for example, flour is made from whole grains and nut butters are unhydrogenated. Meat and dairy products are included only if animals are raised on natural feeds and not treated with drugs or hormones. Part of the health food mystique results from the recommended use of unconventional items such as brewer's yeast, pumpkin seeds, wheat germ, juices from exotic vegetables and herb teas. Protein supplements and megavitamin therapy are frequently pushed as well.

Two claims are fundamental to the marketing approach of the health food industry. The first is that health foods are more nutritious than their supermarket counterparts. The second is that they are safer since they have not been exposed to toxic chemicals. The first claim is nonsense. Health foods are perfectly acceptable nutritionally, but there is not a shred of evidence that they are superior in any way. They are also more expensive. This excess cost can clearly not be justified on nutritional grounds. Is it warranted for safety? The answer cannot be given with certainty, but I strongly suspect that it is no. To the present there is no evidence that plants and vegetables grown in inorganic fertilizers and treated with pesticides are harmful when consumed by humans provided they are washed before being eaten.

The problem of toxins in foods is complicated. Scientists who work in the area distinguish between *toxicity* and *hazard*. *Toxicity* refers to the inherent capacity of a chemical to cause injury while *hazard* refers to the capacity to produce injury under the conditions of exposure. Thus, many chemicals and natural products are toxic but not hazardous because the amount present is too small to be of concern. A classic example is seen in the saccharin controversy. Saccharin in huge amounts can cause bladder cancer in rodents. Yet, long usage of saccharin in modest amounts by humans has not been associated with cancer or any other disease state. Proponents of organic foods focus their attention on external chemicals such as fertilizers and pesticides. Yet, foods eaten every day contain many toxins. For example, the common potato contains around 190 chemicals including the toxins oxalic acid, solanine alkaloids and arsenic. If food chemicals, including those found in natural foods, were subjected to the rigorous screening now required for all drugs and external additives, many would doubtless prove toxic. For these reasons the issue of increased safety with natural foods remains unsettled. My own feeling is that certain risks are inherent in being alive, and it doesn't make much sense to change one's life-style because of the possibility that an insecticide might be present on (or in) a vegetable or fruit. Probably one inhales more potentially harmful substances in an hour of heavy traffic or a few minutes in a smoke-filled room than would occur in a lifetime of eating commercially grown food.

One other point should be made. While most health foods are doubtless prepared and grown as advertised, there are no standard tests to identify organic or natural products. The consumer is therefore forced to rely on the integrity of the farmer and distributor that the products are genuine. Unfortunately, on more than one occasion this has proven not to be the case: repackaged supermarket goods have been sold as natural products. *Caveat emptor.*

SYNDROMES OF
NUTRIENT DEFICIENCY AND
EXCESS

I would now like to review briefly a few of the syndromes caused by deficiency or excess of nutrients. In the past most nutritional diseases were due to deficiencies in the diet. Now many (if not most) nutritional problems are secondary to diseases that interfere with the absorption or utilization of essential nutrients or to the use of drugs which disturb normal nutrient balance. The diminution in primary deficiency disorders is largely due to two factors: the general availability of a wide variety of foods and the practice of fortifying staples such as bread, milk and cereals with minerals and vitamins. Obviously these conditions apply only in developed societies and are not operative in large areas of the world where undernutrition and malnutrition are still rampant. The syndromes to be commented on were chosen either because they are common or because they have special interest for historical or other reasons. Obesity and a peculiar form of undernutrition called anorexia nervosa will be covered in chapter 17. A list of the major abnormalities caused by nutrient deficiency or excess is given in the table at the end of the chapter.

The Classic Nutritional Diseases. As mentioned before, the classic nutritional diseases are now rare except in alcoholics and food faddists. *Vitamin C* deficiency produces *scurvy*. The primary manifestation is hemorrhage. The bleeding is usually into the skin and gums but also occurs in muscle, beneath the membranes surrounding bone and in multiple organs. The basic defect is a fragility of blood vessels due to an inability to form *collagen,* the material that gives strength to tissues. The second of the classic syndromes is *rickets*, caused by a deficiency of vitamin D. The central problem is diminished calcium absorption resulting in faulty bone structure. The limbs become bowed, fractures are common and muscle weakness is profound. Interestingly we now recognize forms of rickets where there is plenty of vitamin D in the body but the tissues are resistant to its action (*vitamin D-resistant rickets*). The final member of the classic triad is *pellagra,* characterized historically by the four D's: diarrhea, dementia (mental illness), dermatitis (skin disease) and death. Originally thought to be due solely to niacin deficiency, it is now known that development of pellagra requires not only combined deficiencies of niacin and the amino acid tryptophan but an excess of the amino acid leucine. This configuration of nutrients is present in certain common types of corn, and thus the disease occurs most often in undernourished individuals who have corn as the major staple in their diet. Altered strains of corn have now been developed with low leucine content and should prevent the appearance of pellagra in those areas of the world where it is still common.

Thiamine Deficiency. Thiamine deficiency is an extremely common accompaniment of alcoholism. Multiple vitamin deficiencies occur in the alcoholic because food intake consists almost exclusively of *empty calories;* by this we mean calories unaccompanied by vitamins and minerals. Alcohol is the prototype of this type of nutrient, but many snack foods (chips, candy, soft drinks) are also "empty." Since snack eaters usually also take in other more balanced foods, vitamin deficiency is rare. In contrast, the alcoholic who derives essentially all calories from alcohol usually has multiple vitamin and nutrient deficiencies. The absence of thiamine produces the most severe disease. Extreme depletion of this vitamin causes one of two types of *beriberi. Wet beriberi* is a form of heart failure with massive fluid retention in the body; untreated it results in vascular collapse (shock). *Dry beriberi* involves the nerves and causes numbness, weakness and pain in the extremities. The gait is abnormal and frank paralysis can occur. Thiamine deficiency, if prolonged, can also affect the brain producing the *Wernicke-Korsakoff syndrome.* The earliest manifestation is inability to control movement of the eyes. *Nystagmus,* a repetitive vertical, horizontal or rotary movement of the eyes, is characteristic. Memory loss is common, often accompanied by *confabulation* (the falsification or fabrication of recent events). Untreated, the disease leads to a semivegetative state.

Folic Acid. Folic acid deficiency is an almost inevitable accompaniment of alcoholism. Its primary manifestation is an anemia which resembles that of vitamin B_{12} deficiency. Folic acid deficiency may also occur in pregnancy, following use of certain drugs and in malabsorptive states.

Vitamin B_{12}. Dietary deficiency of B_{12} never occurs if any significant amount of meat is eaten. It may rarely appear in strict vegetarians or in breast-fed babies of vegetarian mothers. The usual cause of the deficiency state is the disease called *pernicious anemia* in which vitamin B_{12} in the diet cannot be absorbed. The result is severe anemia characterized by very large red blood cells (*macrocytes*) and spinal cord degeneration leading to abnormal gait and/or frank paralysis. Treatment requires administration of vitamin B_{12} by injection. Many normal persons are also treated regularly with injections of B_{12}. While not harmful, the vitamin is simply excreted in the urine if deficiency is not present. It is a classic placebo.

Iron. Iron deficiency is by far the most common cause of anemia throughout the world. Weakness is the primary symptom. Dietary deficiency usually occurs only in infants given a pure milk diet (without vitamin and iron supplementation) and in pregnant women where the growing fetus puts excessive demand on the mother. Most iron deficiency is due to loss of blood. This occurs commonly in women with excessive losses via menstruation, but is also frequent with bleeding lesions of the gastrointestinal tract such as ulcers or cancer.

Potassium. Potassium deficiency is very common in this country. It is primarily due to the use of powerful diuretic agents [12] in the treatment of high blood pressure and congestive heart failure. When severe, potassium deficiency produces profound muscle weakness and predisposes to abnormalities of heart rhythm that may be fatal.

Protein. Protein deficiency is rare in the United States except in alcoholics and families at the lowest poverty level. In parts of Asia, Africa and South America, on the other hand, it is extremely common. Few of us have not been exposed to pictures of children with shrunken faces, wizened extremities, potbellies, discolored hair and ulcerated skin—the classic picture of *kwashiorkor,* now preferably called *protein-energy malnutrition.* With deficiencies of protein calories, muscle mass fades away. Edema and ascites (the accumulation of fluid in the abdominal cavity) are due to drastic falls in plasma albumin, the primary protein in the blood. The cause of death in starvation is almost always the protein deficiency itself which leads to depletion of critical cellular enzymes. Anyone who has ever seen a starving child or adult will never be the same again. That starvation continues to exist in a world where we have the technology to feed every human being adequately is a scandal to men and surely an abomination to God.

Vitamin Toxicities. The only two serious vitamin toxicities are those of vitamin A and vitamin D. They are most commonly caused by the ingestion of excessive quantities of vitamins in the quixotic quest for health that obsesses so many in our society but occasionally result from vitamins given therapeutically

[12] *Diuresis* means excessive urine flow. Diuretic drugs mobilize fluid from the body and produce potassium deficiency as a side effect.

by physicians. Vitamin A toxicity causes headache, nausea, vomiting, vertigo and somnolence if the overdose occurs acutely. Chronic excesses cause bone pain, baldness, mouth sores, coarsening of skin and calcification of tendons. Vitamin D toxicity is manifested by hypercalcemia,[13] nausea, vomiting, coma and death. In chronic overdosage kidney stones may result.

TOTAL PARENTERAL NUTRITION

There are many circumstances in clinical medicine where patients are unable to eat or the absorption of food is drastically impaired. Short periods of food deprivation are extremely common in surgery of any kind, particularly operations on the gastrointestinal tract. More prolonged abstinence from food occurs in patients with strokes either because they are in coma or because the swallowing mechanism is impaired. Finally, there are diseases such as ulcerative colitis or regional ileitis (see chapter 8) where the absorption of food is chronically impaired and where exacerbation of symptoms requires cessation of food intake for "bowel rest." Until fairly recently the only therapy available for such patients was the administration of glucose intravenously. While a minimal number of calories can be given in this way and breakdown of body protein stores can be diminished by glucose, it has long been known that adequate nutrition cannot be sustained by glucose alone. In comatose patients tube feeding is often used: a balanced diet in liquid form is placed into the stomach via a nasogastric tube. In patients with absorptive defects or those needing bowel rest, this approach is not feasible. Two regimens are now available for total sustenance of the individual over prolonged periods by intravenous infusion. These techniques are called *total parenteral nutrition.* (Parenteral means non-oral.) They involve the intravenous administration of amino acids together with a source of calories and the necessary quantities of salt, vitamins and minerals. The older technique provides the nonprotein calories in the form of

---

[13] The prefixes *hyper-, hypo-* and *iso-* are extremely common in medicine. "Hyper" means too much or above normal, "hypo" means too little or below normal and "iso" means normal. The suffix *-emia* means "in the blood." Thus hypercalcemia means elevation of the calcium concentration in the blood.

concentrated (25%) glucose solutions. Because such solutions damage small veins and cause *thrombus* (clot) formation, a catheter has to be placed in the *superior vena cava*, the large vein leading to the heart, in order to deliver the nutrient mixture safely. (Blood flow in the vena cava is so rapid that the infusate is rapidly diluted.) A newer procedure is to give the nonprotein calories as a fat emulsion (Intralipid®). This solution does not cause clot formation and can therefore be given through a peripheral vein. It is now possible to use prolonged periods of total parenteral nutrition in outpatients. The procedure has revolutionized the care of patients with inflammatory bowel disease and shows promise in other areas, such as the treatment of patients wasting away with cancer. The development of total parenteral nutrition represents a major achievement of modern medicine.

TABLE 1
NUTRITIONAL SYNDROMES*

Nutrient	Deficiency State	Excess State
Calories	Undernutrition	Obesity
Water	Dehydration	Water intoxication
Protein	Protein-energy malnutrition	Hepatic encephalopathy, uremia
Essential fatty acids	Skin rash, anemia	—
Vitamin A	Night blindness	Headache, blurred vision, vomiting
Vitamin D	Rickets	Hypercalcemia, vomiting, coma
Vitamin K	Abnormal clotting of blood	—
Vitamin B$_{12}$	Anemia, neurological disease	—
Vitamin C	Scurvy	Burning on urination
Folic acid	Anemia	—
Niacin	Pellagra	Flushing, headache, dryness of skin
Pyridoxine	Skin disease, anemia, convulsions	—
Riboflavin	Sore throat, mouth sores	—
Thiamine	Beriberi, Wernicke-Korsakoff	—
Copper	Anemia	Wilson's disease
Iodine	Hypothyroidism, goiter	Abdominal pain, vomiting, diarrhea
Iron	Anemia, weakness	Hemochromatosis
Magnesium	Low serum calcium, weakness, convulsions	Vomiting, diarrhea, vascular collapse
Pantothenate	Headache, fatigue, insomnia	—
Phosphorus	Weakness, abnormal oxygen transport, renal failure	—
Potassium	Weakness, cardiac irregularities	Cardiac standstill
Sodium	Weakness, shock, renal failure	Edema
Zinc	Slow wound healing	Fever, vomiting, diarrhea

* If an essential nutrient is not listed (e.g., vitamin E) it means that no syndrome of deficiency or excess has been recognized. Clinical syndromes not already described (such as hemachromatosis, Wilson's disease, hepatic encephalopathy) are discussed in subsequent chapters.

3

Principal Manifestations
of Disease

When a person becomes ill the immediate question to be answered is whether the symptoms indicate serious disease, requiring medical evaluation and treatment, or whether they can be assumed to be nonserious and self-limited such that medical intervention is not required. Obviously the majority of illnesses (e.g., colds and viruses) are inconsequential however much they may inconvenience during their acute reign in the body. The symptoms produced are for the most part recognized as trivial—a stuffy nose, mild headache, a day or two of muscle aches and perhaps a few hours of diarrhea or vomiting. Conversely, there are symptoms and signs that are highly suggestive of the possibility of serious illness. These signs and symptoms have been called the *principal* (or *cardinal*) *manifestations of disease* and are, with rare exceptions, absolute indication for medical evaluation. A few of the cardinal manifestations may be caused by either serious or nonserious disease. For example, fever may be due to a common cold or potentially fatal spinal meningitis. For these symptoms the context in which they appear is often helpful in assessing significance. In this chapter the principal signs will be discussed and the major diseases that have to be considered with each indicated. Guidelines will be provided as to when medical advice should be sought in those cases where there is a question. Emphasis will be placed on those manifestations of disease that develop acutely although serious illness may also be heralded by signs and symptoms that develop gradually (almost imperceptibly) over many months. These symptoms will be discussed in later chapters under the individual diseases that produce them.

PAIN

The preeminent signal of potentially serious disease for most people is pain. Yet, it has long been known that pain—even severe pain—can occur in the absence of major illness or even any illness at all. Furthermore, the perception of pain differs widely among individuals and in the same individual at different times. Thus, a chronic backache may be a minor annoyance when other aspects of life are going well and incapacitating in times of emotional stress. How does one determine if pain is serious or nonserious? The answer depends partly on location and partly on the character of the pain.

Musculoskeletal Pain. Pain in the bony structures, joints and muscles may be severe, even excruciating, but only rarely requires acute medical consultation. Aching backs and extremities are so common to the human experience that they should routinely be treated with rest and analgesics (aspirin or acetaminophen) for a few days before seeking medical help. Three exceptions should be noted. The first is a *traumatic injury* where fracture is suspected. The second is the sudden appearance of *pain, heat* or *swelling in the joints* suggesting an acute arthritis of the type associated with *gout, rheumatic fever, rheumatoid arthritis* or a *septic* (caused by bacteria) joint disease. The most common cause of the latter is gonorrhea. The third is the presence of *thrombophlebitis,* a clot with inflammation[1] in the deep veins of the legs. Thrombophlebitis is usually accompanied by swelling of the thigh or calf with heat and tenderness in the involved area. The thrombosed vein is often felt running cordlike through the inflamed region. The danger of thrombo-

---

[1] Inflammation is a word much used in medicine. The outward signs of inflammation are redness, heat, swelling and pain. Microscopically inflammation means the tissue is infiltrated with white blood cells (inflammatory cells) which migrate in to fight the disease process.

phlebitis is that the clot will break off and travel to the lung (*pulmonary embolus*).

Headache. Greater than 95 percent of all pain in the head is due to nervous tension. As a consequence headache is rarely an indication for early medical evaluation. Clues to the possibility of serious headache include the following: (1) new headache of a severe nature in a patient who has never had headache before; (2) headache associated with fever and a stiff neck (meningitis); (3) headache coupled with blurring of the vision, nausea and vomiting (migraine, high blood pressure); (4) headache that is worse lying flat than sitting or standing (brain tumor, high blood pressure); (5) headache that wakens one from sleep (brain tumor, high blood pressure); and (6) headache associated with neurological symptoms, such as weakness in an arm or leg or altered mental function (bleeding into the brain or subarachnoid space, brain tumor).[2]

Pain in the Chest. In contrast to headache and musculoskeletal pain, pain in the chest frequently means serious disease and is often a signal for emergency care. The presence of a heavy, squeezing or pressing sensation in the center of the chest (beneath the *sternum* or breastbone) is strongly suggestive of *coronary artery disease.* The pain may or may not radiate into the arms, neck or abdomen. If the pain is brought on by exertion or emotion and relieved within a few minutes by rest, *angina pectoris* is the likely diagnosis. More prolonged and severe pain of the same quality, particularly if it is associated with sweating, faintness, pallor and a sense of impending doom, should be considered a heart attack (*myocardial infarction*) until proven otherwise. Emergency evaluation is absolutely required. Sharp pain in the chest that is made worse by respiration (the pain is diminished by holding the breath or breathing shallowly but accentuated by deep inspiration or coughing) should also be taken seriously. Such pain is called *pleurisy* and is due to inflammation of the membranes (*pleurae*) surrounding the lungs. While pleuritic pain may be due to a benign viral illness called *pleurodynia,* it often heralds the presence of

---

[2] For the physician the *affect* (outward appearance) of the patient is also important. Individuals with tension headache often describe their pain as excruciating but continue to talk freely and carry out activities and movement. In contrast, a patient with a subarachnoid hemorrhage or a brain tumor often holds the head completely motionless and speaks only as necessary: their affect reflects the seriousness of the illness.

pneumonia or *pulmonary embolus.* If the pleuritic pain is associated with high fever and sputum production, the diagnosis is probably the former. Pulmonary embolism causes the abrupt onset of shortness of breath, faintness, collapse and sometimes the coughing of blood. If thrombophlebitis can be identified the diagnosis is easy, but often the site of origin of the clot is not apparent. Occasionally *pericarditis,* an inflammation of the membranous sac surrounding the heart, may extend to the chest cavity and cause typical pleuritic pain. More commonly pericarditis causes nonpleuritic central chest pain that is made worse by lying down and is relieved by sitting up or leaning forward.

While substernal chest pain and pleurisy represent potentially dangerous illnesses, there are other forms of chest pain that are very common and not serious. Sharp or sticking pains in the left side of the chest ("over the heart, doctor") are usually psychosomatic in origin and represent anxiety. Often such pain occurs in the context of generalized weakness, fatigue, sighing respiration or frank hyperventilation. In the past this syndrome was called *neurocirculatory asthenia,* but most physicians now simply label it as anxiety neurosis with a cardiac focus. A second common cause of nonserious chest pain is the *Tietze syndrome.* The pain is substernal in location and may thus suggest heart disease. The problem is actually an inflammation at the junction of the ribs with the sternum—a *costochondritis.* The cause is unknown, but the key to diagnosis is identification of one or more trigger points that when pressed reproduce the pain.

Abdominal Pain. Abdominal pain may or may not be serious. Transient sharp pains are a common experience and quite insignificant. Their cause is not known although they are often attributed to intestinal "gas." Cramping abdominal pain frequently occurs in association with the acute onset of diarrhea and mild fever—the infamous (but entirely benign) 24- or 48-hour intestinal "virus." On the other hand if cramping pain occurs in the absence of diarrhea, is severe, prolonged and accompanied by abdominal distension, *mechanical intestinal obstruction* is suggested. Obstruction may be due to adhesions in a patient who has had previous abdominal surgery, cancer or regional ileitis. If obstruction continues to the point of bowel death, the pain may abate despite the fact the patient is becoming sicker, resulting in a tricky diagnostic problem. Pain due to *peptic ulcer* is burning or gnawing in nature, and is usually located in the upper abdomen. Its fundamental characteristic is relief by food with recurrence several hours after the meal (as the stomach empties and gastric acid levels increase). Burning pain following heavy alcohol intake is due to *gastritis*. Both ulcer and gastritis may cause vomiting of blood in association with abdominal pain. Pain that begins around the *umbilicus* (navel) and migrates to the right lower quadrant of the abdomen over a several-hour period, especially if accompanied by anorexia (loss of appetite) and vomiting, is strongly suggestive of *appendicitis*. The sudden onset of severe pain followed in a few hours by rigidity and tenderness of the abdominal wall indicates the possibility of a *perforated intestine* and *peritonitis*. A history of ulcer disease increases the likelihood that perforation is present. Deep, boring pain in the center or upper middle portion of the abdomen radiating through to the back is the hallmark of pancreatic pain. If it occurs during or after heavy alcohol intake, the diagnosis is almost certainly *acute pancreatitis*, a potentially fatal illness. Chronic pain of this type is suggestive of *cancer of the pancreas*. A peculiar characteristic of pancreatic pain is that it is often relieved by sitting up and leaning forward or by assuming a crawling position (on all fours). The pain is made worse by lying on the back. Cramping or steady pain in the right upper quadrant of the abdomen, sometimes radiating to the right shoulder or around the right side to the back is characteristic of *cholecystitis* (gallbladder disease). Acute attacks are almost always accompanied by nausea and vomiting. Persistent pain in the left lower quadrant of the abdomen suggests the possibility of *diverticulitis, cancer of the sigmoid colon* or *spastic colon*. Severe generalized abdominal pain in a young black person may be due to *sickle cell crisis*. A sudden, steady, tearing pain, which may extend from chest to abdomen, raises the possibility of *dissecting aneurysm of the aorta*. In this illness the walls of the aorta, the main blood vessel leading from the heart, become separated or split. The pain is often accompanied by signs of shock or vascular collapse. Extreme pain that radiates from the flank around the abdomen to the inner thigh or the testis signals the presence of a *kidney stone* which has passed into the ureter. Severe pain in the lower portion of the abdomen (on one or both sides) in young women raises the possibility of *pelvic inflammatory dis-*

ease due to gonorrhea. Vaginal or cervical discharge may or may not be present. This syndrome is extremely common in sexually active women who are promiscuous. Severe abdominal pain in women at the time of menstruation suggests the possibility of *endometriosis,* a syndrome in which uterine tissue is located aberrantly outside the uterus. The pain is usually more severe than ordinary menstrual cramps. Sudden, extreme pain in the pelvis early in pregnancy raises the possibility of a *ruptured ectopic pregnancy.* In this illness the fetus has become implanted in the fallopian tube rather than in the normal site in the uterus. A rare cause of excruciating abdominal pain without localizing signs is *acute intermittent porphyria.* The pain often follows use of sedative drugs (which precipitate the acute attack) and may be accompanied by urine that turns dark on exposure to light.

It is obvious from this partial listing that there are many serious causes of abdominal pain. Basically all severe pain in the abdomen, especially if it lasts more than a few hours or is accompanied by other signs, requires medical consultation.

WEIGHT LOSS AND WEIGHT GAIN

Weight Loss. Under normal circumstances body weight is maintained at a stable level despite moderate day-to-day variations in food intake. Loss of weight in the absence of deliberate dieting is almost always a sign that organic disease is present. The seven most common causes are occult malignant disease, diabetes mellitus, gastrointestinal disease, infections, endocrine disease, uremia and psychiatric illness. *Occult malignancy* is the number one worry when weight loss occurs in the absence of other signs and symptoms. The most frequent sites of hidden cancer are the gastrointestinal tract, liver and pancreas. *Diabetes mellitus* causes weight loss primarily through wastage of glucose in the urine. It is the only one of the seven characterized by excessive urine flow. A wide variety of *gastrointestinal diseases* have weight loss as a major component of the initial clinical presentation. Steatorrhea, the inability to absorb fat, is notorious in this regard. It can be caused by chronic pancreatitis, cystic fibrosis or a condition called sprue. Bulky, greasy stools which float in the water because of their high fat content characterize the illness. Chronic diarrhea due to inflammatory bowel disease (ulcerative colitis, regional ileitis) or parasites such as amoebae almost always causes major weight loss. *Infections* inevitably have to be considered in the differential diagnosis. The infection could be a systemic illness such as tuberculosis, fungal disease or bacterial endocarditis (bacterial infection on the heart valves) or a localized collection of pus (abscess) in the liver, abdomen or chest cavity. Certain *endocrine diseases* are associated with loss of tissue mass. By far the most common is thyrotoxicosis (overactivity of the thyroid gland) which causes weight loss in the face of a voracious appetite and markedly increased food intake. Panhypopituitarism (failure or destruction of the pituitary gland) and adrenal insufficiency may also cause significant wasting. *Kidney failure* may present with weight loss as a major complaint because of its propensity to cause anorexia. However, diminution of tissue mass may not be reflected in body weight because of retention of fluids by the diseased kidneys. Finally, *psychiatric illness* may be associated with significant weight loss. The classic example is anorexia nervosa, a syndrome in which young women starve themselves to a degree equivalent to that seen in the concentration camps of World War II (see chapter 17). Anorexia also frequently accompanies chronic depression and schizophrenic states.

An important general rule can now be given: if weight loss occurs in the face of *increased* food intake, the diagnosis will usually be diabetes mellitus, thyrotoxicosis or steatorrhea. All other types of weight loss are accompanied by *decreased* food intake.

Weight Gain. Weight gain is only rarely a sign of underlying illness. Most patients gain weight simply because they overeat. In children, certain congenital diseases such as the *Prader-Willi* abnormality and the *Laurence-Moon-Biedl* syndrome can cause obesity. Both are probably due to abnormalities in the hypothalamic region of the brain where centers controlling food intake are located. *Tumors* in the hypothalamic region can also cause pathologic obesity. In the adult, *Cushing's disease* (overactivity of the adrenal gland) results in a peculiar truncal obesity which spares the arms and legs. *Hypothyroidism* (underactivity of the thyroid gland) may cause modest weight gain, and rarely, *insulin-secreting tumors* of the pancreas produce an obese state. All these causes represent only a tiny fraction of 1 percent of patients presenting to the doctor with obesity.

FEVER

Ordinarily body temperature is maintained within quite narrow limits despite environmental temperatures that range from below 0° to more than 100° F. The body temperature varies in normal persons throughout the day; it may be as low as 97° F orally early in the morning and rise to as high as 99° F in the afternoon.[3] In general a temperature above 99° F is considered abnormal if obtained in the nonexercising state and usually indicates that disease is present. Most persons immediately think of infection when a temperature elevation occurs. While infections probably do represent the commonest cause, many other conditions are febrile in character. These include *rheumatoid arthritis* (and other connective tissue diseases), *cancers, leukemias, lymphomas, inflammatory bowel disease, hemolytic anemia, drug reactions* and even *strokes*.

Since fever may accompany both minor and major illnesses, the question is: when should fever be considered worrisome? Absolute answers that are universally applicable cannot be given. The general rule is that mild temperature elevation lasting for a few days and accompanied only by general malaise[4] or other minor symptoms is probably benign and of little concern. The common cold and the incredible number of transmissible viral illnesses that afflict the human species fit these criteria. In other circumstances fever is an indication for early medical consultation. A summary of these situations follows:

1. *Fever above 103°.* Most nonserious illnesses are accompanied by mild elevations of body temperature. While benign viral disease can produce temperature levels as high as 105°, one worries about the possibility of serious illness at levels greater than 103°. I prefer to see the patient who has spontaneous high temperatures even if no other signs or symptoms are present.

---

[3] Rectal temperatures are 0.5° to 1.0° F higher than oral temperatures.
[4] Malaise implies the absence of a sense of well-being rather than specific symptoms. It is a general feeling of discomfort, uneasiness or out-of-sortness and may be the first sign of illness.

2. *Fever associated with shaking chills.* It is important to distinguish between chilliness and chills. *Chilliness* is a sensation of coldness. With *chills* the sense of coldness is accompanied by chattering of the teeth and rhythmic, uncontrollable muscle contractions throughout the body. While viruses and other illnesses can occasionally produce chills, their presence usually signifies that bacteria or bacterial products have entered the bloodstream (*septicemia*), requiring antibiotic therapy.

3. *Fever associated with severe headache, stiff neck or altered consciousness.* This constellation of symptoms raises the possibility of bacterial meningitis or other infection of the central nervous system. Since one form of meningitis, *meningococcal meningitis* (usually called "spinal meningitis" by the lay public), is fatal within a matter of hours, the need for consultation with these symptoms is urgent. An additional sign suggesting the possibility of meningococcal meningitis is the presence of bleeding into the skin. The bleeding, which may initially resemble a rash, may be pinpoint in nature (*petechial hemorrhages*) or may present as spreading areas of hemorrhage within the skin, called *purpura.*

4. *Fever in conjunction with pleuritic chest pain or coughing of blood.* This symptom complex suggests the presence either of *pneumonia* or a *pulmonary embolus,* as previously discussed. *Pulmonary tuberculosis* and *fungal diseases* may also manifest themselves in this fashion.

5. *Fever coupled with pain on urination, urinary frequency and/or flank pain.* These symptoms are the hallmark of *infections of the urinary bladder or kidney.* Such infections are extremely common, particularly in women. While they are usually not life-threatening, they require prompt treatment. In men similar symptoms are produced by *prostatitis,* an inflammation of the prostate gland.

6. *Fever associated with acute pain and swelling of the joints.* A variety of illnesses may begin in this way including *acute rheumatic fever* in children, *drug reactions, septic arthritis,* and *connective tissue diseases* such as rheumatoid arthritis or lupus erythematosis.

7. *Fever with sore throat and lymph node enlargement in the neck.* This would be the picture of the common streptococcal sore throat. A minor illness in itself, if not properly

treated it may lead to late complications such as *acute rheumatic fever* or *glomerulonephritis,* a serious disease of the kidneys. It is also not uncommon for *acute leukemia* to present with fever, chills and sore throat, although when one considers the overall incidence of sore throats, the percentage due to this type of illness is very small. Finally, *infectious mononucleosis,* a disease that afflicts many young adults, is notorious for producing the sore throat-fever-lymph node triad.

8. *Fever in a patient with previous known rheumatic heart disease.* Damage to the heart valves by a previous episode of rheumatic fever makes them extremely vulnerable to implantation of bacteria, resulting in a life-threatening disease called *subacute bacterial endocarditis.* If rheumatic heart disease has been previously diagnosed, any episode of fever requires medical consultation to rule out this greatly feared complication.

9. *Fever in illicit drug users.* An increasing problem in today's society is infection acquired by the injection into the bloodstream of illicit drugs that are contaminated with bacteria and other chemicals. If the staphylococcus is injected, an *acute bacterial endocarditis* can be produced. In contrast to subacute bacterial endocarditis, previous damage to the heart valves is not required. Acute bacterial endocarditis will destroy the affected valves in a matter of days. *Viral hepatitis* also occurs in almost epidemic proportions in the drug subculture where common use of the same needle is standard procedure. The hepatitis virus is transmitted by contaminating blood in the needle. Street drugs can also cause *pneumonia, lung abscesses* and *acute pulmonary edema* (the sudden filling of the lungs with fluid), all of which may be accompanied by fever.

10. *Fever after exposure to high environmental temperatures.* An extremely high body temperature following exposure to a hot, humid environment is called *heatstroke.* It is a grave, frequently fatal illness that requires *immediate* hospitalization. Athletes, military recruits and the elderly are particularly vulnerable. Often the victim has exercised excessively prior to the onset of symptoms. Progression from health to death may occur rapidly over a matter of hours.

HYPOTHERMIA

Hypothermia, or low body temperature, is much less commonly a manifestation of disease than is fever. Any temperature below 97° F represents hypothermia. Since clinical thermometers do not register below 95° F, accurate determination of the level of hypothermia below this range requires use of a thermocouple or a laboratory thermometer with a lower scale. The only common disease causing serious depression of the body temperature under spontaneous circumstances is *myxedema*, the clinical syndrome produced by inadequate function of the thyroid gland. In *myxedema coma*, the end stage of hypothyroidism, the body temperature may fall into the eighties. Milder degrees of hypothermia can occur with *hypoglycemia* (low blood sugar) and occasionally a *stroke* produces it. By far more common is *accidental hypothermia* where the body temperature becomes very low because of exposure to environmental cold. Alcoholics, users of other depressant or consciousness-altering drugs and the elderly ill constitute the population at risk. Body temperatures below 80° F invariably cause coma. The prognosis under such circumstances is grim.

ALTERATIONS IN CONSCIOUSNESS

Loss of consciousness (and the preliminary symptoms that warn of impending loss of consciousness—dizziness, confusion, altered vision and weakness) is another of the cardinal manifestations that may be due to either trivial or serious abnormalities. Five common syndromes can be identified: vasovagal syncope, orthostatic hypotension, cardiac syncope, convulsions and coma.

Vasovagal Syncope. Syncope, the technical name for fainting, implies a loss of consciousness that is transient and self-limited. It usually occurs at a time of emotional stress. That stress may be as minor as having blood drawn or being in a hot, crowded room. The mechanism appears to be sudden dilation of peripheral blood vessels such that blood drains away from the brain into the lower extremities under the influence of gravity. It is an entirely benign condition, consciousness being recovered as soon as the patient is supine.

Orthostatic Hypotension.[5] This syndrome, also called *postural hypotension* or *postural syncope,* is similar in mechanism to vasovagal syncope except that it occurs following assumption of the standing position rather than as a response to stress. Under ordinary circumstances when a person stands there is a reflex (automatic) contraction of the blood vessels in the legs that prevents a gravity-induced drainage of blood away from the upper body and head. When this reflex is impaired, dizziness or fainting results. The symptom most often occurs as a side effect of *drugs used to treat high blood pressure.* It may also be due to *arteriosclerosis* (hardening of the arteries) where degeneration and calcium deposition in the muscle layer of the arteries impairs their response to the reflexes described above. *Neuropathies*[6] such as those of diabetes mellitus, alcoholism, vitamin B_{12} deficiency and tabes dorsalis may also cause the syndrome. Here the reflex itself is interrupted by nerve disease. Finally *hemorrhage* and *dehydration* may produce postural symptoms because of shrinkage in the blood volume that cannot be compensated for in the upright position even by maximal reflex constriction in the lower extremities.

Cardiac Syncope. Cardiac syncope is due to a sudden reduction in the output of blood from the heart. The most common form (known as *Stokes-Adams attacks*) is due to an extremely slow heart rate secondary to a block in conduction of the electrical impulses that normally trigger cardiac contractions. Very rapid heart rates or irregular rhythms can also cause fainting. The critical rate on the low side is about 25–30 beats per minute while on the high side the danger point is somewhere between 150 and 200 beats per minute. It is characteristic of cardiac syncope that the attacks begin very suddenly, usually with few premonitory symptoms. Unlike vasovagal or postural syncope, consciousness does not return on assumption of the supine po-

[5] The terms hyper- and hypotension are very confusing to many lay persons because it is assumed they refer to nervous tension. In fact hypertension means high blood pressure and hypotension means low blood pressure.

[6] The suffix "-pathy" means "disease of." Thus neuropathy means a disease of nerves, retinopathy means disease of the retina and nephropathy means disease of the kidney. The term is nonspecific and does not identify the underlying disease process without the addition of a descriptive term; if one wishes to attribute a neuropathy to diabetes mellitus, the phrase "diabetic neuropathy" would be used.

sition. Unless the attack terminates quickly, neurological signs due to *ischemia*[7] or sudden death may occur. Other causes of cardiac syncope include a *sensitive carotid sinus* and *stenosis* (narrowing) *of the aortic valve* (which separates the left ventricle of the heart from the aorta). The former is due to a reflex center in the neck (*the carotid sinus*) becoming oversensitive to external pressure. When this happens a tight collar or turning the head causes dramatic slowing of the heart rate and syncope. Aortic stenosis causes fainting only after exercise; the block to outflow means the heart cannot meet the demands of the exercising muscles which dilate their vessels and thus steal blood away from the brain.

Convulsions. The presence of convulsions always indicates a disease state. A new seizure should be considered a *brain tumor* until proven otherwise. Other causes of convulsions include *brain abscess, hemorrhage into the brain* and *metabolic disorders* such as hypoglycemia, hypocalcemia, low magnesium concentrations in blood and hypoxemia (low oxygen content of blood). Seizures are common during an alcoholic debauch (*rum fits*) or following alcohol withdrawal (*delirium tremens*). Withdrawal from barbiturates and tranquilizers may also induce convulsions. If no cause for the convulsive disorder can be found, the diagnosis will be *idiopathic*[8] *epilepsy*. Epilepsy usually begins early in childhood but may be acquired in later life as a consequence of head injury or surgery on the brain. I want to emphasize as critically important the dictum that *convulsions should not be assumed to be idiopathic epilepsy until careful search has ruled out brain tumor.*

Physicians recognize several types of convulsions. The *grand mal seizure* begins with a sudden loss of consciousness, often accompanied by a cry, followed by a fall to the ground. Sustained contraction of the muscles followed by repetitive jerking movements then occurs, often with spontaneous urination or defecation. When the convulsion is over, an unconscious state may last for an hour or so followed by confusion and drowsiness for longer periods (the *postictal state*). *Petit mal epilepsy* is characterized by momentary loss of consciousness without con-

[7] *Ischemia* means inadequate blood supply to a tissue.

[8] *Idiopathic* means the cause of a disorder is not known. It is not implied that a specific cause does not exist, only that the cause has not yet yielded to the inquiry of medical science.

vulsions while *Jacksonian seizures* are rhythmic jerking movements limited to one side of the body. A peculiar syndrome is *psychomotor epilepsy* which is characterized by hallucinations or perceptual illusions and a dreamy state of separation from reality.

Coma. The term coma refers to a loss of consciousness in which the patient is totally unarousable by external stimuli for prolonged periods of time (as opposed to syncope which is transient). True coma always implies the presence of serious disease in the central nervous system. The common causes are *stroke, trauma to the head* (with or without bleeding into the brain or surrounding tissues), *increased intracranial pressure* (tumors, abscesses), *metabolic disorders* (such as deficiencies of glucose or oxygen) and *drug intoxications*. The latter is now the most common cause of coma in young people. (These disorders will be discussed in chapter 5.)

PARALYSIS

The causes of paralysis are numerous. The most common syndrome is loss of consciousness associated with paralysis of one side of the body. This coupled sequence almost always signals the presence of a *stroke* due to clot formation in a major vessel of the brain or hemorrhage from such a vessel. Motor weakness or paralysis due to a stroke can also occur in the absence of altered consciousness. *Brain tumors* can produce paralysis with altered consciousness resembling a stroke but are statistically much less frequent. *Spinal cord injury,* the sad but frequent consequence of traumatic injury to the cord as a result of automobile, sport and other accidents, produces permanent, usually total paralysis below the level of the lesion. A similar syndrome of total paralysis can occur spontaneously due to clot formation in the *anterior spinal artery.* The onset is rapid and usually totally unexpected. *Tumors of the spinal cord* develop much more slowly but may produce the same clinical picture. A variety of *neuropathies* including those due to alcohol, thiamine deficiency, lead intoxication, arsenic poisoning and diabetes may cause motor deficits in one or more extremities. *Poliomyelitis* was a dread cause of permanent paralysis prior to development of the polio vaccine. In the *Landry-Guillain-Barré syndrome* paralysis usually starts in the lower extremities and ascends to involve the whole body. Its cause is unknown. *Acute intermittent porphyria* produces a similar picture. *Tetanus* and *botulism* are infectious diseases that may result in total body paralysis. Tetanus is due to contamination of wounds or puncture sites with *Clostridium tetani* in a nonimmunized subject. Botulism results from ingestion of improperly heated canned foods that are contaminated with the toxin of *Clostridium botulinum*. A very interesting illness is *familial periodic paralysis*. In this disease otherwise normal persons develop partial or complete paralysis that may involve only the legs or extend to the whole body, lasting for minutes to several days. Attacks tend to be precipitated by exercise or high carbohydrate meals. The mechanism is not entirely clear, but the initial event is usually a profound drop in the potassium concentration of the blood. Periodic paralysis may also occur in nonhereditary fashion in association with hyperthyroidism. Two diseases that usually cause only muscle weakness but can lead to frank paralysis are *myasthenia gravis* and *multiple sclerosis*.

It is important to note that in the paralytic syndromes mentioned here, paralysis occurs initially in the absence of muscle atrophy. Primary muscle disease can also result in functional paralysis but usually only after considerable atrophy has developed (e.g., *muscular dystrophy*).

BLEEDING

The appearance of bleeding in the absence of injury must always be taken seriously. If the bleeding occurs in multiple sites, it is safe to assume that a disorder of the clotting system is present. The cause may be *thrombocytopenia*, a deficiency of the blood platelets, or low levels of clotting chemicals in the blood. One always worries about the presence of *leukemia* when generalized bleeding appears spontaneously, but *liver disease, kidney failure* and *reactions to drugs* are also high on the list of possibilities. If bleeding is localized, the site of the blood loss usually gives a good clue to the nature of the problem. A brief summary of the major types of hemorrhage and their causes follows.

Epistaxis (Nosebleeds). Nosebleeds may occur spontaneously without apparent disease, particularly in children. In the adult the most common associated cause is *high blood pressure.*

Hemoptysis (Coughing of Blood). Hemoptysis almost always means disease in the lungs. The major worry in smokers is *cancer of the lung. Tuberculosis, fungal disease, pneumonia, pulmonary embolus* and *acute bronchitis* can also cause the symptom. One form of heart disease, a narrowing of the mitral valve called *mitral stenosis,* causes hemoptysis in association with shortness of breath.

Hematemesis (Vomiting of Blood). A variety of lesions may lead to vomiting of blood. It is important to recognize that this blood may or may not be bright red. If gastric acid levels are high, blood appears dark and particulate, resembling coffee grounds. The most common cause by far is bleeding from an *ulcer* in the stomach or duodenum. Alcoholics with *cirrhosis of the liver* hemorrhage from large, dilated veins in the esophagus (the tube connecting the oral cavity and the stomach) called *esophageal varices. Cancers* and *lymphomas* of the stomach and esophagus also bleed and lead to vomiting. *Gastritis,* an inflammation of the stomach lining due to alcohol, is another frequent offender. Occasionally prolonged vomiting produces a tear at the junction of the stomach and esophagus, causing major hemorrhage (the *Mallory-Weiss syndrome*).

Bleeding in the Stool. Bleeding in the stool (or from the rectum) demands early investigation. The number one suspect is always *cancer of the colon,* now the second most common form of neoplastic disease in the United States. Other causes include: *hemorrhoids, diverticulosis, bacillary dysentery* (usually an acute illness which is not a diagnostic problem), *ulcerative colitis* and *regional ileitis* (the so-called inflammatory bowel diseases), *amebiasis* and, in older people, *mesenteric thrombosis* (clot formation in vessels supplying blood to the intestine).

Blood in the stool may be bright red or, alternatively, the fecal material can be black in color (*melena*). Melena implies that the bleeding has occurred high up in the gastrointestinal tract, allowing the hemoglobin of the red cells to be broken down by intestinal juices and bacteria during its passage to the colon. Melena thus implies a lesion in the stomach, small intestine or initial part of the colon while red blood suggests a lesion lower down. Many cancers do not bleed heavily but leak only small amounts of blood that are not visible to the eye (*occult blood*). Such blood can only be detected by chemical testing. Every person over 40 should have a test for occult blood in the stool at the time of annual physical examination. It is also possible that home test kits will be available in the near future.

Hematuria (Bleeding into the Urine). The most common cause of hematuria is bladder infection (*cystitis*). Other etiologies include *kidney stones, bladder polyps* and *cancers of the bladder and kidneys.* Occasionally severe hematuria may occur in patients with abnormal hemoglobins, particularly *sickle cell anemia* or the milder *sickle cell trait.* If blood in the urine is associated with pain or a burning sensation on voiding, urinary frequency and fever, the chances are so high that the cause is a bladder or kidney infection that treatment with antibiotics can be carried out without additional workup. Persistent or recurrent bleeding, on the other hand, always demands direct examination of the bladder by cystoscopy and X-ray evaluation of the kidneys.

Bleeding into the Skin. Bleeding into the skin essentially always means the presence of systemic disease. The major categories are *clotting defects, infections* (meningococcal meningitis, systemic gonorrhea, bacterial endocarditis, Rocky Mountain spotted fever) and *primary disease of the blood vessels* (scurvy, periarteritis nodosa).

SHORTNESS OF BREATH

Shortness of breath (*dyspnea*) is a sign of disease only when it occurs inappropriately. Since a subjective sense of air hunger occurs normally after severe exertion even in the trained athlete, dyspnea can be considered pathological only when it occurs at rest or after mild exertion. The two common causes are *heart failure* and *pulmonary disease.* The term *heart failure* refers to all situations in which the pumping function of the heart is inadequate. As a result blood pools in the lungs (see chapter 6) resulting in stiffness, increased work of breathing and, in the end, filling of the air spaces with fluid (*pulmonary edema*). The usual sequence is for exertional dyspnea to appear first, followed by episodic shortness of breath at night (*parox-ysmal nocturnal dyspnea*) and finally shortness of breath when-ever the patient lies flat (*orthopnea*). In acute pulmonary edema the patient gasps for breath and pink-tinged froth pours from the mouth. The nails and skin are blue from lack of oxygen (*cyanosis*).

A variety of acute and chronic pulmonary diseases cause dyspnea. Episodic wheezing respiration is characteristic of *bronchial asthma. Pneumonia, pulmonary embolism* and *pleural effusions* (the accumulation of fluid in the chest cavity surrounding the lungs) can all account for the rapid appearance of dyspnea in a previously normal person. Chronic dyspnea is usually due to *bronchitis* and *emphysema* in patients who have been heavy smokers. *Cancer of the lung* may also cause short-ness of breath, but usually this does not occur until late in the course.

While shortness of breath at rest usually indicates disease, this is not true in one commonly encountered clinical situation, the *hyperventilation syndrome.* A manifestation of anxiety, the syndrome consists of overbreathing, rapid heart rate, numbness and tingling around the mouth and in the fingers, an involun-tary drawing together of the fingers (*tetany*), tightness or pain in the chest and, in the extreme case, loss of consciousness. These symptoms are due to rapid lowering of the carbon diox-ide content of the blood by the hyperventilation. All are rapidly reversible if the respiration is voluntarily slowed or if the pa-tient breathes into a paper bag (which traps the expired carbon dioxide for rebreathing). It is an extraordinarily common afflic-tion of our time and if not recognized frequently leads to exten-sive (and unnecessary) workup for cardiac or pulmonary disease.

FATIGUE AND WEAKNESS

While patients often use the terms fatigue and weakness syn-onymously, and while both symptoms may coexist, they actually refer to different abnormalities. *Fatigue* means tiredness, lack of energy or loss of the sense of well-being while *weakness* refers to loss of strength. Fatigue after strenuous exercise or prolonged mental effort is expected and considered normal. A high percentage of patients seeking medical help, on the other hand, complain of tiredness in the absence of any reason for fatigue. In almost all such cases careful questioning reveals evidence of emotional stress, anxiety or depression, and in the majority no underlying illness is found. Indeed, it can be said without equivocation that the overwhelming cause of persistent tiredness is not physical disease but mental distress. Nevertheless, fatigue can be caused by organic disease, and the wise physician will not diagnose a functional (psychosomatic) illness until he has excluded other possibilities.

The list of organic diseases that can cause *fatigue* is quite long. In fact probably almost any chronic illness can produce the symptom. When fatigue is the paramount complaint, certain *infections* need to be ruled out. In young persons the viral disease called *infectious mononucleosis* is a prime suspect. While it may produce other symptoms, fatigue, which may last weeks to months, is outstanding. *Infectious hepatitis* is another cause of major fatigue, and the bacterial infections *tuberculosis* and *brucellosis* are also characterized by this symptom. A second major category of diseases to be considered is *metabolic* and *endocrine illness. Hypothyroidism, adrenal insufficiency* and *hypopituitarism* are classic examples. Patients with *diabetes mellitus* often complain of fatigue. In the uncontrolled diabetic state, patients must urinate frequently during the night, and probably the major cause of fatigue is simply loss of sleep. Finally, severe *anemia* of any kind can result in a persistent sense of tiredness and should be considered in any patient presenting with fatigue as a chief complaint.

When *weakness* appears in a previously well patient, the primary focus of the physician will be on muscle or nerve disease. In children and young persons, one of the *muscular dystrophies* may be present. Common causes of muscle disease in adults are the so-called *collagen* or *connective tissue diseases,* and of these *polymyositis* and *dermatomyositis* exhibit the greatest propensity to cause weakness. A number of endocrine diseases also cause serious myopathies with muscle weakness. In *hyperthyroidism* weakness of the thigh muscles becomes so great in many patients that they are unable to rise from a squatting position. *Cushing's syndrome,* which is due to overproduction of adrenal hormones, commonly produces marked weakness in the extremities. Cortisonelike drugs given in high doses for therapeutic reasons do the same thing. *Hypokalemia,* a decrease in potassium levels in the blood, causes muscle weakness in a high percentage of cases. Certain *poisons* can also profoundly impair muscle function. Organic phosphates used in agricultural insecticides are notorious in this regard. The chlorinated insecticides such as DDT, chlordane and dieldrin, in addition to producing hyperexcitability of the central nervous system, cause muscle tremors and weakness. An extremely interesting disease that causes an unusual type of muscle weakness is *myasthenia gravis.* Patients with this illness have good strength on initial muscle use but with repetitive exercise (such as sequential handshakes) become progressively weaker.

A number of diseases involving the *nerves* can cause muscle weakness but many of them are quite rare. The two most dreaded acquired illnesses are *multiple sclerosis* and *amyotrophic lateral sclerosis* (sometimes known as "Lou Gehrig's disease"). These diseases are described in chapter 5. All the secondary neuropathies previously mentioned (e.g., those due to diabetes, alcoholism) can cause muscle weakness on the way to frank paralysis.

JAUNDICE

Jaundice is the medical term for yellow discoloration of the skin and eyes due to the accumulation in the blood of a chemical substance called *bilirubin.* Bilirubin is a breakdown product of hemoglobin, the oxygen-carrying chemical of the red blood cells. It is produced in significant amounts every day from the destruction of red blood cells that have reached the end of their normal life span (ordinarily about 100–120 days). In the liver bilirubin is conjugated with a chemical called glucuronic acid to form *bilirubin glucuronide,* the form that is excreted into the bile. Jaundice can be due to *abnormal breakdown of blood (hemolytic anemia), primary disease of the liver* (which interferes with the conjugation of bilirubin) or *obstruction of the bile ducts* (which blocks bilirubin excretion). Hemolytic anemia is rare. The most common diseases of liver causing jaundice are *viral hepatitis* and *cirrhosis.* The former is a disease primarily of young people while cirrhosis most often is the consequence of alcoholism. (One form of cirrhosis, called *postnecrotic*, is not due to alcohol but is a complication of viral hepatitis.) Obstructive jaundice has two major causes: *gallstones* occluding the common bile duct, or blockading *cancers* arising in the pancreas, intestine or bile ducts themselves. Certain drugs can also cause obstructive jaundice by inducing *cholestasis*, an impairment of bile flow in the small bile channels inside the liver.

It must be emphasized that jaundice never occurs in the absence of disease. It is always an indication for immediate medical consultation.

VOMITING

Vomiting accompanies such a vast array of illnesses that it is of little value by itself in distinguishing benign from serious disease. It is another of the cardinal manifestations of disease that can only be evaluated by the presence or absence of other signs and symptoms. In general if vomiting occurs by itself or in association with diarrhea and is accompanied by nothing more than mild fever and muscle aches, it can be presumed to be due to a viral gastroenteritis that will rapidly pass. Such illnesses are usually of no consequence except in infants or the very elderly where dehydration may become a problem. Conversely, early medical evaluation is indicated if vomiting is associated with severe abdominal pain, distension and failure to pass feces or gas by rectum, a sequence suggesting *intestinal obstruction*. Vomiting that precedes or accompanies pain in the area of the umbilicus or right lower quadrant of the abdomen suggests *appendicitis*. Pain in the right upper quadrant of the abdomen coupled with vomiting indicates the possibility of *gallbladder disease*. Vomiting associated with headache, stiff neck and fever may herald the onset of *meningitis* or *stroke*. Headache, visual difficulties, excessive tear formation, nausea and vomiting constitute the syndrome of *migraine headache*. If fainting or shock occurs with vomiting, the possibility of a crisis due to *adrenal gland insufficiency* must be considered. Vomiting followed by deep, rapid respiration and altered consciousness is characteristic of *diabetic acidosis*. In children the possibility of *accidental poisoning* has to be kept in mind when the onset of vomiting is rapid. Many *drugs* produce vomiting as a side effect and alcohol is notorious in this regard. Nausea and vomiting are very frequent in *early pregnancy*. *Chronic vomiting*, not infrequently seen in young women, is usually psychogenic. Occasionally patients with *diverticulae* (outpouchings) of the esophagus or *hiatal hernia* (a partial protrusion of the stomach through the *diaphragm*, the muscle that separates the abdominal cavity from the chest) complain of vomiting. In actuality these two illnesses cause regurgitation rather than true vomiting. With regurgitation small amounts of fluid and food are returned to the oral cavity, but there is no nausea and no forceful contraction of the abdominal musculature and diaphragm as is the case with vomiting.

DIFFICULTY IN SWALLOWING (DYSPHAGIA)

The complaint of dysphagia in a patient should always be taken seriously and is almost invariably an indication of organic disease. Two major syndromes can be identified. In the first, difficulty in swallowing is due to an abnormality of the swallowing mechanism itself. When this is the case the swallowing act may be followed by regurgitation of fluid into the nose or aspiration into the lung. These symptoms indicate *incoordination* in the complex series of events required to close off the airway to the lungs and the passages from the posterior throat into the nose during the propulsion of food into the esophagus. By far the most common cause of this difficulty is a *stroke* involving areas of the brain or brain stem that control the tongue and pharyngeal muscles. *Myasthenia gravis, poliomyelitis, diphtheria, polymyositis* and the *muscular dystrophies* can produce the same symptom complex.

The second major cause of dysphagia is *obstruction* to passage of food from the mouth to the stomach. When obstructive dysphagia occurs in a person who has been previously healthy, the number one possibility is *cancer of the esophagus. Achalasia* (failure of relaxation of muscles in the lower esophagus) and *scleroderma*, one of the collagen diseases, can also cause obstructive symptoms. Rarely a large goiter or cancer of the thyroid produces external compression of the esophagus with dysphagia. Not infrequently patients complain of a "lump in the throat" which interferes with swallowing, but the most careful examination fails to show any abnormality. In this case the diagnosis is likely to be *globus hystericus,* a manifestation of severe anxiety or hysteria.

DIARRHEA

Diarrhea refers to the presence of two or more defecations per day where the stool is qualitatively or quantitatively abnormal: it is watery, bulky, greasy, mucus-containing or bloody. *Viral gastroenteritis* affects almost every individual at some time of life. It is a self-limited illness of no major consequence (but considerable discomfort). *Bacterial dysenteries* are more serious. Here the diarrhea is explosive and accompanied by high fever, abdominal pain and pus, blood or mucus in the stool. In the United States the usual causes are *Salmonella* or *Shigella* species, but in much of the world *cholera* is the major problem. The diarrhea in the latter is violent and life-threatening. *Parasites* may cause diarrhea and amoebic dysentery is the classic example. Recent travel to any area of the world where sanitary facilities are inadequate should raise the index of suspicion for amebiasis. *Traveler's diarrhea* ("turista") is usually not due to parasites but to toxin-producing strains of normal bowel organisms.

Chronic diarrhea can be caused by several different illnesses. These include: *ulcerative colitis; regional ileitis; a deficiency of the enzyme lactase* (which breaks down milk sugar); *sprue, cystic fibrosis* and *chronic pancreatitis* (all of which cause steatorrhea, the inability to absorb fat from the diet); *certain endocrine diseases* (hyperthyroidism, adrenal insufficiency, hypoparathyroidism); *hormone-producing tumors of the pancreas* and an unusual tumor of the rectum called a *villous adenoma.* Surprisingly, *self-induced diarrhea* is a common problem faced by physicians. For ill-understood psychiatric reasons, such patients surreptitiously take laxatives to produce a diarrheal syndrome.[9]

---

[9] Diseases produced by the deliberate ingestion of drugs and hormones are called *factitious.* They are often difficult to detect. Insulin, thyroid hormone and laxatives top the list of offenders, producing the clinical pictures of insulin-secreting pancreatic tumors, hyperthyroidism and chronic diarrhea respectively.

CONSTIPATION

For reasons that are unclear to me, most Americans appear to be obsessed with the idea that good health requires a regular bowel movement each day. In actuality there is no physiologic basis for this feeling since many normal persons require only one elimination every 4–7 days to feel healthy and comfortable. This variation makes a definition of constipation difficult. The term should probably be defined as a diminution in the frequency of defecation accompanied by increased hardness of stool, diminished caliber of the fecal mass or the inability to defecate in the absence of external assistance such as a laxative, suppository or enema. The necessity to strain at stool is implicit in the definition. When constipation represents a manifestation of underlying disease, the cardinal sign is a change in evacuation patterns; lifelong constipation is not worrisome while the appearance of constipation for no apparent reason in a previously normal person is. The critical diagnostic issue under these circumstances is whether a *cancer of the rectum* or *left side of the colon* is present. Constipation is much more commonly due to *poor dietary habits* with insufficient intake of fiber. Another frequent cause is *chronic laxative use* which, if prolonged, always produces a syndrome where spontaneous evacuation is impossible. In very elderly persons a *fecal impaction* may lead to cessation of bowel movements. Incomplete evacuation of stool from the rectum leads to formation of a mass of feces too large to pass through the anal exit. *Irritable (spastic) colon* refers to a syndrome of lower abdominal pain and constipation, sometimes alternating with diarrhea, which is most often seen in women between the ages of 15 and 45. It is generally considered to be a psychosomatic manifestation of stress or anxiety.

CHANGE IN URINE VOLUME

A sudden change in the daily urine volume, either up or down, is usually indication of disease. The most common cause of increased urine flow (*polyuria*) in the adult is *diabetes mel-*

litus. Polyuria may also be produced by destructive lesions in the posterior part of the pituitary gland which result in deficiency in the secretion of antidiuretic hormone (*diabetes insipidus*). The most common cause is a *tumor*, but impaired blood supply and a disease called *sarcoidosis* may also be involved. Certain chemical imbalances can also produce polyuria, with long-standing *deficiency of potassium* in the blood being the outstanding example. *Hypercalcemia* can produce the same clinical picture. Some patients drink massive amounts of fluid and produce huge amounts of urine because of a psychiatric disorder. Such persons are called *pathologic water drinkers.*

The outstanding cause of diminished urinary output (*oliguria*)[10] is *dehydration.* When body fluids are short, the kidney rigidly conserves water by slowing urine formation. *Acute* and *chronic kidney failure* from any cause may result in oliguria or anuria. In the former, recovery is accompanied by a marked increase in urine output following the anuric period (before function returns to normal). Decreased urination with difficulty starting the stream is a common symptom in middle-aged and elderly men who have developed *enlargement of the prostate gland.* The enlargement is usually due to benign hypertrophy but can also be caused by cancer of the prostate. A fall in urinary volume may be a late consequence of *cancer of the cervix* in women and is due to obstruction of the ureters (the tubes leading from kidneys to bladder) by the tumor.

COUGH

The causes of cough are multitudinous and vary from a nervous habit to cancer of the lung. The most common causes are trivial—colds and allergy. Evidence that a cough may be associated with serious disease includes: cough persisting for prolonged periods (more than a month after an upper respiratory infection); cough associated with significant sputum production, particularly if the sputum is foul-smelling or contains blood or pus; cough associated with weight loss, especially in a smoker; and cough associated with chest pain or shortness of

[10] *Oliguria,* meaning scanty urine, usually refers to a 24-hour urine volume of less than 500 milliliters. *Anuria* means no urine output. In practice, urine volumes of less than 100 milliliters are frequently called anuria.

breath. Any one of these associations is an indication for workup to rule out *pulmonary infections* (bacterial or fungal), *noninfectious inflammatory disease, cancer, pulmonary embolism, chronic bronchitis* or *emphysema.*

EDEMA

Edema refers to the accumulation of excess amounts of fluid in the body. It is usually first seen as swelling around the ankles and lower legs. It is often described as being pitting in nature, meaning that firm pressure with the fingertip leaves a depression in the swollen area which only slowly refills. There are two prevalent benign causes of edema. The first is *varicose veins,* a condition in which the valves of the leg veins become destroyed, leaving knotted, dilated and cosmetically unattractive vessels visible in the lower extremities. The second is severe *obesity* which causes obstruction to lymph drainage from the legs. An uncommon syndrome is that of *cyclic* or *periodic edema,* most often seen in women. For reasons that are not clear, fluid retention sufficient to cause abdominal distension and a several pound increase in weight occurs at recurrent intervals.

Leg edema, particularly if accompanied by the accumulation of fluid inside the abdomen (*ascites*), chest cavity (*pleural effusion*) or over the back can also be a sign of serious systemic disease.

The chief causes are *congestive heart failure, cirrhosis of the liver* and *kidney disease.* The latter includes both end-stage kidney failure and a distinct constellation of abnormalities called the *nephrotic syndrome.* The nephrotic syndrome may be benign and self-limited or accompany chronic renal disease. It consists of generalized edema, marked loss of protein in the urine, low levels of protein in the plasma and elevation of the serum cholesterol concentration. *Hypoalbuminemia* (low plasma protein) due to liver disease is also a common cause of generalized edema. *Lymphedema* is a specialized form of edema due to direct blockage of lymph channels. The swelling is much firmer than ordinary edema and pits with difficulty if at all. Eventually the overlying skin becomes pigmented and brawny in texture. It can occur in women for no apparent reason

(*Milroy's disease*) or be due to blockage of lymphatics by cancers or lymphomas. Lymphedema of the arm is very frequent in women who have undergone radical mastectomy for cancer of the breast because all the lymph nodes and vessels draining the upper extremity are removed at surgery. In some parts of the world *filariasis,* a parasitic disease in which worms lodge in lymphatics, causes lymphedema which can become massive in nature. The extreme form is called *elephantiasis* and results in gigantic enlargement of legs, penis and scrotum. Some 15,000 American servicemen contracted the parasite in World War II.

VERTIGO

The terms *dizziness* and *vertigo* are often used synonymously although they are distinct. Both may be associated with feelings of lightheadedness, faintness and blurring of the vision, but vertigo, in addition, indicates a feeling that the surroundings are rotating in space. Occasionally the symptom is interpreted as a pull or veering of the body to one side or to the floor. With true vertigo, nausea, vomiting and nystagmus accompany the attack. Vertigo occurring suddenly in a previously normal person usually means disease of the *labyrinth of the inner ear.* The labyrinth (or semicircular canals) detects movement and monitors balance assisted by impulses from the eyes and the position-sensing nerves of joints and muscles, particularly those of the neck. Labyrinthine disease may be the consequence of *trauma* (a blow to the head), *infection in the ear* or occur *spontaneously* without apparent cause. If vertigo occurs in association with deafness and *tinnitus* (a buzzing or whistling sound in the ears) it is called *Ménière's syndrome.* Unfortunately tumors of the auditory nerve (the 8th cranial nerve) also cause both deafness and vertigo. These tumors, called *acoustic neurinomas,* are a worrisome possibility when vertigo and deafness are the primary symptoms of disease and must be ruled out before a diagnosis of idiopathic labyrinthitis or Ménière's syndrome can be made with confidence. Some otherwise normal persons have vertigo whenever there is a change in posture but especially on extending or turning the neck. This is called *positional vertigo of Bárány. Strokes* or ischemic lesions in the brain stem (and possibly the cerebellum) can cause vertigo as may tumors in these areas. *Multiple sclerosis* may also begin with vertigo as the initial complaint.

ABNORMAL GROWTHS

The discovery of an abnormal mass or growth anywhere in the body requires evaluation, and a biopsy to rule out malignancy is frequently indicated. The classic example is the breast mass in women, but lymph node enlargement or new skin lesions should likewise never be ignored. Masses over the back, buttocks and extremities are usually lipomas (fatty tumors) or sebaceous cysts, both benign lesions, but even these should be evaluated and removed. Any change in a previously stable lesion such as a mole should be considered suspicious.

CONCLUDING REMARKS

Now that the major symptoms of disease have been outlined, a philosophic word is in order. The appearance of any nontrivial symptom is distressing not only because of its direct physical effects but because it brings to surface the worry that serious disease may be present. This anxiety is entirely normal. The problem comes when consultation is delayed because of fear about what may be found (a phenomenon seen repeatedly by every physician).[11] The simple fact is that anxiety about health can only be dispelled after proper medical examination. The quickest way to have fear vanish is to hear the words, "I don't find anything serious," or "You've got a problem and this is how we're going to handle it." If a serious or potentially life-threatening disease is found, three things can be said. First, knowing the enemy somehow makes it easier to deal with. The unknown is sometimes more fearsome than even the worst of knowns. Second, therapy is available for a large majority of the

[11] If some persons delay consultation because of fear, others, overly anxious, see life-threatening illness in the most minor symptoms and visit physicians continually. In our society, bombarded by sensationalized medical reports, it is easy to become a hypochondriac and psychosomatic illness is rampant. Such patients are particularly difficult for the physician because even if multiple examinations show nothing wrong, there is always the possibility that the next time a symptom will be real.

major diseases (including many cancers). Even when cure is not possible, prolongation of useful (and comfortable) life is frequently obtainable. Third, it helps to share the burden of serious illness with the physician, presuming he or she is both kind and competent. Family and friends can provide love and derivative supportive measures, but the patient needs someone more objective to answer questions, assess progress and indicate prognosis. The bottom line is simply this: If a cardinal symptom is present in a context suggesting the possibility of serious illness, stay calm but act promptly.

4

Genetics and Disease

From time to time in the remainder of this book, it will be necessary to refer to genetics and modes of inheritance of various diseases. There has been an explosion of knowledge in this area over the past three decades, and the new information has revolutionized biological and medical science. A review of these advances will form the basis of this chapter.

It is quite remarkable that from a strictly chemical point of view human life is initiated by the merger of a tiny amount of genetic material from the father with an equivalent quantity derived from the mother. That genetic material is transported to the site of fertilization in the form of an egg and spermatozoon so small as to be invisible to the naked eye. Yet all that the individual will ultimately be flows from these initial genetic determinants and their interaction with environmental and cultural modifiers. Physical structure, intellectual capacity, susceptibility to disease, possibly even the stability of emotional and social life is determined, at least in part, by the nature and quality of the inherited genes.

The genetic machinery is complex, beautiful and incredibly efficient as evidenced by the fact that a high percentage of all conceptions proceed normally with production of healthy human organisms. It can be damaged, however. When that occurs a genetic disease is produced, meaning that the offspring of the affected parent is at risk for inheriting the abnormality. Sometimes the effect of the inherited abnormal gene is trivial;

in other cases it is lethal. For literally hundreds of defects it is somewhere in between. Before turning to the problem of mutations and mechanisms of inheritance in genetic disease, I want to summarize the normal process by which genetic information is translated into those biochemical processes that allow life to proceed.

CHROMOSOMES, GENES AND DEOXYRIBONUCLEIC ACID

Genetic information is carried in a type of chemical molecule called *deoxyribonucleic acid (DNA)*. Deoxyribonucleic acid, in turn, is composed of long strings of smaller molecules called *nucleotides* arranged in linear sequence. Some have likened the arrangement to boxcars in a train, each car being attached to the car in front and behind. The entire DNA molecule is constructed from only 4 nucleotides: *adenine* (A), *cytosine* (C), *guanine* (G) and *thymine* (T). DNA molecules are among the largest of naturally occurring compounds with up to 100,000 nucleotides linked together in one DNA chain. Weights can be as high as 10^9 daltons.[1] Deoxyribonucleic acid is contained within the nucleus of the cell where it is bound to specialized proteins called *histones*. The DNA-histone complexes form rodlike bodies in the nucleus called *chromosomes*. Chromosomes are the storage vault for all the genetic information possessed by the cell. Discrete portions of each DNA strand within the chromosome carry the information necessary for the synthesis of a single protein molecule[2] which might be an enzyme, hormone, transport protein or structural component of the cell. It is an extremely important concept that the genetic information carried in DNA can only be expressed through the synthesis of a protein which is the ultimate mediator of the genetic message. Thus if one is to inherit blue eyes, the initial step is

---

[1] The *dalton* is the mass of the hydrogen atom (1.67 x 10^{-24} grams). In the laboratory scientists, for convenience, often use *gram molecular weights* in which the dalton is assigned a value of 1 gram. The gram molecular weight of water (H_2O) is thus 18: one gram for each hydrogen and 16 grams for oxygen. The relative hugeness of some DNA molecules becomes apparent when it is considered that the gram molecular weight of a molecule the size of 10^9 daltons is 1 billion grams (over 2 million pounds).

[2] Protein as used here includes all molecules that are made up of chains of amino acids.

the production of a protein which initiates the biochemical sequence leading to formation of the necessary pigment in the iris. Some proteins exert their effects directly while others act by influencing intermediate steps to achieve the genetically determined goal. The genetic information necessary for the coding of *one* protein is called a *gene*. Each chromosome contains thousands of genes. In fact, it has been estimated that there is sufficient DNA in the nucleus of every cell to account for more than 100,000 genes.

In humans each cell contains 46 chromosomes. These chromosomes are arranged in pairs with one of each pair coming from the mother and the other from the father. Twenty-two of the pairs are *autosomal* (non-sex-determining) chromosomes while the 23rd pair determines the *sex* of an individual. If two X chromosomes are present, the genetic sex is female while the XY configuration represents a genetic male. It is now possible to isolate and examine under the microscope the chromosomes from human cells, a procedure that is called *karyotyping*. Ordinarily white blood cells are the source, but cells isolated from tissues such as testis and ovary can also be tested. Geneticists frequently use a shorthand code to indicate the chromosomal makeup found by karyotyping. For example, a normal male would be coded *46, XY* while a normal female would be *46, XX*. The number always refers to the total number of chromosomes in the cell while the X's and Y's indicate genetic sex. In a variety of disease states, chromosomal abnormalities exist and they would be coded according to the abnormality present; thus, *45, XO* indicates a mutation in which the total number of chromosomes is one less than normal. The letter O reflects the deletion of a sex chromosome. This configuration is characteristic of *Turner's syndrome*, a common congenital disorder in girls causing short stature, webbed neck, absent breast development and amenorrhea (absence of menstrual periods).

Each gene is normally always located at a specific site on a given chromosome whether that chromosome comes from the mother or the father. That site is called the *gene locus*.[3] When the chromosomes are lined up in pairs, a gene from one parent

[3] A surprisingly large number of human genes can now be reliably assigned to a specific chromosome. In species such as the mouse, it has been possible to go even further and identify the approximate location of many genes within the chromosome itself. Geneticists call this localizing procedure *mapping*.

is located opposite its equivalent from the other parent; each chromosome with all its multiple genes is thus a mirror image of its partner. A variety of genes may be found at the same locus, but each variant at that locus codes for the same characteristic (e.g., color of the eyes). If the genes at a given locus on the two chromosomes are identical, the individual is said to be *homozygous* for that trait. If the genes are nonidentical, the person is described as being *heterozygous*. A gene that is not identical to its counterpart at the same locus on the opposite chromosome is called an *allele*.

The genetic material carried on chromosomes is passed down to daughter cells by two mechanisms. When a *somatic* cell (cells not concerned with reproduction) divides, the process is called *mitosis;* in this process the chromosomes split in two and when the two daughter cells separate, each receives an identical complement of genetic material from the parent cell. *Germ* cells (reproductive cells) also reduplicate by mitosis, but when it is necessary to produce an egg or spermatozoon for purposes of conception, another process, called *meiosis,* is activated. In meiosis the daughter cells receive only one-half the genetic material of the mature germ cell. This is necessary in order to allow the union of a spermatozoon and ovum to result in a fertilized egg with a normal complement of chromosomes. If reduction did not occur, the product of fertilization would contain 92 chromosomes and would not survive. It is important to note that the chromosomes of parent cells split randomly during meiosis. The new daughter cells will thus contain some chromosomes originally derived from the mother and others from the father. This means that eggs and sperm produced in the same meiotic division will have differing genetic makeups relative to each other and to the parent cell. The random distribution of genetic material accounts for the fact that children of the same parents differ from one another. Only identical twins receive exactly the same genetic inheritance.

THE GENETIC CODE AND GENE EXPRESSION

As noted before the gene-bearing DNA molecule consists of long chains of nucleotides arranged in linear sequence. The arrangement of the nucleotides in DNA is not random. Rather,

groups of 3 nucleotides function as code words (*codons*) that
direct the incorporation of specific amino acids into the protein
which is the gene product. For example, the codon adenine-
adenine-adenine (symbol AAA) always codes for the incorporation of the amino acid phenylalanine while adenine-adenine-
thymine (AAT) codes for leucine. This nucleotide-amino acid
incorporation system is called the *genetic code*. Its discovery
and elucidation was one of the great scientific achievements of
all time.

Since the system is a little complicated from a biochemical
standpoint, I will give only a simplified summary here. Basically the DNA of human chromosomes is arranged in two
strands twisted into a ribbonlike form called a *double helix*.
When genetic information needs to be translated (a continuing
process in the cell, although different genes are active or inactive at any given time), the helix opens up so that its nucleotide
sequences can be *transcribed*. In this process a second nucleo-
tide-containing molecule called *messenger RNA* is formed.[4]
What this means is that nucleotide triplets in the DNA attract
complementary nucleotides attached to ribose and construct an
RNA molecule under the influence of an enzyme called DNA-
dependent RNA polymerase. The newly formed messenger
RNA then passes out of the nucleus and becomes attached to
protein-synthesizing particles called *ribosomes* located in the
cytoplasm (the extranuclear protoplasm) of the cell. The amino
acids from which protein is to be made by the ribosome are
attached to a second type of RNA called *transfer RNA*. Each
transfer RNA is specific for one amino acid and has a characteristic terminal nucleotide triplet. What happens is that each triplet of the messenger RNA selects the proper transfer RNA
through its attraction for the latter's terminal nucleotide triplet.
Basically the ribosome moves down the messenger RNA chain
"reading" its nucleotide sequence like a computer; as it senses

[4] RNA stands for *ribonucleic acid*. Deoxyribonucleic acid (DNA) contains a sugar
called *deoxyribose* while the sugar of RNA is named *ribose*. Each nucleotide contains
one or the other of these two sugars to which is attached a phosphoric acid molecule.
The sugars are linked to one another by the latter (so that one phosphoric acid is located
between every pair of riboses or deoxyriboses) to form the chains of DNA and RNA.
Three of the four nucleotides in DNA and RNA are identical: adenine, guanine and
cytosine. The fourth is different. DNA contains thymine while RNA contains uracil.
The genetic code is based on the fact that these nucleotides are chemically attracted to
each other. Thus, adenine always attracts thymine (DNA) or uracil (RNA), cytosine
attracts guanine, guanine attracts cytosine, and thymine and uracil attract adenine.

a nucleotide triplet for a given amino acid, it then attaches the transfer RNA carrying the proper amino acid and couples it to the amino acid which was coded for by the immediately preceding triplet (hooking the amino acids together almost like a zipper). When all the triplets of the messenger RNA have been read (*translated*), the new protein molecule, containing as many amino acids as there were nucleotide triplets in the message, comes off the ribosome and is ready to carry out its function. To reiterate, the nucleotide triplets of DNA are transcribed to a chain of complementary nucleotide triplets in messenger RNA. The latter is then used by the ribosome as a pattern to attach the transfer RNAs, each of which has a unique terminal nucleotide triplet that recognizes the complementary triplet in the messenger RNA (and is equivalent to the original codon in DNA). For the amino acid phenylalanine, the sequence can be represented schematically as follows:

AAA (DNA)
↓
UUU (messenger RNA)
↓
AAA (transfer RNA)
↓
phenylalanine

If biochemical reactions can ever be legitimately called beautiful (and I think they can), this is a consummately beautiful process.

MUTATIONS

A mutation represents an alteration of DNA which disturbs the genetic message that it normally transmits. Mutations occurring in somatic cells are thought to result in cancer while those affecting germ cells in the testes or ovaries produce inheritable disease. Germ cell mutations may be *silent* (nonapparent) if the gene product is not essential for life and if no biochemical marker is available for its detection. Alternatively, the mutation may be *lethal:* the defect produced is so severe as to be incompatible with life. A high percentage of miscarriages (spontaneous abortions) probably reflect such lethal mutations.

Finally, the mutation may be *expressed,* meaning that it produces disease or a measurable biochemical abnormality. While most genetic diseases are rare, it is staggering to realize that over 1,200 disorders have now been identified. It has been estimated that genetic disease accounts for more than 5 percent of all hospital admissions.

The nature of the agents causing mutations is not known with certainty. Suspicion has centered on radiation (particularly cosmic radiation originating in outer space), viruses and chemicals. It is thought that mutagenic events occur commonly in all persons, but that efficient chromosomal repair processes active in the nucleus delete most of them. Only when the repair system breaks down does a permanent mutation occur.

Mutations can cause visible damage or alteration of whole chromosomes (in which case multiple genes are involved) or produce changes in one nucleotide of a triplet codon. When the change involves one nucleotide, it is called a *point* mutation. Usually this means that the normal nucleotide present at a given location in the gene is replaced by another resulting in the incorporation of a wrong amino acid when the gene is transcribed and translated. An excellent example of a point mutation is *sickle cell anemia,* a common disease of blood in blacks. It is caused by the substitution of the amino acid valine for glutamic acid in the 6th position of the β-chain of hemoglobin. In the gene coding for the β-chain of hemoglobin, the 6th position is normally occupied by 1 of 2 triplets, CTT or CTC, both of which code for glutamic acid.[5] When the sickle cell mutation occurred centuries ago, an adenine replaced the thymine in position 2 of 1 of these 2 triplets, producing either CAT or CAC, both of which code for valine. Diseases produced by point mutations (also called simply inherited or *Mendelian disorders*) are much more common than those produced by chromosomal abnormalities. A third category of genetic disease is much less well understood. Called *multifactorial disorders,* these diseases represent conditions that tend to occur in families but do not follow simple rules of inheritance. The assumption is that multiple genes are involved and that environmental factors also play a role.

[5] The genetic code is made up of 64 triplet codons despite the fact that there are only 20 amino acids available for incorporation into protein. This means that some amino acids are coded for by more than one codon. The reason for this redundancy is not completely understood.

CHROMOSOMAL DISORDERS

Chromosomal syndromes may be due to the presence of too many, too few or abnormally structured chromosomes. The majority appear to be new mutations since it is usual for both parents of an affected child to be normal. It is probable that most mutations involving a whole chromosome are lethal. This follows from the observation that if karyotypes are done on unselected newborn infants, the incidence of chromosomal defects is about 1 in 200. In spontaneous abortions, on the other hand, the incidence may be as high as 1 in 2, a finding compatible with the thesis that high rates of lethality result from these disorders. In infants who survive gestation, three common diseases due to chromosomal defects are found: *Turner's syndrome*, the 45, XO disorder mentioned earlier in this chapter,[6] *Klinefelter's syndrome* and *Down's syndrome* or *mongolism*. The karyotype in *Klinefelter's syndrome* is usually 47, XXY; that is, the patients have an extra X chromosome which appears to diminish the masculinizing efficiency of the Y (male) chromosome. The disorder, which occurs once in about 450 live male births, is characterized by tall stature, sterility, extremely small testes and gynecomastia (breast development in the male). In *Down's syndrome* there are 3 copies of the 21st chromosome (called *trisomy 21*) instead of the normal 2. These children have the characteristic mongoloid facies (recognizable by anyone who has ever seen such a patient), mental retardation, curved little fingers, poor muscle development and a variety of congenital defects. The incidence of Klinefelter's syndrome increases with advancing age of the father while mongolism is associated with increasing maternal age. The risk of producing a child with Down's syndrome is less than 0.1 percent in women under the age of 30. Above the age of 35 that risk rapidly rises to 1 percent or higher.

Chromosomal abnormalities have also been associated with four forms of neoplastic disease in humans. In *chronic myelo-*

---

[6] While the 45, XO karyotype may be present in all cells, it is possible to have two lines of cells in the body, one normal and the other abnormal. This condition is called *mosaicism*. The designation of the Turner mosaic is 45,XO/46,XX, reflecting the presence of some cells with deletion of an X and others with the normal female complement of 2 X's. Mosaicism also exists in Klinefelter's syndrome.

genous leukemia chromosome 22 is abnormal. Called the *Philadelphia chromosome*, it is present in over 90 percent of the abnormally dividing cells in the leukemic bone marrow. *Meningioma,* a tumor of the meninges (the membranes covering the brain), is also associated with a deletion or deficiency of chromosome 22. *Burkitt's lymphoma,* a common lesion in Africa, is due to abnormalities in chromosomes 8 and 14. In 1979 a family was described in which 10 members in 3 generations had *renal* (kidney) *cancer.* In these patients chromosomes 3 and 8 appeared abnormal, the suggestion being that there had been an exchange of material between the two. It is of great interest that cancer was sought in three of the members (who were completely asymptomatic) because chromosomal analysis showed the same abnormality that was present in other members who had been demonstrated to have cancer. In each case cancer was found at operation. The findings in this family raise the exciting possibility that genes predisposing to cancer may ultimately be identified.

MENDELIAN DISORDERS

The simply inherited disorders fall into three categories: (1) autosomal dominant, (2) autosomal recessive, and (3) X-linked. *Autosomal disorders* are due to gene defects in one of the 22 pairs of autosomal chromosomes while *X-linked diseases* are due to change on the X chromosome. There is no Y-linked category for reasons which are not clear. The Y chromosome carries the genetic information that imparts maleness, but details about its other functions (if any) are unavailable.

Most readers will have heard the terms *dominant* and *recessive* used in the genetic sense. Unfortunately there is a widespread misconception about their meaning. That misconception holds that a dominant gene is somehow stronger than its normal counterpart and that it therefore overpowers the latter, always expressing itself. In fact, all genes express their activities in the same way; none is more powerful than another. Dominant simply means that a defect will be expressed even if only 1 copy of the abnormal gene is present. In a recessive defect 2 copies of the abnormal gene must be present for full expression of the disorder: the abnormal gene must be present on both the maternally and the paternally derived chromosomes. If only 1 copy of the recessive gene is present, the subject is called a *carrier* and does not have overt disease (although careful search may reveal minor physical or chemical defects due to the presence of the gene). Rarely an individual does inherit 2 copies of an abnormal dominant gene. The disease produced by the homozygous dominant state is generally more severe than that of the heterozygous form. Dominant mutations are usually associated with synthesis of an abnormal gene product (e.g., an enzyme that has lost its normal control mechanisms) while in recessive defects the general problem is that the gene product is not made at all. Thus, deficiency of an enzyme would be a classic expression of recessive disease. Earlier in this chapter it was pointed out that a single gene directs the production of only one protein. That point must be re-emphasized here. All the multiple symptoms of a genetic disease are believed to flow directly or indirectly from the absence of or abnormality in 1 protein. In many cases the mechanism by which a single defect causes the multiple manifestations (secondary events) of a genetic disease is not known.

AUTOSOMAL DOMINANT DISORDERS

When a dominant disorder is heterozygous (as is usually the case), the abnormal gene is paired with a normal gene at the allelic site of the matching chromosome from the other parent. As a consequence, during meiosis (the process by which germ cells reduce their chromosomes by half preparatory to fertilization) one daughter cell will receive the abnormal gene and one the normal. This means that in dominant disorders only half the offspring of an affected parent will be expected to inherit the defect.[7] The characteristics of a dominant disorder can be summarized as follows:

1. Each affected individual has a parent with the same disorder (see following paragraph for exceptions).

---

[7] The distribution of chromosomes in daughter cells occurs randomly. Therefore genetic statements are *statistically* true but do not necessarily hold in small samples. It is statistically true that offspring of a father with a dominant disease will show 50 percent affected children since half of his spermatozoa will be carrying the abnormal gene. By chance, however, the egg of the mother in 3 successive pregnancies might be fertilized by one of the normal spermatozoa. Thus one could have 3 normal children from a parent with a dominant disease. Conversely, all the children might inherit the disease if the number of children were few. If the family had 10 or 12 children, the distribution would approach the expected 50 percent.

2. Affected subjects have normal and abnormal offspring in equal proportions.
3. The offspring of unaffected children will be normal since their parent has not inherited the defective gene.
4. Males and females are affected equally and each can transmit the defect to offspring of either sex.
5. The defect is seen in each successive generation provided a significant number of children are produced.

Characteristic (1) may not hold under two circumstances. A known dominant disease may appear in the face of a negative family history if it is the result of a new mutation. In this case the rules of inheritance just outlined become operative in the progeny of the new mutation, and a characteristic family history will subsequently be established. The other alternative for the appearance of a dominant trait in the absence of a family history of the disease is extramarital paternity: the gene is introduced by a father who is not the husband. Tests of large numbers of newborn infants suggest that extramarital paternity is responsible for 3–5 percent of all births in the United States.

AUTOSOMAL RECESSIVE DISORDERS

As noted before, in recessive disorders both genes at the affected site must be abnormal to produce a clinical syndrome. This means that both father and mother have to be carriers of the trait although they are themselves clinically normal. When this is the case, distribution of the abnormal gene in the offspring will be as follows: 25 percent of the children will be normal, 50 percent will be carriers of the gene (heterozygotes) and 25 percent will be homozygous and thus express the abnormality. (In the rare circumstance of marriage between two persons who actually have the same recessive disease—that is, are homozygotes—all children will also have the disease since neither parent has a normal gene at the affected locus.) The characteristics of a recessive abnormality can be summarized as follows:

1. Both parents are clinically normal.
2. One-fourth of the children of carrier parents inherit the abnormality while half will carry the abnormal gene.
3. Offspring of affected subjects are not affected since the child will receive the abnormal gene from the afflicted parent but

a normal gene from the other parent (unless the parent happens to marry a carrier of the same gene).
4. Males and females are equally affected.

For reasons that are not precisely clear, recessive disorders tend to appear earlier in life than do dominant diseases; a high percentage are diagnosed in childhood while dominant defects frequently do not manifest themselves until after adult life has been reached.

Most recessive diseases are rare because the gene does not occur frequently enough in the population to make likely the possibility that carriers will marry. The chance that both parents will be carriers of any trait increases dramatically if mother and father are related. If a common ancestor bore an abnormal recessive gene, the chance of its presence in descendants who are cousins, say, will be far higher than the prevalence of the gene in the general population. Ancient taboos against marriage between relatives reflected awareness that genetic disease is often the consequence of such mating. It is for this reason that physicians probe for evidence of consanguineous marriage whenever a patient is discovered to have a recessive disease. The rarer the clinical disorder, the more likely is the possibility of consanguinity, although in general rates of marriage between relatives are very low in the United States.

A variant recessive disorder is called a *compound genetic abnormality*. It is due to the fact that 2 different abnormal genes occupy the same allelic site in the affected individual. Perhaps the most common example in the United States is *sickle cell C disease*. In this illness the patient inherits the gene for the abnormal C hemoglobin from one parent and the gene for sickle hemoglobin from the other, causing a disease with mixed features. Compound disorders are quite rare.

X-LINKED DISORDERS

X-linked inheritance is more complicated than that of autosomal dominant and recessive diseases. Recall that the female has two X chromosomes in every cell while the male has unpaired sex chromosomes, an X and a Y. It follows that a female can be either heterozygous or homozygous for an abnormal gene exactly analogous to the situation in autosomal chromosomes. For recessive genes no disease would be expected in the heterozygous state since the abnormal X-linked gene would be balanced by a normal allele on the paired chromosome. On the other hand if the male inherits an abnormal X-linked gene from the mother—*even if that gene is recessive in nature*—it will be expressed because the unpaired Y chromosome cannot neutralize the presence of the abnormal gene on the X chromosome (its genetic material is separate and distinct from that carried by the X). Since the male contributes his Y chromosome to all of his sons, it follows that male-to-male transmission of X-linked disorders does not occur. Conversely, an affected father contributes the abnormal gene on the X chromosome to all his daughters, each of whom becomes a carrier. The characteristic features of X-linked recessive transmission can be summarized as follows:

1. Mothers of affected males do not have the disease.
2. Male offspring of carrier women have a 50 percent chance of being affected, and 50 percent of female children are carriers.
3. All female offspring of affected males are carriers while all male offspring are free of the abnormal gene.
4. Females develop the disease in question only when an affected male marries a carrier female such that female offspring are homozygous.

Examples of sex-linked recessive disorders are: colorblindness, a benign condition; and hemophilia, the bleeding disease.

X-linked dominant traits are less common than X-linked recessive diseases. In these conditions the trait is expressed in both mother and offspring since only one abnormal gene is required; the normal X chromosome of the mother does not protect her. The characteristics of X-linked dominant transmission are as follows:

1. An affected mother transmits the gene to half her sons and half her daughters.
2. An affected male transmits the disorder to all his daughters and none of his sons.
3. The disease is more variable in affected females than affected males.

The explanation for point 3 is given by what has come to be called the *Lyon hypothesis*. It is now recognized that early in embryonic life one of the two X chromosomes in each somatic cell of the woman becomes inactivated in random fashion. Thus each woman is actually a *mosaic*—half of her cells have an active X chromosome derived from the father and half an X chromosome coming from the mother. For this reason half (and sometimes, by chance more than half) of the X chromosomes containing the abnormal gene are inactivated during development. This inactivation accounts for the fact that a dominant abnormal X in the female may produce less severe disease than the same gene in the male. Conversely, a woman who is heterozygous for a recessive gene and who ordinarily would be expected to be an asymptomatic carrier may develop symptoms if by chance more of the normal than abnormal X chromosomes are inactivated during fetal development. Inactivation of the X chromosome occurs only in somatic cells. In germ cells both X's remain active.

The inactivated X chromosome is of interest from another standpoint. It was recognized early that somatic cells of women, when examined under a microscope, had a visible mass of chromatin (nuclear material) at the periphery of the nucleus. This chromatin mass was called a *Barr body*. It is now known that the Barr body is the inactivated X chromosome. In the days before karyotyping was available, it was common to test for genetic sex by taking smears of the lining of the mouth and looking for Barr bodies in the cells so obtained. If Barr bodies were not found, it was assumed that the genetic sex was male. (Readers will doubtless remember the uproar that developed when women performing in the Olympic games were required to be tested for Barr bodies to prove that they were true females.) A table listing some of the common genetic diseases and their pattern of inheritance is appended to the end of this chapter.

MULTIFACTORIAL DISEASES

This category of genetic disease is much less well defined than those previously described. It has long been known to clinicians that certain diseases have a predisposition to run in families even though a precise pattern of inheritance is not possible to ascertain. For example, such diverse conditions as coronary artery disease, diabetes mellitus, schizophrenia and cleft palate occur more commonly in certain families than in the population as a whole. Most geneticists now believe that certain combinations of genes (rather than an abnormality in a single gene) may predispose to these disorders, probably in combination with environmental or nongenetic factors. Much remains to be learned about these diseases and the gene–gene interactions that cause them.

GENES AND ENVIRONMENT

While this chapter has emphasized the role of genetics in causing disease, it should be recognized that nongenetic (environmental) factors often determine the seriousness of the clinical presentation in genetic diseases or even whether symptoms will appear. Drugs are common offenders. For example, *acute intermittent porphyria* is a disease resulting from an abnormality in the biochemical pathway leading to hemoglobin synthesis. Acute exacerbations of the illness lead to excruciating abdominal pain and muscle paralysis. These crises are frequently produced by the ingestion of drugs such as barbiturates or certain tranquilizers. Thus, even though one could not have the disease in the absence of the gene abnormality, expression of the defect is dramatically worsened by an environmental factor, in this case drugs. Dietary components may act in the same way. For example, mental retardation in *phenylketonuria* can be prevented if the amino acid phenylalanine is removed from the diet, while avoidance of milk may prevent the cataracts and other abnormalities seen in *galactosemia,* a disease in which the sugar galactose cannot be metabolized normally.

If environmental factors can influence diseases considered to be primarily genetic, the converse is also true: genes play a role in diseases that on the face would appear to be purely environmental. For example, a car turns a corner rapidly and hits a boy on a bicycle, breaking his leg. That could hardly be considered anything but disease due to an environmental agent. Yet another boy in the identical situation but with genetically determined better hearing might have perceived a warning sound earlier and jumped out of the car's path, escaping injury. The difference in the two outcomes depends on the genes. Few (if any) diseases are purely genetic or purely environmental. While one or the other may be primary, every genetic disease is influenced by environmental factors and every externally induced disease is modified by the genetic makeup of the affected subject.

PREVENTION OF GENETIC DISORDERS

Basically four methods are available for prevention of genetic disease. The first is *genetic counseling*. If a disease is known to exist in families and if the inheritance patterns of that disease are clear, advice as to whether to have children can sometimes be given with fair assurance. If a disease is known to be present in a family but the parents desire children despite the risk, a second approach is the use of *amniocentesis*. In this technique a sample of the amniotic fluid which surrounds the fetus is taken by a needle inserted into the womb through the abdomen. In certain diseases the fluid can be tested directly for the presence or absence of the abnormality, but more commonly cells floating in the fluid (which are derived from the fetus) are isolated and grown in culture outside the body. The cells are then tested for the genetic disease in question (e.g., trisomy 21 in mongolism). If the diagnosis is confirmed, a therapeutic abortion can be carried out (presuming this to be acceptable to the parents). A third approach is to *screen* all infants for common genetic diseases at birth. This is now done routinely for phenylketonuria but is obviously not possible for all known genetic disorders. In a high percentage of inherited diseases, either the primary defect is not known or there is no easily testable marker of its presence. Moreover, the expense of such screening is formidable. The fourth approach is to *treat* the defect as soon after birth as possible in order to avoid permanent damage from the lesion. This is most effective in diseases where avoidance of drugs or certain dietary constituents prevent the clinical manifestations. The importance of taking a detailed family history from prospective parents resides in the fact that the physician can then be alert to possible genetic defects and attempt to minimize their impact.

A WORD ABOUT THE RECOMBINANT DNA DEBATE

No chapter on genetics would be complete without a brief discussion of the recombinant DNA debate since no scientific issue in memory has stirred such great emotional response. Recombinant DNA techniques allow the insertion of genetic material from any source (including humans) into bacteria or viruses which can then be programmed to produce the gene product of the transplanted genetic material. The methodology involves use of certain enzymes (called *restriction nucleases*) isolated from bacteria. These enzymes have the capacity to clip open double-stranded DNA in such a way as to leave the ends chemically "sticky." This is done most commonly in a bacterium called *Escherichia coli,* a common gut inhabitant. The next step is to insert foreign genetic material (such as a purified gene) into the opened DNA strand.[8] The grafted material is then reinserted into *E. coli.* The *E. coli* multiply and, under proper conditions, make the gene product coded for by the genetic material inserted by the recombinant technique. The potential for making rare biological chemicals, such as enzymes and hormones, is unlimited. For example, children with a deficiency of pituitary growth hormone are doomed to short stature unless treated. Human growth hormone can be laboriously extracted from pituitary glands collected at autopsy, but supplies are insufficient to meet current demands. As a consequence treatment must stop when the child reaches 5 feet in height. If the gene for human growth hormone were inserted in *E. coli* by recombinant techniques and if it could be activated to transcribe, the problem of inadequate supplies of growth hormone would be solved. Similarly, scientists fear that there will be a worldwide shortage of insulin within the next few years. This too could be solved by genetic engineering in bacteria. Indeed, the insulin gene has been inserted successfully in *E. coli* and human insulin has been produced. Note that the power of the recombinant DNA techniques has been enormously increased by other recent advances in molecular biology which not only

---

[8] *E. coli* contains one large chromosome and several smaller loops of DNA called *plasmids.* It is usually the plasmid that is used for gene splicing.

allow the structure of specific genes to be deduced but make possible their actual synthesis in the laboratory.

Why the concern about recombinant DNA research? The answer is that a number of people, including some of the leading scientists working in the field, feel that the possibility of harm —grave harm to the universe as a whole—from this type of research is very real. Anxiety from the very beginning was expressed at two levels. The first was a rather general feeling that it is possible to know too much. Often cited was the example of the breakthrough in nuclear physics immediately before and during World War II which ended up as hydrogen bombs. Some have felt that this research might lead to tampering with the life process itself. As one scientist asked, "Do we want to assume the basic responsibility for life on this planet? To develop new living forms for our own purposes?" Along similar lines the specter of genetic engineering in humans for less than honorable purposes has hovered in the background of many discussions. The second possible danger was more immediate and more real. *E. coli,* the standard organism used in these experiments, is an occupant of every human intestinal tract. If by accident (or, perish the thought, design) genetic information coding for a lethal toxin were introduced into the organism and it was somehow released into the environment, an epidemic new disease might be produced. Similar arguments have been mobilized against the use of viruses as vehicles for genetic manipulation. Even if an altered virus did not affect man, would it attack animals or plants destroying the ecologic balance?

Because of these concerns an unprecedented event in the world of science occurred in 1974. A group of leading investigators in recombinant DNA research called for a voluntary moratorium on certain types of experiments considered to be of high risk until answers about safety could be obtained. The moratorium was generally followed for the next 2 years. In 1976 the federal government, through its chief research agency, the National Institutes of Health, released a set of guidelines for recombinant DNA research and the moratorium was rescinded. These guidelines were derived from a "worst-case" type of analysis which attempted to assess the risk if the worst possible accident occurred. Certain types of experiments were entirely proscribed under the guidelines while others were considered to constitute little risk. Critics did not accept the NIH assessment and claimed that potential hazards were underplayed. Whatever the validity of the arguments on either side, it is clear that no untoward event has ever resulted from recombinant DNA research, and great strides have been made in reducing the risks, including development of new strains of *E. coli* which contain genetic deficiencies such that the organism would not likely survive outside the laboratory. Still, the critics—who, incidentally, are acting with the very high motive of protecting mankind and environment—are not satisfied. Dr. Robert L. Sinsheimer of the California Institute of Technology, a leading spokesman for those wishing to limit this type of research, has been quoted as saying, "There are certain matters best left unknown, at least for a while."[9]

Despite the eloquence of the critics, at the present time the consensus is that this type of research should go forward. I am personally in accord with this view. I do not believe it possible to limit the acquisition of new knowledge or the exploration of the unknown even if that were desirable. Somewhere, somehow, inquisitive minds will ask the questions and find the answers. I prefer to have this done openly under rigid guidelines and in the face of peer examination, which is an extremely powerful deterrent to unwise and unethical behavior in the scientific community. Above and beyond the philosophical arguments, I believe it highly likely that recombinant DNA research will produce benefit for mankind as a whole and for those who are ill with a variety of genetic diseases in particular. Indeed, it is not inconceivable that all genetic diseases may one day be treatable by these approaches. That there is risk goes without saying. But there are very few things of value that can be attained without risk.

[9] For those interested in a good lay summary of the debate, see Grobstein, "The Recombinant-DNA Debate," *Scientific American* 237: 22, (July) 1977.

TABLE 2
SOME COMMON GENETIC DISORDERS

1. *Autosomal Dominant*
   Acute intermittent porphyria
   Adult polycystic kidney disease
   Familial hypercholesterolemia
   Hemochromatosis
   Hereditary hemorrhagic telangiectasia
   Hereditary spherocytosis
   Huntington's chorea
   Idiopathic hypertrophic subaortic
     stenosis
   Marfan's syndrome
   Neurofibromatosis
   Noonan's syndrome
   Osteogenesis imperfecta tarda
   Tuberous sclerosis
   von Willebrand's disease

2. *Autosomal Recessive*
   Albinism
   β-thalassemia
   Cystic fibrosis
   Deafness
   Familial Mediterranean fever
   Friedreich's ataxia
   Hereditary emphysema
   Homocystinuria
   Phenylketonuria
   Sickle cell anemia
   Wilson's disease

3. *X-linked Recessive Disorders*
   Colorblindness
   Fabry's disease
   Glucose-6-phosphate dehydrogenase
     deficiency
   Hemophilia A
   Hypophosphatemic rickets
   Ocular albinism
   Testicular feminization

4. *X-linked Dominant Disorders*
   Pseudohypoparathyroidism
   Vitamin D resistant rickets

5

Diseases of the Nervous System

The nervous system of the human being is so complex that despite decades of intensive study, only a tiny fraction of its secrets have yielded to the inquiry of neuroscientists. Every organ system in the body is dependent on its direction, and the integration of their multiple individual functions into a coherent whole requires its continual and unimpaired activity. It is, perhaps, not too difficult at this stage of scientific development to understand how an impulse is transported down a peripheral nerve to result in the contraction of a muscle or how a peripheral sensation like the prick of a pin initiates a signal that passes from a receptor in the skin through the spinal cord to the pain recognition site in the brain. In stark contrast is the apparently impenetrable mystery of how the specialized nervous tissue we call the brain generates rational thought, the emotions which characterize human life, the capacity to create originally in music, art and written word, the ability to act against instinctual (animal) drives for survival or self-fulfillment and the conception of right and wrong.[1] In this chapter the basic structure and function of the nervous system will be described, and modern diagnostic techniques for identification of neurologic disease

[1] I once heard Dr. Jerome Y. Lettvin of the Massachusetts Institute of Technology give a faculty seminar at my medical school which was entitled (as I recall) "Why I am leaving neurobiology." After years of experimentation designed to reveal how visual images might be transmitted to and interpreted by the brain, he was saying, somewhat tongue-in-cheek, that the system appeared so complicated that it could be beyond dissection.

reviewed. Finally, the major diseases of the nervous system will be outlined.

STRUCTURE AND FUNCTION OF THE NERVOUS SYSTEM

The nervous system is made up of two large divisions, the *central* and *peripheral nervous systems*. The *central nervous system* consists of the brain, the brain stem and the spinal cord. The *peripheral nervous system* is made up of the cranial nerves, which pass from the brain stem to various portions of the head; the spinal nerves, which run from the spinal cord to all parts of the body except the head; and the autonomic nervous system, which innervates viscera, blood vessels, glands and smooth muscle throughout the body. Traffic over the nervous system is two way. *Afferent* fibers transmit sensations such as pain, touch, pressure, temperature and position sense centrally to the brain from the periphery. *Efferent* fibers transmit in the opposite direction, from brain to peripheral tissues. An important principle is that nerve connections between brain and peripheral tissues cross from their side of origin at some point in their course; that is, the right side of the brain is connected to and controls the left side of the body while the left side of the brain is connected to and controls the right side of the body.

Brain. The brain proper consists of paired *cerebral hemispheres* (sometimes called the *cerebral cortex*), each the mirror image of the other, and the single *cerebellum*. The complex network of cells that make up the *cortex* are responsible for all of what we generally consider to be intellectual function (including memory) and the myriad of feeling responses or emotions that make up the personality of each individual. The cerebral hemispheres are also responsible for sensory perception and for the initiation of voluntary movement (*motor activity*). The cortex is divided into four lobes or divisions called *frontal, parietal, occipital* and *temporal*. The first three occupy the anterior, middle and posterior portions of the upper brain, respectively, while the temporal lobes are below and to the side. Each lobe carries out specific functions and damage to that lobe will result in the loss of those functions. The *frontal lobe* is responsible for motor activity on the opposite side of the body, speech,[2] coordination of head-eye movements and normal emotional responses. The *parietal lobe* is the primary area of sensory perception. It is also the seat of normal reading, writing and calculating skills as well as the ability to use symbolic concepts. The *occipital lobe* contains the visual area and is responsible for the perception and interpretation of images. The *temporal lobe* is concerned with memory, space perception and sleep; in addition it contributes to normal vision, speech and hearing. Many other functions of the cerebral cortex cannot be precisely localized to any one anatomic site. These include orientation to time, place and person; maintenance of spontaneity, interest and humor; the ability to smell and taste; the capacity to think and speak coherently; generation of sexual drive; and the ability to preserve modest and civilized behavior patterns.

The *cerebellum* is best conceived as a kind of regulatory computer that assures the capacity to carry out motor activity in smooth and coordinated fashion. Damage to the cerebellum does not cause paralysis, but muscle movements are crude and unbalanced, gait is abnormal, tremor and nystagmus appear and the ability to gauge distances is lost in the absence of its input.

Brain Stem. The brain stem connects the brain and the spinal cord, transmitting nerve impulses between the two. It has four divisions (from above down) called the *diencephalon, midbrain, pons* and *medulla oblongata.* It is the seat of specialized centers that control automatic functions such as respiration and circulation as well as those governing food and water intake. The *hypothalamus,* located in the diencephalon, is an extraordinarily important area since it releases hormones that control the activity of the pituitary gland and thereby regulates endocrine function throughout the body. The brain stem is also responsible for maintenance of consciousness, and lesions in the pons, particularly, cause deep coma. Finally, the cranial nerves arise from this portion of the central nervous system.

The Spinal Cord. The spinal cord merges imperceptibly into the medulla oblongata and the boundary between the two is indistinct. It consists of bundles of nerve cells and fibers that

---

[2] While each hemisphere can be considered to be basically identical to its opposite partner, it is characteristic for one side to dominate. The left hemisphere is dominant in right-handed persons while the right is dominant in left-handed persons. Some functions, like the control of speech, are localized to the dominant hemisphere.

transmit impulses between the peripheral nervous system and the brain. The cord has no original activity; by that I mean that impulses are normally not initiated in its fiber tracts but only transmitted through them. Lesions damaging the cord block communication from below upward and from above downward. The spinal cord is enclosed by the vertebral bodies of the bony spine and the spinal nerves emerge between adjacent vertebrae. The latter arrangement accounts for the fact that disease or displacement of vertebrae or vertebral discs may cause pain or weakness in that part of the body serviced by the involved nerve.

Peripheral Nerves. Three types of nerves emerge from the central nervous system. All are paired, one of each pair supplying the left side of the body and the other the right. The 12 *cranial* nerves provide sensory and motor innervation for the head and face. The 31 *spinal* nerves supply the remainder of the body. The spinal nerves are designated by their relation to the vertebral section from which they emerge: *cervical* (neck), *thoracic* (chest), *lumbar* (back), *sacral* and *coccygeal* (lower spine). In general the cervical nerves innervate the neck and arms, the thoracic nerves the chest and abdomen, the lumbar nerves the legs and the sacral and coccygeal nerves the perineal area, including the genital organs, bladder and rectum. Physicians often use an easy shorthand in describing the nerves. To illustrate, the nerve that exits at thoracic vertebra 5 is called T_5, that emerging at lumbar vertebra 4, L_4 and so on. The third category of nerves makes up the *autonomic system*. Their function is automatic and is not directed voluntarily. Heart rate, blood pressure, intestinal motility and sweating are examples of functions under autonomic control. The system is divided into *sympathetic* and *parasympathetic* divisions, which tend to be antagonistic; for example, parasympathetic nerves slow the heart rate while sympathetic fibers accelerate it.

Neurons and Synapses. The fundamental unit of the nervous system is the *neuron* (nerve cell). Each neuron consists of a cell body from which extend short receiving processes called *dendrites* and an elongated, fiberlike transmitting unit called the *axon.* The axon is surrounded by a thin sheath or membrane (*Schwann sheath*) which in some nerves produces a second internal layer, the *myelin sheath.* The latter is arranged in segments and appears to function like an electrical insulator for the axon. A number of diseases, such as multiple sclerosis, cause

damage to the myelin sheath and thus are classified as *demye-*
linating diseases.

In simple terms the nervous system consists of vast quantities
of interconnecting neurons together with certain support cells
not directly involved in neural transmission. It is important to
recognize that single neurons do not connect the brain and peripheral tissues. Rather, signals are transmitted through chains
of neurons. The point where one neuron connects to the dendrites of the next neuron or to the specific receptor area in a
target organ is called a *synapse*. The transmission of an impulse
along a nerve is an electrical event generated by movement of
chemical ions across the cell membrane. When the impulse
reaches the synapse, it causes release of one of a variety of
chemicals called *neurotransmitters*.[3] The neurotransmitter
then moves across the synaptic gap and initiates a new electrical impulse in the next link of the chain.

Cerebrospinal Fluid (CSF). The brain and spinal cord are
surrounded by a clear, cell-free liquid called the *cerebrospinal*
fluid. It is similar in composition to plasma but not identical.
Three membranous layers of tissue called *meninges* enclose the
brain, brain stem and cord (from out–in, the *dural, arachnoid*
and *pial* membranes). The CSF is contained in a space between
the pial and arachnoid layers (the *subarachnoid space*) which
is in communication with the hollow core of the brain known
as the *ventricular system*. The cerebrospinal fluid can be obtained for examination by a procedure called *spinal tap* (see
following section). Since the fluid is in immediate proximity to
the major structures of the central nervous system, it frequently
reveals abnormalities such as infection or hemorrhage occurring in the tissues themselves.

Diagnostic Procedures

In addition to routine X-rays, a number of specialized procedures are utilized for neurological diagnosis. It should be help-

---

[3] Recent research has made clear that much of what goes on in the brain is mediated
by chemical transmitters and modifiers. The old idea that neurologic regulation was
solely the result of electrical activity over complex networks of neurons acting like
computer wires is no longer tenable. The fact that the brain has been found to produce
many hormones has even led some to label it an endocrine organ. In truth its function
is mediated through both the traditional neuronal circuits (electrically) and the newly
discovered hormones and chemical transmitters.

ful to review these before discussing the diseases that will require their use.

Lumbar Puncture (Spinal Tap). Lumbar puncture is a common and important procedure. A needle is inserted between the vertebrae of the lumbar region into the subarachnoid space. The pressure of the fluid is measured, and sufficient volume is removed for microscopic examination (blood, white cells, bacteria), culture (bacteria and fungi) and chemical tests (protein, glucose, serologic test for syphilis). Many lay persons have a great fear of lumbar puncture, but this fear is entirely unwarranted. (I speak from experience, having had the procedure myself.) A mild post-tap headache may occur but is not inevitable. Spinal tap is not done if increased intracranial pressure is present or suspected because of the danger of herniating the brain stem through the *foramen magnum* (the opening between the intracranial cavity and spinal column) when pressure is lowered from below by removal of cerebrospinal fluid.

Electroencephalogram (EEG). In this procedure the electrical activity of the brain is measured by placing a series of electrodes over the head. It is entirely painless. Abnormal electrical activity is seen in epilepsy and a variety of other diseases. The EEG is the final arbiter of brain death since no patient has ever returned to functional life if electrical activity of the brain has ceased (even if the heart continues to beat and respiration is preserved).

Angiogram (Arteriogram). Angiography involves the injection of special dyes that are *radiopaque* (they do not allow X-rays to pass through) into the carotid and/or vertebral arteries to allow visualization of the blood vessels of the brain. Blocked arteries and vascular malformations are readily diagnosed. Mass lesions such as tumors, abscesses, intracerebral hemorrhages and accumulation of blood beneath or outside the meninges can also be identified by their capacity to push or displace vessels from their normal course. Tumors, in addition, often exhibit a "blush," a sort of smudging of the dye in the area of the mass. Angiography is a relatively safe technique with a complication rate of about 5 percent. Rarely the procedure itself can produce a strokelike picture.

Brain Scan. The brain scan is an extremely safe test in which radioactive isotopes are injected intravenously and their distribution over the brain determined. Areas of increased uptake indicate an abnormality. The greater the blood supply to a lesion the higher the likelihood that it will be picked up by brain scan. Many physicians use the scan as a screening procedure for brain lesions, but most would not dismiss the possibility of serious disease on the basis of a negative brain scan alone in a patient who has objective neurological findings.

Computerized Axial Tomography (CAT or CT scan). Computerized axial tomography, which was first introduced in 1972, represents an astonishing advance in diagnostic radiology. Its greatest use has been in the evaluation of brain lesions, but whole-body scanners are also available. The instruments used are too complicated to be described in detail here. Basically the procedure involves projection of a narrow beam of X-rays through the area to be tested with measurement of the degree of absorption of the beam by a series of detectors on the other side. In effect, over a period of only a few minutes, thousands of images are obtained and these images are merged by a sophisticated computer into a composite, photographlike projection of the internal structures of the head or body. Modern CAT scanners can identify hemorrhages, abscesses, tumors and swelling of the brain with ease.

Pneumoencephalography. In pneumoencephalography a lumbar tap is performed, spinal fluid is removed and air is injected into the subarachnoid space. This air moves upward and fills the ventricular cavities of the brain. Because air is radiotransparent, the cerebral hemispheres and other parts of the brain are clearly outlined, and mass lesions can be identified by their distorting features. Pneumoencephalography is generally a painful procedure, and severe headaches during and after injection of the air are extremely common. Since the same information can be obtained better by CAT scanning, pneumoencephalography is now rarely used except in certain cases where a pituitary tumor is suspected.

Myelography. The myelogram is a test used when one suspects the presence of a herniated (slipped) vertebral disc or a spinal cord tumor. In this procedure a spinal needle is inserted into the subarachnoid space exactly as is done in a routine lumbar puncture. Radiopaque dye is injected, the patient is tipped on a tilt table and the flow of the dye is followed under fluoroscopic observation. Blockade or deviation of the dye column indicates the site of obstruction.

Electromyography (EMG). Electromyography is a procedure

used for the objective demonstration of muscle or nerve disease. A needle electrode is inserted into one of several muscles, and electrical activity is measured during rest and contraction. The technique can usually differentiate between primary muscle disease and abnormalities of the nerves supplying the muscle.

DISEASE OF THE BRAIN

An important characteristic of brain tissue is its fragility. Permanent damage occurs after only a few minutes if the blood supply is interrupted and regenerative capacity is almost nil. In general, therefore, when tissue death occurs the loss is permanent. Eight major categories of disease affect the brain. These are: stroke, tumors, infections, metabolic disorders, degenerative disease, nutritional deficiencies, trauma and epilepsy.

STROKE

The term *stroke* refers to the sudden appearance of a neurological deficit due to disease in the blood vessels of the brain. The deficit may be trivial, such as a slight slurring of the speech, or it may result in death. The most frequent picture is that of a sudden loss of consciousness coupled with a paralysis over one-half of the body (*hemiplegia*). Occasionally symptoms appear and disappear rapidly in which case they are called *transient ischemic attacks* (*TIAs*). Usually transient attacks are a harbinger of more severe and permanent disease. An important concept is that neurological deficits due to stroke develop over a short period of time—minutes to hours. If a neurological loss appears gradually over days to weeks, it can be assumed with fair certainty that the cause is not a stroke and that one had best look for a brain tumor, abscess or other lesion.

There are three general causes of the stroke syndrome: *thrombus, embolus* and *hemorrhage. Thrombus* refers to *in situ* clot formation. It is by far the most common form of stroke and is due to atherosclerosis of the cerebral vessels. *Cerebral embolism* refers to blockade of blood flow by a clot breaking off elsewhere in the body and lodging in a vessel of the brain. The usual source of the embolus is the heart, and the most frequent mechanism is an abnormal heart rhythm called *atrial fibrilla-*

tion. The major cause of *cerebral hemorrhage* is high blood pressure although disease or drugs interfering with the clotting mechanism also predispose to bleeding in the brain. Structural abnormalities of the cerebral vessels, particularly weakened arterial outpouchings called *aneurysms,* can likewise cause massive bleeding in the head. Cerebral hemorrhage usually produces rapid loss of consciousness, often coupled with vomiting and convulsions. The latter are rare in stroke due to thrombus or embolus.

The course and prognosis of stroke syndromes are difficult to predict. With minor deficits full recovery is possible. If coma is profound a high percentage of patients die either from the brain injury itself or a delayed complication such as pneumonia. Mortality is particularly high with cerebral hemorrhage. The general rule is that the longer recovery is delayed the less likely will be restoration of function. If no recovery has begun by 1–2 weeks, the outlook is gloomy. Once started, function may continue to improve over a period of 5–6 months but not much beyond.

Treatment of strokes is divided into acute and chronic phases. Initially one must try to maintain respiratory function. In the common forms of stroke with unconsciousness and paralysis, impairment of the swallowing mechanism tends to cause aspiration of secretions from the mouth into the lungs. As a consequence, frequent suctioning of the trachea (the tube leading from throat to lungs) is required to prevent aspiration pneumonia. Should the blood pressure be high, acute measures to lower it have to be taken. Since stroke patients usually cannot eat, fluids must be given intravenously. It is general policy to use intravenous glucose for about one week following which feeding by stomach tube is usually undertaken. The patient is turned frequently to avoid pooling of secretions in the lungs and to prevent the development of bedsores (*decubitus ulcers*). If bladder control has been lost, a catheter (a rubber tube passed into the bladder through the urethra) has to be placed to drain the urine. Keeping the patient clean and dry is critical (and very difficult to do in most hospitals because of insufficient nursing help). It is not very glamorous to clean feces and urine off a comatose body, to repeatedly turn a dead weight in bed or to suction thick mucus from the trachea, but it means the difference, often, between life and death.

Neurosurgical intervention following stroke is indicated in two circumstances. The first is when CAT scan shows an intracerebral accumulation of blood (*hematoma*) and the patient is deteriorating. In such circumstances evacuation of the blood should be attempted. Second, ruptured aneurysms should be tied off.

The chronic phase of therapy is essentially rehabilitative in nature. Physical and speech therapists play the primary role as an attempt is made to get the patient to walk and talk again.

BRAIN TUMORS

All brain tumors, whether benign or malignant, are life-threatening. This is true because the intracranial cavity is fixed in size by the bones of the skull, and any expanding mass can increase intracranial pressure sufficiently to cause death. Brain tumors generally identify their presence by one or more of a triad of symptoms: *headache, change in mental function or convulsions.* Headache, mild at first, becomes increasingly severe as intracranial pressure rises. Early on the patient may have a sense of giddiness—an ill-defined sense that "something is wrong," especially when the head is turned. Change in mental function may occur gradually and not be apparent to the person himself. Convulsions are common. They may be generalized or localized to one arm or leg. The appearance of seizures in the absence of a known cause should be considered a brain tumor until proven otherwise.

Tumors may involve any part of the brain. Within the brain substance, the two most common forms are *glioblastoma multiforme* and *astrocytoma.* The former is malignant and fast growing. The outlook, even with surgery, is grim and 2-year survival is less than 10 percent. Astrocytomas, in contrast, grow very slowly and may run a course of years even if not treated. *Meningiomas* are tumors of the covering of the brain. They usually can be cured if in an accessible site since they do not invade the brain tissue itself. *Craniopharyngioma* is an interesting tumor of young people that may cause endocrine changes such as obesity, delayed growth, impaired sexual development and diabetes insipidus when localized in or near the hypothalamus. *Tumors of the pituitary gland* also cause endocrine disease of a variety of types (see chapter 15). *Acoustic neurinomas* are tumors of the auditory or 8th cranial nerve. They cause loss of hearing, vertigo and tinnitus (noise in the ear). Unfortunately exactly the same symptoms may be produced in the absence of tumor in a condition of unknown cause called *Ménière's syndrome.* Differentiation is difficult. Lastly, brain tumors may be *metastatic* (meaning that they arise elsewhere in the body); lung and breast are the most common primary sites from which secondary spread occurs.

Diagnosis of brain tumors requires CAT scanning and angiography. These two procedures allow identification and localization of even very small lesions. Treatment is surgical removal. Regrettably, normal tissue must often be destroyed to reach and remove the growth. Tumors deep within the brain or located in vital areas may not be surgically approachable at all. Chemotherapy is not helpful with primary brain tumors, but radiation to the head may be of palliative value.

Before leaving brain tumors I want to say a word about a peculiar syndrome called *pseudotumor cerebri.* It is usually found in young women who consult the physician for headache. They are found to have increased intracranial pressure with *papilledema* ("choking" or elevation of the optic nerve head in the back of the eye) but no tumor is found. They respond to treatment with dexamethasone, a powerful cortisonelike drug, and repeated spinal taps. The cause is not known.

INFECTIONS OF THE BRAIN

The central nervous system is susceptible to several types of infectious processes. The most common is *meningitis; encephalitis* and *brain abscess* are much less frequent. *Tertiary syphilis* is in a category by itself. It may present either as dementia (*paresis*) or a strokelike illness (*meningovascular syphilis*). The clinical picture of meningitis consists of fever, severe headache, stiff neck, stupor and occasionally coma or convulsions. The symptoms are due to infection of the covering membranes and surfaces of the brain and spinal cord as well as the cerebrospinal fluid. Meningitis may be due either to bacteria or viruses. Three organisms, *Neisseria meningitidis* (the *meningococcus*), *Hemophilus influenzae,* and *Streptococcus pneumoniae* (the *pneumococcus*), account for over 90 percent of the bacterial forms. The most serious is *meningococcal meningitis* which can kill in a matter of hours. Primarily a disease of young adults, it is highly contagious. Extensive bleeding into the skin accompanies the neurological symptoms in over half the patients. *He-mophilus* is the leading cause of meningitis in children while the *pneumococcus* ordinarily causes disease in older adults. These organisms reach the central nervous system either by invasion of the bloodstream or by direct extension from infections in the throat, sinuses or ears. More indolent forms of meningitis are those due to *tuberculosis* or *fungal infections*. With these fever is less marked, and weight loss and night sweats are prominent accompaniments of the headache and stiff neck. *Viral meningitis* is usually a benign illness in which symptoms last only a few days. It is often called *aseptic meningitis* because no bacteria are found when the cerebrospinal fluid is examined and cultured. Usually the virus involved is never identified.

Some viruses invade the brain tissue in preference to the surface membranes in which case *encephalitis* is produced. Stiff neck is not so prominent in encephalitis as in aseptic meningitis, and stupor or coma tend to dominate the picture. Mortality rates are much higher than in viral meningitis. Mosquito-borne epidemics of encephalitis still occur in the United States. The causative organisms are the *Eastern* and *Western equine*, the *St. Louis* and *California encephalitis viruses*. Other viruses causing encephalitis are those of the childhood illnesses: measles, mumps, chicken pox and rubella. Up to 20 percent of children may have some sign of encephalitis following these illnesses if carefully examined. *Rabies*, the greatly feared disease transmitted by animal bite, is another form of viral encephalitis.

Brain abscess refers to a localized collection of pus in the brain. It is usually due to *anaerobic organisms* (bacteria that do not grow in the presence of oxygen) originating in the lungs, ears or sinuses. Occasionally *staphylococcus* is the infecting agent. Abscess is suggested whenever a clinical picture of fever, headache, altered consciousness, convulsions and a neurological deficit (e.g., hemiplegia) is seen. Basically abscess behaves like a brain tumor except that the presence of fever reveals its infectious nature.[4]

Diagnosis of meningitis and encephalitis is made by exami-

---

[4] Fever is characteristic of the early stages of abscess formation but disappears later. At this stage differentiation from tumor is difficult.

nation of the cerebrospinal fluid while brain abscess is revealed by CAT scan or arteriography. The CSF in meningitis shows increased numbers of white blood cells with or without an increase in pressure and protein content. The key issue in separating bacterial meningitis from aseptic meningitis or encephalitis is the glucose (sugar) concentration. In bacterial meningitis the glucose content is low while it is normal in viral disease. At times bacteria can also be seen by direct smear but confirmation requires culture of the fluid. The type of white cell present may also help; bacteria attract neutrophilic leuko-cytes while lymphocytes predominate in viral disease. If the spinal fluid is suggestive of bacterial meningitis, treatment with antibiotics is started even before the causal organism has been identified. *However, no patient with fever, headache or stiff neck should receive antibiotics before the CSF has been examined and cultured.* The reason is that even one shot of antibiotic can mask the spinal fluid picture of bacterial meningitis and make it appear like that of aseptic meningitis, thus confusing therapy. The usual sequence is for a patient (often a college student or military recruit since meningococcal disease is most common in institutions) to be given a shot of penicillin for fever, then sent to a hospital when they do not improve. The consulting physician does a spinal tap and finds the picture of aseptic meningitis (a few cells, normal glucose, no bacteria). Antibiotics are withheld (since they do not work in viral men-ingitis or encephalitis) and the patient dies. Autopsy then re-veals the presence of bacterial disease.

Bacterial meningitis and brain abscess are treated with mas-sive amounts of antibiotics given intravenously. The antibiotic chosen will vary depending on the organism suspected but usu-ally is penicillin, ampicillin or chloramphenicol (often two drugs are given). Tuberculosis and fungi require other drugs. Abscesses may require surgical drainage as well as antibiotics. No specific treatment is available for aseptic meningitis or en-cephalitis. Immediate contacts of patients with meningococcal meningitis should be given prophylactic antibiotics in view of its highly contagious nature.

METABOLIC DISORDERS

A large number of illnesses originating elsewhere in the body produce secondary changes in the metabolism of the brain.

They ordinarily do not cause paralysis or localizing signs but induce disordered function, stupor, coma or convulsions. The operative mechanism is usually a chemical abnormality in the blood that interferes with brain function; e.g., too little oxygen or glucose, too much carbon dioxide or ammonia. A whole host of drugs also produce altered brain function, the tranquilizers, narcotics and CNS stimulants being most prominent. All of these must be considered in evaluating the unconscious or convulsing patient.

DEGENERATIVE DISEASES

The degenerative diseases represent a set of illnesses in which there is a gradual deterioration of function in the brain for reasons that are in many cases not yet understood. The major syndromes are senility, Creutzfeldt-Jakob disease, Huntington's chorea and Parkinson's disease.

Senility. The term senility refers to a clinical state in which there is failing memory and deterioration of intellectual function in an elderly person. Characteristically, events of the distant past are remembered while recent memory is blurred or totally nonfunctional. Repetitive statements, neglect of social niceties and depression are common. In late stages recognition of family and friends disappears and frank dementia supervenes. Symptoms are worsened by fever, dehydration or other intercurrent illness. The underlying cause of senility is atherosclerosis in the brain vessels with diminished blood flow and tissue atrophy.[5] Patients with this problem are a difficult burden for the family, particularly if they stay in the home. The only advice that can be offered is to remember how one treats a child: with patient firmness, good humor, kindness and love.

Creutzfeldt-Jakob Disease. Creutzfeldt-Jakob disease is characterized by signs and symptoms of senility developing in men between the ages of 40 and 60. *Myoclonus*, the spontaneous contraction of various muscles in nonpurposeful fashion, accompanies the loss of memory. Hallucinations, gait disorders, difficulty in speaking, muscle atrophy and convulsions complete the syndrome which leads to death in less than a year for most affected subjects. It has now been shown that the disease

---

[5] Senility can occur in middle life. The premature form is called *Alzheimer's disease* or diffuse cerebral atrophy. Its cause is unknown.

is due to one of a peculiar group of viruses (*slow viruses*) that have extremely long incubation times: months to years.[6] The concept is that the virus infects the tissue for prolonged periods before producing symptoms. This truly exciting discovery suggests that other neurological illnesses of unknown etiology (such as multiple sclerosis) may also be caused by such viruses. While antiviral agents are not now available, hopefully they will be developed in the near future, rendering these diseases susceptible to treatment.

Huntington's Chorea. This disease is inherited as a dominant trait and usually makes its appearance around the age of 40, although earlier onset is possible. It is characterized by involuntary movements of face and limbs (*chorea*) and progressive loss of mental function. Facial grimacing may be almost constant, and the legs or arms may suddenly shoot out in unexpected directions as though being out of control. The course is always downhill but prolonged survival is possible. The cause is thought to be a deficiency of an inhibitory neurotransmitter called *gamma aminobutyric acid* that normally keeps the abnormal movements from occurring. No treatment is available.

Parkinson's Disease. Parkinson's disease is due to chemical abnormalities in the brain stem and the specialized areas called *basal ganglia.* It begins in middle or late life and runs a slow but progressive downhill course until death. The disease is characterized by stiffness of muscles, rhythmic tremor of the hands and legs, a peculiar gait in which the patient moves progressively faster with each step, stooped posture and loss of facial expression. The voice is flat and spontaneous movement is limited. The skin is greasy from increased activity of the sebaceous glands. In the late stages there is drooling from the mouth, and eventually the patient is unable to care for himself.

It is suspected that the disease is due to deficiency of a neurotransmitter called *dopamine.* In accord with this hypothesis is the observation that administration of *L-dihydroxyphenylalanine* (L-dopa), a precursor of dopamine, markedly improves symptoms in a majority of patients. The primary effect is on muscle rigidity but tremor may also improve in some cases. A variety of other drugs can be used in combination with L-dopa

---

[6] Slow viruses were originally found to cause a disease called *Kuru* in natives of New Guinea. Kuru is characterized by gait disturbances, tremor and nystagmus. It is contracted by the cannibalistic ingestion of infected human brain.

to further enhance control. Some patients respond dramatically to brain surgery. Using sophisticated instrumentation, the neurosurgeon places destructive lesions in the *thalamus* or *globus pallidus* (two of the basal ganglia) by freezing or other techniques. The operation is particularly useful in stopping tremor.

NUTRITIONAL DISEASE

The primary nutritional disease of the brain, the *Wernicke-Korsakoff syndrome,* is essentially limited to alcoholics and is due primarily to thiamine deficiency. The fundamental characteristics include nystagmus and/or paralysis of eye movements, abnormal gait and mental disturbances that range from apathy to frank psychosis. Memory loss is almost constant. If treated early with thiamine, reversal is possible, but once the disease is fully established the changes are usually permanent.

TRAUMA (HEAD INJURIES)

In modern society head injuries are extremely common. Trauma to the head may be *penetrating* or *blunt.* With a penetrating injury the neurological loss is due to direct destruction of brain tissue. Blunt trauma can produce a loss of consciousness without structural damage (*concussion*) or result in *hemorrhage.* The latter may be in the brain substance itself or between the bony skull and the brain. Accumulations of blood are called *hematomas;* if the hematoma is in the brain it is called *intracerebral* while locations beneath or outside the dura mater are designated *subdural* and *extradural,* respectively. Symptoms produced by head injuries are due either to increased intracranial pressure or to specific neuronal losses secondary to lacerations and bleeding. While neurological damage may be immediately apparent, it is also possible for symptoms to occur hours to weeks after the original injury. The mechanism is complicated, but basically a relatively small hematoma (insufficient to be dangerous in itself) swells with time as the trapped blood breaks down. The swelling is due to movement of fluid from plasma into the lesion because of an increase in osmotic pressure secondary to the degradation of blood. (The osmotic pressure is a measure of the attractive force for water induced by molecules that are surrounded by a membrane they cannot cross.) In essence the hematoma becomes an expanding intracranial mass. Availability of the CAT scan has greatly simplified diagnosis. If a hematoma is identified, neurosurgical drainage will usually be required.

EPILEPSY
The various types of epilepsy are described in chapter 3.

SPINAL CORD DISEASE

Trauma. The leading cause of spinal cord disease is trauma. Automobile accidents and athletic injuries are the most common precipitating events. The immediate mechanism is usually fracture or dislocation of one or more vertebrae leading to bruising, hemorrhage or laceration of the cord. Complete paralysis and loss of sensation is found below the level of injury. A high cervical cord lesion will cause paralysis of all four extremities and the muscles of respiration while a lesion lower down will spare the arms. Immediately following injury all reflexes are lost (a condition called *spinal shock*). After 2–3 weeks reflex activity returns and involuntary spasms of the muscles develop. Such activity may falsely encourage the patient to believe that function is returning. If the spinal cord is only bruised, improvement or recovery may occur. Hemorrhage or transection produces permanent damage. Any defect remaining after 6 months will likely be permanent.

Patients with permanent spinal cord injuries in the neck need lifetime care. Life expectancy is shortened for at least three reasons. First, the need for chronic catheter drainage of the bladder (which is paralyzed) predisposes to urinary tract infection. Second, decubitus (pressure) ulcers develop in the skin and lead to infection of underlying bone or the bloodstream. Third, poor respiratory excursion and general debility facilitate the development of pneumonia.

It cannot be stressed too strongly that the only effective treatment for transection of the spinal cord is prevention. In automobiles, seat belts should be worn and defensive driving practiced. Trampolines are very dangerous and should only be used under formal guidance by a trained instructor. No one should ever dive into the shallow end of the swimming pool or into waters of unknown depth. Spinal cord injuries will always occur in football, but the frequency will be lessened if players avoid use of the head and neck in tackling and blocking. One has to see only a single person with total paralysis to learn these lessons forever.

Multiple Sclerosis. Multiple sclerosis is a puzzling disease in which neurologic symptoms come and go over prolonged periods of time. Called a demyelinating disease, the myelin sheath of the nerve fiber disintegrates without damage to the axon itself, at least in the early stages. Later scar formation occurs as axonal tissue is destroyed. The etiology is not known, but a virus (possibly a slow virus) is suspected. Clinically the disease produces a wide spectrum of symptoms. A common initial event is an episode of blurred vision or blindness in one eye (*optic neuritis*) which generally improves or disappears over a short period of time leaving the patient symptom free. Some subjects who develop optic neuritis as an initial symptom never develop other signs; others progress through the full syndrome. Spinal cord or brain stem signs rather than visual difficulties may be the initial manifestation in some patients. Numbness or weakness of a leg or arm, nystagmus, tremor or bladder paralysis may occur. Paralysis of ocular muscles with double vision is not unusual. Symptoms may disappear as rapidly as they developed, leaving slight or no residual, only to return at a subsequent time. After years of remission and exacerbation, the disease usually becomes progressive with exaggeration of symptoms, paralysis and death. As is common with all forms of progressive neurological disease, pneumonia is the leading cause of death. Life expectancy is actually quite good for the majority of patients and in some may extend up to 30 years after the onset. Occasionally an acute progressive form of the disease occurs with the period from onset to death being a matter of months.

No specific tests are available for multiple sclerosis and the diagnosis is based on clinical presentation. Treatment is ineffective, although adrenocorticotrophic hormone (ACTH) is often administered intravenously during acute episodes.

Amyotrophic Lateral Sclerosis. Amyotrophic lateral sclerosis, infamous as the illness that took the life of baseball star Lou Gehrig, is a rapidly progressive illness involving motor nerve cells in the spinal cord and even in the cortex of the brain itself. Muscle atrophy and weakness are accompanied by characteristic twitching (*fasciculations*) which makes the diagnosis obvious. Usually the hands, arms and shoulders are first involved. Reflexes become exaggerated and spasticity of the muscles is usual. Occasionally involuntary laughter or crying occur, probably secondary to brain stem disease. There is no treatment and death from pneumonia or respiratory failure occurs in less than 5 years from the onset of symptoms, sometimes in less than 1 year.

Syringomyelia. Syringomyelia is a peculiar disease in which a patient has loss of pain and temperature sensation in the arms, shoulders and neck while the sense of touch in the same areas is preserved. Muscle atrophy occurs, and often there is an accompanying curvature of the spine in the thoracic region due to weakness of the paraspinal muscles. With time the face and lower body may also be involved. The disease is caused by a destruction or cavitation of the inner portions of the spinal cord. The etiology is unknown and there is no treatment.

Degenerative and Intervertebral Disc Disease of the Spine. Pain and/or weakness over the distribution of a spinal nerve may result from disease of bony spine. Two major causes account for most of the problems. *Degeneration* of vertebrae with age (a wear-and-tear process that is inevitable) results in bony overgrowth which compresses the nerve roots as they emerge from the spinal cord. Any part of the spine may be involved. The problem is particularly common in obesity since the extra weight places great stress on the vertebral column. The pain usually responds to large doses of aspirin but no specific treatment is available. Weight loss is imperative. The second cause of the syndrome is a *herniated intervertebral disc.* The intervertebral disc is a cushionlike structure between each pair of bony vertebrae that functions like a shock absorber. It also can degenerate and protrude or herniate, impinging on nerve roots. Like degeneration, herniation can occur at any level, but it is most common in the lumbar region. The clinical picture of a lumbar disc is back pain coupled with pain, numbness, weakness or paralysis of the foot or leg on one side. Diagnosis requires myelography. If conservative treatment with bed rest, traction, sedatives and physical therapy does not relieve the pain, surgery may be necessary. In the past disc removal was often coupled with spinal fusion, a procedure in which a section of the spine was surgically immobilized by bone grafting. Fusion is rarely done at the present time.

Other Lesions. The spinal cord is subject to a number of other lesions similar to those described for the brain. *Tumors, abscesses* and *occlusion of the blood supply* can all produce paralysis and sensory changes. In the past by far the most common disease of the spinal cord was *poliomyelitis,* which occurred in epidemic form prior to the development of the polio vaccine. Physicians are greatly concerned about the return of poliomyelitis since the number of persons receiving proper immunization has been declining rapidly, and new cases are appearing with worrisome frequency. *Tabes dorsalis,* a disease characterized by lightninglike pains in the legs and loss of position sense, is due to syphilis. Untreated *pernicious anemia* leads to destructive lesions which may end in complete paralysis. A rare form of spinal paralysis is due to the presence of a *tick* on the body. Apparently the tick injects a paralyzing neurotoxin at the time it is sucking blood. The paralysis is rapidly reversed by removal of the tick.

DISEASE OF THE CRANIAL NERVES

The most common cause of cranial nerve defects is stroke, but the nerves may also be secondarily involved in generalized neuropathies caused by diseases such as diabetes. Two primary syndromes deserve comment. *Bell's palsy* (facial or 7th cranial nerve paralysis) refers to the sudden appearance of paralysis over one side of the face. The face sags on the affected side, the corner of the mouth droops and the eyelid will not close. About 80 percent of patients recover spontaneously over a period of a few weeks while the remainder have residual damage that may be partial or complete. Occasionally facial paralysis is caused by *tumors* compressing the 7th nerve. The previously mentioned acoustic neurinoma can involve the facial nerve as can tumors of the parotid gland (the salivary gland at the angle of the jaw, best known for its involvement in mumps). Rarely *herpes zoster virus* affects the facial nerve and causes paralysis. *Trigeminal neuralgia (tic douloureux)* is a striking syndrome of facial pain over the distribution of the trigeminal (5th cranial) nerve. Excruciating, lightninglike flashes of pain occur at repetitive intervals. The cause is unknown. Therapy consists of the administration of carbamazepine, an anticonvulsant drug. Should this fail the nerve may have to be destroyed surgically.

DISEASE OF THE PERIPHERAL NERVES

Peripheral Polyneuropathy. Many diseases lead to abnormalities of the peripheral nerves. The symptoms produced may be purely motor or purely sensory, but frequently both motor and sensory components are involved. With motor disease there is weakness, muscle atrophy and absence of reflexes, while the sensory abnormalities include pain, anesthesia and loss of position sense. The extremities are involved more often than the trunk, and the legs are generally affected to a greater extent than the arms. Many of the polyneuropathies are reversible if the primary disease or precipitating event can be controlled or removed. The major causes are diabetes mellitus, alcoholism, uremia, heavy metal poisoning (arsenic, lead), organic chemicals of a variety of types, the infectious diseases diphtheria and leprosy, certain types of cancer (especially lung), vascular diseases such as periarteritis nodosa and a few genetic disorders.

Landry-Guillain-Barré Syndrome. The clinical picture in this disease is remarkable. Over a several day period, muscle weakness and paralysis begins in the distal extremities and progresses in ascending fashion to involve the abdomen, chest and eventually the face, such that the patient is completely paralyzed. On occasion progression of paralysis stops before the face is reached. Numbness and paresthesias occur but pain is unusual. The cerebrospinal fluid is characteristic in that protein concentrations are high, but pressure is normal and no cells are seen. The cause is unknown in most cases, though the syndrome has been seen in the context of *infectious mononucleosis.* It has also followed immunizations and was the reason for the recall of the swine influenza vaccine during the recent epidemic. Some have suggested that it represents a form of allergy to foreign proteins, but this is unproven. Most patients recover completely over a period of a few weeks, but courses lasting for months have been observed. The problem is keeping the patient who has respiratory paralysis alive until recovery sets in. Hospitalization in a pulmonary unit is usually required.

Porphyrias. The porphyrias are a group of diseases in which abnormalities exist in the enzymes leading to the synthesis of heme, the functional component of the hemoglobin molecule. As a consequence precursors called porphyrins accumulate in the body. Two forms of the disease, *acute intermittent porphyria* and *variegate porphyria*, are associated with reversible neurologic impairment in a high percentage of cases. Neurological findings include wrist drop (when the arm is extended the hand sags passively and cannot be voluntarily lifted), foot drop, numbness, tingling or even an ascending paralysis resembling the Landry-Guillain-Barré syndrome. The patients also exhibit excruciating abdominal pain, fever and tachycardia (rapid heartbeat), symptoms that are likely due to involvement of autonomic nerves. A number of drugs, particularly barbiturates, precipitate porphyric crises, and patients with either of the above variants of the disease should be given medications only with caution. Diagnosis depends on demonstrating abnormal amounts of porphyrins or porphyrin precursors in the urine. Treatment is not satisfactory although a high-carbohydrate diet may help. Avoidance of precipitating drugs is mandatory. During the acute phase the intravenous administration of *hematin,* a derivative of heme, seems to block production of the offending porphyrin precursors and shorten the attack.

Nerve Injury. Injury to a single nerve or groups of nerves may be due to pressure, stretching or transection. After pressure or stretching recovery is possible while with transection regeneration is problematical unless careful surgical re-anastomosis is undertaken rapidly. An example of stretch or pressure injury is dislocation or fracture of the shoulder with damage to the *brachial plexus,* the large nerve complex serving the arm. Following such an injury the arm hangs loosely at the side, internally rotated with the elbow extended. Similarly, ill-fitting crutches may cause damage to the radial nerve leaving the axilla and cause wrist drop. The *carpal tunnel syndrome* is due to thickening of the ligaments on the inner aspect of the wrist, trapping the median nerve. It causes weakness of the hand muscles, loss of sensation over the outer ⅔ of the palm and pain. Carpal tunnel syndrome may appear spontaneously or be secondary to systemic disease such as *hypothyroidism* or *acromegaly.* Treatment is surgical freeing of the trapped nerve.

DISEASE OF THE AUTONOMIC NERVOUS SYSTEM

Disease states in which the primary manifestations focus on the autonomic nervous system are rare. *Familial dysautonomia* is an illness found primarily in Ashkenazi Jews. It is characterized by feeding problems in infancy, orthostatic hypotension, intermittent hypertension, impaired perception of pain, temperature and taste, gait disturbances and clearly demonstrable deficiency in the control of blood vessels and heart rate. Lack of tear formation in the eyes leads to corneal ulceration. The disease is inherited in an autosomal recessive pattern. *Idiopathic orthostatic hypotension (Shy-Drager syndrome)* is similar in many respects to familial dysautonomia. Patients exhibit hypotension on standing (sometimes with fainting) and elevated blood pressure when lying down. They do not sweat. Impotence is common in males and bladder dysfunction may be present. Some patients develop cerebellar signs with ataxia or the picture of Parkinson's disease later in life. The nature of the underlying defect that specifically affects autonomic nerves in these two conditions is not known.

6

Diseases of the
Heart and Circulation

Heart disease is the leading cause of death in this country. By the age of 65, 50 percent of Americans have significant narrowing of at least one coronary artery and are thus at risk to develop a heart attack. When one adds diseases affecting the valves, heart muscle and peripheral vessels, the prevalence of heart and circulatory problems becomes quite astounding. Tremendous advances have been made in the diagnosis and treatment of these disorders, yet much remains to be learned. In particular, the cause of atherosclerosis continues to be obscure. Importantly, however, a number of risk factors under the control of the patient have been identified, elimination of which would sharply curtail the deadly toll now levied by atherosclerosis in the coronary circulation. Since heart disease due to rheumatic fever, syphilis and hypertension can be completely prevented by proper treatment of the causal illness, it follows that aggressive prophylaxis is an essential first step if deaths from heart disease are to be reduced. The elements of such a prophylactic program will be outlined in this chapter following a discussion of the major circulatory diseases and contemporary methods of therapy.

STRUCTURE AND FUNCTION OF THE CIRCULATORY SYSTEM

The circulatory system is commonly divided into *central* and *peripheral* divisions; in actuality the two divisions are coterminous parts of a single closed network of vessels, separated only for convenience in discussing their physiological function. The *central circulation,* located in the chest cavity, consists of the heart, the pulmonary vessels and the great arteries and veins that serve as conduits to and from the peripheral system. The *peripheral system* consists of all the vessels outside the chest cavity and is responsible for the delivery of oxygen and other nutrients to the various tissues of the body. Blood vessels in both systems are divided into three types: arteries, capillaries and veins. The peripheral arteries carry oxygenated blood to the capillaries, which represent the nutrient exchange site; the veins pick up deoxygenated blood from the capillaries and return it to the heart.[1] The arterial network is a high pressure system (when blood pressure is measured on physical examination, it is arterial pressure that is being assessed) and that pressure is the driving force that assures movement of blood through the multiple vessels of the body. It is developed primarily by the pumping action of the heart but is also partially determined by contraction and relaxation of the muscular layers in large and medium-sized arteries: when the vessels contract blood pressure rises and when they relax pressure falls. The state of contraction or relaxation is called the *peripheral resistance.* Peripheral resistance is regulated by pressure receptors located in the vessel walls; their purpose is to maintain the blood pressure in the range required for adequate circulation throughout the body. If pressure falls the receptors signal arterial constriction; if it rises relaxation is induced. Inappropriate increase in the contractile response leads to *hypertension* (high blood pressure) while blockade of the constrictive reflex causes

---

[1] The type of blood carried in arteries and veins is reversed in the central circulation. Pulmonary arteries transmit deoxygenated blood to the lungs while pulmonary veins return oxygenated blood to the heart. Peripheral and central capillaries function identically.

a fall in blood pressure or frank *shock* (vascular collapse).[2] Contractile tissue in small arteries (*arterioles*) functions not to regulate blood pressure but to direct flow to and from specific areas: if the arterioles in one area contract while those of another relax simultaneously, blood flow shifts to the latter, moving along the path of least resistance. Pressure in capillaries and veins is very low compared to arteries. Veins can contract, but the response is far weaker and less important than that of their arterial counterparts.

Oxygen and nutrients inside vessels are of no use unless they can reach the cells of the body. Transport from the blood to the *interstitial fluid* which surrounds the cells (but is outside the vessels) is possible because the capillaries are extremely thin walled and thus permeable to oxygen and small nutrient molecules. The interstitial fluid, which really is a cell-free, low-protein derivative of plasma, leaves the arterial side of the capillary and returns (with accumulated waste products) into the distal segment immediately before the capillaries join the small veins for the return journey to the heart. Part of the interstitial fluid (called *lymph*) returns centrally by an alternative system of delicate vessels (the *lymph ducts*) that eventually empty into the great veins of the chest prior to entry of the latter into the heart. Under certain circumstances (especially heart disease) the volume of the interstitial fluid becomes expanded. When this happens the patient is said to have *edema*. The signs of edema are rapid increase in body weight, swelling of the feet and ankles and a pitting reaction of the skin when it is depressed by a finger.

The heart, a powerful muscular organ, consists of four chambers linked in series. There are two *atria* (singular, *atrium*) which receive blood from the veins, and two *ventricles* which pump blood into the lungs and the arteries of the peripheral circulation. From the periphery venous blood passes through the very large *inferior* and *superior vena cavas* into the right atrium and thence into the right ventricle which pumps it into

---

[2] *Shock* refers to blood pressure sufficiently low that vital tissues are not perfused adequately. It may be due to paralysis of the arterial contractile response (bacterial invasion of the blood, hypoxemia, drugs), hemorrhage, dehydration or failure of the heart as a pump following a myocardial infarction. The signs of shock include low or unmeasurable blood pressure, pallor, sweating, fast heartbeat, cyanosis (a blue color of skin and nail beds caused by decreased oxygen content of blood) and altered central nervous system function varying from confusion to loss of consciousness.

the pulmonary arteries and lung capillaries. Following oxygenation in the lungs, the blood returns to the left atrium via the pulmonary veins. It then enters the left ventricle and from there exits into the *aorta* and peripheral circulation. Each chamber has an exit valve which functions something like a swinging door that opens outward but cannot be pushed inward. The valve between the right atrium and right ventricle is called the *tricuspid valve* and that between the right ventricle and pulmonary artery, the *pulmonic valve*. The valve between the left atrium and ventricle is the *mitral valve* while that separating the left ventricle and aorta is called the *aortic valve*. When pressure in a chamber becomes higher than pressure on the other side of the valve, the valve leaflets swing open and blood flows through. Once pressure on the distal side exceeds that present proximally, the valve slams shut. To illustrate, when the left ventricle contracts, pressure in the ventricular cavity rises, closing the mitral valve (preventing back flow) and opening the aortic valve (allowing egress of blood into the aorta). Disease of the valves can cause narrowing of the valve opening (*stenosis*), leading to obstruction of blood flow from the chamber or inadequate closure (*insufficiency*), in which case back leakage occurs, diminishing forward flow in degree equivalent to the backward leak.

Contraction of the heart muscle occurs in response to an intrinsic electrical impulse generated from a specialized center called the *sinoatrial* node located in the right atrium. The electrical impulse is carried throughout the heart over a specialized conduction system distinct from the muscle itself. The rate at which the sinoatrial node discharges is determined by a variety of factors both physiological and emotional. Thus a fast heart rate may be produced by both exercise and fright. Signals controlling heart rate arise in the brain, from reflex receptors located in the blood vessels or from hormonal discharge by the adrenal gland. The first two can either speed or slow the heart rate while the adrenal gland, acting via the release of epinephrine (adrenalin), can only speed it.

Blood supply to the heart is provided by the two *coronary arteries* which arise directly from the aorta. The *left coronary artery* divides shortly after its origin into a *left anterior descending branch* and a *left circumflex branch*. These vessels supply the left side of the heart while the *right coronary artery* carries blood to the muscles of the right chambers.

The heart is surrounded by a two-layered membrane called the *pericardium*. The space between the two layers contains a small amount of fluid that serves as a lubricant minimizing friction as the heart contracts. Inflammation of the membrane (*pericarditis*) causes chest pain and excessive fluid accumulation can severely impair cardiac function. Diseases such as tuberculosis can cause scarring of the pericardium and lead to the syndrome of *constrictive pericarditis* wherein venous return to the heart is greatly restricted.

From this brief description it is apparent that cardiac disease may involve the muscle of the heart (*myocardium*), the conduction system which regulates its rate and rhythm, the valves which direct blood flow, the blood vessels which supply the heart with its oxygen and nutrients or the pericardial sac which surrounds it. In view of these multiple vulnerable sites, it is perhaps not surprising that heart disease is common. What seems remarkable is the fact that it functions normally for so long in most people. Considering the average heart rate to be 70 beats per minute, over a 70-year life span the organ contracts 2,575,440,000 times without rest or respite.

DIAGNOSTIC PROCEDURES

Cardiac diagnosis is quite precise—perhaps more so than for any other organ system in the body. A variety of sophisticated techniques allows quantitative assessment of the state of cardiac function and accurate identification of pathologic defects. While auscultation (listening with a stethoscope) and other forms of physical examination continue to be important in the initial evaluation of the cardiac patient, one or more of the procedures described in the following pages are essentially always used when heart disease is suspected or known to be present.

Electrocardiography. The electrocardiogram (*ECG* or *EKG*) measures the electrical impulses generated by the heart during its rhythmic contractions. Usually twelve different recordings (called *leads*) are taken during the test. The tracing indicates the type of rhythm present and identifies the site of origin of abnormal impulses. The electrocardiogram can also provide evidence of strain or hypertrophy of the heart muscle due to increased work loads and shows characteristic patterns with angina pectoris or a heart attack. Since the electrocardiogram may be perfectly normal at rest (despite severe heart disease), it is also frequently recorded during an *exercise stress test*.[3] In this test the patient is exercised on a bicycle or by walking on a treadmill, usually for 3-minute periods with increasing levels of difficulty. The electrocardiogram is recorded continuously and oxygen uptake and blood pressure are also assessed. The stress of exercise frequently brings out symptoms (chest pain, shortness of breath) or electrocardiographic evidence of diminished blood flow that was not present at rest. While stress testing is in general quite safe, it should not be done unless a physician is present since the exercise itself may (rarely) induce an abnormal rhythm or produce a heart seizure.

Cardiac Series. This term refers to a multiple set of routine chest X-rays taken from different angles. Some of the films are taken after barium is swallowed. The technique usually allows determination of the size of the individual cardiac chambers.

Cardiac Catheterization. In this technique a small tube (catheter) is passed into the heart through a peripheral artery or vein under direct visualization with a fluoroscope. In *right heart catheterization* the right atrium, ventricle and pulmonary artery are entered, while in *left heart catheterization* the two left chambers are evaluated. At each site pressure and the oxygen content of blood are measured. Cardiac output (the amount of blood pumped by the heart) is routinely assessed. Often radiopaque contrast material is infused to test valve competency; for example, if dye injected in the left ventricle flows back into the left atrium during contraction, it is clear that the mitral valve is incompetent. The dye also allows visualization of heart wall movement. In addition pressures taken in each chamber tell whether the muscle is contracting normally. Similarly an abnormally elevated pressure gradient across a valve indicates the presence of stenosis. In congenital heart disease, where abnormal openings in the heart are common, oxygen measurements are extremely helpful. Thus, if the blood sample from the left ventricular chamber (which should be completely oxygenated) shows an oxygen saturation of only 85 percent (instead of 98–

---

[3] It is not unheard of for a person to die suddenly from a heart attack within hours after having a normal electrocardiogram. An abnormal ECG almost always means cardiac disease, but a normal resting tracing does not rule out cardiac pathology. If the stress electrocardiogram is normal, on the other hand, the chances are good that the heart is healthy.

100 percent), it is clear that deoxygenated venous blood from the right side of the heart has passed through an abnormal opening into the left side without first traversing the lungs. Conversely, a higher than normal value in right atrium or ventricle indicates a left to right shunt, since oxygenated blood has reached the venous side of the heart.

When cardiac catheterization is recommended by the physician, most people immediately wish to know about safety. There is a small risk involved, but this is minimal in experienced cardiac catheterization laboratories. The procedure may lead to abnormalities of cardiac rhythm, breaking off of a clot from inside the heart, perforation of a cardiac chamber or loss of blood supply in the arm through which the catheter is passed. All of these are uncommon. The risk for death is generally stated to be 0.1 percent with right heart catheterization and 1 percent for left. Most deaths, however, occur in patients who are already seriously ill at the time of catheterization; in these cases the procedure is usually being done preparatory to an attempt at life-saving cardiac surgery. Since the information gained by catheterization is usually critical for therapy, there should be no hesitation in having it done when indicated. Hospitalization is always required for cardiac catheterization, the stay ordinarily being 48 hours.

Coronary Angiography. Coronary angiography is a technique in which a catheter is passed retrograde through a peripheral artery to the point where the coronary vessels arise from the aorta. Radiopaque dye is injected and the flow of the dye through the right and left coronary arteries is recorded on film. The procedure is utilized to identify and localize atherosclerotic blockade of the coronary circulation. It has become of major importance with the advent of coronary bypass surgery. The risks are similar to those of left heart catheterization.

Echocardiography. The advantage of this relatively new technique is that it is noninvasive. No catheter has to be placed inside the body. Sound waves (*ultrasound*) are beamed into the heart from a transducer placed on the chest wall and the "echo" or reflection of that sound is converted to a visual image and recorded. The principle is identical to that of sonar used for the detection of submarines and other underwater objects. A properly done echocardiogram allows estimation of ventricular wall thickness, evaluation of valve anatomy and function, definition of great vessel structure and detection of fluid in the pericardial sac. It is a procedure devoid of risk.

Phonocardiography. Phonocardiography refers to the recording of heart sounds and murmurs. Obtained with simultaneous pulse and electrocardiographic recordings, it allows the timing of murmurs and other abnormal heart sounds. Timing is important since some valve lesions produce murmurs during *systole* (the contraction period of the cardiac cycle) while others lead to abnormal sounds during *diastole* (the relaxation or filling phase of the cycle). With rapid heart rates the differentiation is sometimes difficult with bedside auscultation.

Radionuclide Imaging (Isotopic Scans). The use of radionuclides (radioisotopes) for scanning purposes in the brain has already been mentioned. Basically a radioisotope is injected into the bloodstream, and the radioactivity over the heart is recorded and converted to a visual image by *isotopic cameras.* Two types of scans are used in cardiology. *Dynamic scans* allow estimation of cardiac output and regional blood flow in the heart muscle without the need for cardiac catheterization. They are performed by injecting tiny radioactive particles (*microspheres*) or radioactive gases such as krypton 85 or xenon 133 and sequentially recording the isotopic image from the heart. The technique also gives an estimate of cardiac muscle strength and function. In *static imaging,* isotopes are injected that localize either in normal heart muscle or in devitalized tissue. Such scans allow direct visualization of the dead area of the myocardium after a heart attack. By combining the two types of isotopic examination, one can both confirm the fact that a heart attack has occurred and assess the impact of that attack on heart function. With scanners in the coronary intensive care unit, the progress of a myocardial infarction can be monitored several times each day if necessary. The direct visualization provided by radionuclide imaging has been important in research studies of heart function after occlusion of a coronary artery but also provides information of value in the ordinary clinical situation.

THE MANIFESTATIONS OF CARDIAC DISEASE

A very large number of diseases affect the heart either directly or indirectly. The cardiac response to such disease is, however, quite limited. Three major syndromes are commonly seen: ischemia of the myocardium leading ultimately to a heart attack (*myocardial infarction*), irregularities of rate or rhythm (*arrhythmias*) and failure of the heart as a pump (*congestive heart failure*).

ISCHEMIC HEART DISEASE

Clinical Picture. Ischemic heart disease refers to disease of the coronary arteries leading to impairment of blood flow to heart muscle. For practical purposes the cause is atherosclerosis of the vessels, and atherosclerotic heart disease is a synonymous term. The involvement of the coronary arteries by other forms of arterial disease is exceedingly rare. The primary symptom of insufficient blood supply to the myocardium is chest pain. If the pain is short lived and does not result in death of heart tissue, it is called *angina pectoris*. The pain of angina is usually located beneath the sternum in the center of the chest; it is heavy, pressing or squeezing in nature (almost never sharp or cutting). Frequently the patient holds a closed fist over the center of the chest to describe it (the *Levine sign*). The pain may radiate to the arms, neck or abdomen, but more frequently is localized to the chest alone. The patient is usually aware that the pain is serious (even on its first appearance) and often there is a sense that death is imminent.

Angina is produced whenever the oxygen demands of the heart are greater than can be met by blood flow through the narrowed coronary arteries. The most common precipitating event for anginal pain is exercise. Some patients have pain only on strenuous exertion while others may develop it after walking a few steps. Excitement, anger, fear, exposure to cold and eating a heavy meal are other precipitating factors. Angina may also occur spontaneously in the absence of known inducing events. When pain occurs exclusively (or mostly) at rest or during the night, the syndrome is called *variant* or *Prinzmetal's* angina. In contrast to ordinary angina, variant angina is not associated with atherosclerosis. Rather, such patients have been shown to have intense spasm of a segment of the artery, the spasm being the mechanism of impaired blood flow.

The pain of angina lasts only a few minutes if the precipitating event is removed: a patient developing pain on walking finds that the pain disappears rapidly if he stops and rests. The pain can also be aborted by nitroglycerin tablets placed under the tongue. If pain lasts for more than a few minutes following rest or nitroglycerin, it is called *coronary insufficiency*, indicating that more serious myocardial ischemia is occurring. *Unstable angina* refers to an unexplained increase in frequency of chest pain or a diminution in the amount of exercise or stress that will bring it on. Coronary insufficiency and unstable angina often indicate that a heart attack is about to occur. *Myocardial infarction* occurs when oxygen deficiency becomes so severe that a portion of the heart muscle dies. The pain of myocardial infarction is similar in quality to that of angina but is much more severe. Weakness, sweating, nausea, vomiting, pallor and fainting often accompany the pain. While this constellation of symptoms constitutes the usual picture of infarction, it should be noted that 10–20 percent of heart attacks are silent; they produce no pain.

Ischemic heart disease is responsible for almost all *sudden death* in this country. Sudden death is defined as rapid, unexpected demise occurring before the patient can be taken to a hospital.[4] It may occur without warning or follow the onset of chest pain typical of angina pectoris or myocardial infarction. The usual mechanism is for oxygen deficiency to induce an aimless (noncoordinated) rhythm of the ventricles called *ventricular fibrillation*; fibrillation is then followed shortly by cardiac standstill (*asystole*). The patient loses consciousness within 15 seconds after cessation of cardiac function. At this point a seizure may occur. Respirations become slow and shallow, then cease. A bluish color settles over the skin and the pupils of the eyes widely dilate, failing to constrict when exposed to light. Pulse and blood pressure are not detectable. Resuscitation requires reinitiation of cardiac function within 4–6 minutes following the onset of arrest if survival is to be possible. Four to six hundred thousand sudden deaths occur in the United States each year.[5]

[4] Sudden death due to external events such as shootings, accidents or other forms of trauma are not considered *medical* sudden deaths.

[5] Most communities offer free courses in cardiopulmonary resuscitation for lay persons. Ideally the entire population should be trained in these techniques. Briefly the method involves mouth-to-mouth respiration and chest compression. If two persons are available, one tilts the head posteriorly, pinches off the nasal passages and breathes into the victim's mouth very sharply 12 times a minute. With successful ventilation the chest should be seen to rise. The second resuscitator briskly compresses the chest by placing the long axis of one hand parallel to and over the lower sternum with the

Diagnosis. The diagnosis of ischemic heart disease is usually first suggested by the history of typical pain. Confirmation requires the demonstration of abnormal electrocardiographic findings during or after a symptomatic episode. If the patient has a normal ECG at rest, exercise stress testing is carried out. A positive test is indicated by the appearance of symptoms and/ or development of an abnormal electrocardiographic pattern in association with exercise. Coronary angiography is usually reserved for patients known to have coronary artery disease who are being considered as candidates for bypass surgery, but occasionally angiograms are obtained for diagnostic purposes in puzzling cases where chest pain is atypical or heart failure has occurred without obvious cause.

The diagnosis of myocardial infarction can usually be made from the presenting symptoms, but confirmation requires electrocardiographic demonstration of tissue death or elevation in blood levels of *cardiac enzymes.* Heart muscle cells, like all cells in the body, contain many enzymes. When tissue death occurs some of these enzymes leak into the blood where their concentration can be measured. Significant elevations strongly suggest the presence of myocardial infarction. *Creatine phosphokinase (CPK), lactic dehydrogenase (LDH)* and *serum glutamic-oxaloacetic transaminase (SGOT)* are the enzymes ordinarily tested. In larger centers additional confirmation is obtained by radionuclide imaging which allows direct visualization of the infarct.

Medical Treatment. The primary treatment for angina is *nitroglycerin,* a drug that causes dilation of blood vessels. The tablet is placed under the tongue with the onset of pain and usually relieves symptoms over a 3–5 minute period. Occasionally more than one tablet is required to stop an attack. (Nitroglycerin tablets deteriorate rapidly. They should be kept tightly capped and replaced every few months.) Longer-acting vasodilators that can be taken by mouth are also available. Nitroglycerin paste that can be rubbed into the chest for longer action is favored by a number of patients, particularly at night. Side ef-

---

second hand on top of the first. Pressing vertically downward, the sternum should be depressed about 2 inches at a rate of 60 compressions a minute. The victim must be on the ground or a firm surface (not a bed). In this sequence 1 respiration is carried out for every 12 compressions. If only one person is available, 15 chest compressions (rate, 80 per minute) are followed by 2 quick lung inflations over a 5-second interval. This 15:2 ratio is maintained until additional help can be provided.

fects of these drugs include lightheadedness, flushing, a pounding heart and headache. A second agent that has proved extremely helpful is *propranolol*. It acts to block the effects of epinephrine and norepinephrine on the heart, thereby slowing the rate of contraction and decreasing oxygen demand. It is ordinarily prescribed in any patient who cannot be controlled by nitroglycerin alone.

The critical first step in treatment of myocardial infarction is to get the patient to the hospital. If a cardiac arrest has occurred, resuscitative efforts should be carried out and continued in transit. Morphine or meperidine (Demerol) should be given for relief of pain and oxygen started in the ambulance if possible, otherwise immediately after arrival in the emergency room. Electrocardiographic monitoring is mandatory. Irregular rhythms are treated with various intravenous drugs that vary depending on the nature of the arrhythmia. If the irritable focus is in the ventricle, *lidocaine* is the drug of choice. Should ventricular fibrillation supervene, electric shock with a defibrillating instrument is carried out. Falling blood pressure or shock is treated with *dopamine*, a relatively new drug that has the capacity to increase the strength of cardiac contraction. It is a major addition to the armamentarium of the cardiologist. If shock is not present, *digitalis* may be used in place of dopamine to enhance cardiac contractility. Fluid accumulation in the lungs as a consequence of pump failure is treated by powerful diuretic agents such as *furosemide* that remove water and salt from the body by markedly increasing urine output.

Most patients who die from myocardial infarction never reach the hospital (they are victims of sudden death). The prognosis for life in patients with uncomplicated myocardial infarction who are admitted to intensive care units is quite good—greater than 70 percent in almost every reported series.[6] The first 3–4 days are critical, and death, when it occurs, is usually due to abnormal rhythms or pump failure; rupture of the infarcted wall is less common but invariably fatal. In general the patient is kept in the coronary care unit for 96 hours and remains hospitalized for a total period of 3 weeks. Return to work is allowed after 6 weeks. Following recovery a major effort is made to

[6] In England it is quite common to treat uncomplicated myocardial infarctions in the home. This regime has not been widely accepted in the United States because of the feeling that an uncomplicated infarction may become complicated rapidly and unpredictably.

restore the patient to previous levels of activity and to eliminate risk factors predisposing to another infarction. If the patient survives the heart attack for 1 year, there is a 75 percent chance he will live 5 years longer. If he survives 5 years, the chance of living 15 years is 50 percent. These figures are very encouraging.

Coronary Bypass Surgery. The surgical treatment of angina pectoris and coronary artery disease has become increasingly popular in recent years. If a blood vessel is blocked off by an atherosclerotic plaque or clot, it would seem quite logical to try to remove the obstruction or devise a way to transport blood around the block. In large vessels of the legs and abdomen, it is often possible for the vascular surgeon to ream out the obstructed vessel or place an artificial graft to re-establish flow. In the coronary circulation this is not feasible. As a consequence cardiac surgeons have opted for a procedure in which a normal vessel from elsewhere in the body is anastomosed (surgically connected) between the aorta and a portion of the coronary artery located beyond the obstructing lesion. Most often the bypass vessel is the *saphenous vein* taken from the leg. For the procedure to be successful, the involved vessel must have a relatively normal segment distal to the major obstruction. Several grafts may be required if more than one obstruction is present. An artery that is narrowed or occluded throughout its length is not surgically correctable. This means that coronary angiograms are absolutely required to localize and evaluate the type of lesion present in any potential candidate for surgery. The bypass procedure involves opening the chest but it is not open-heart surgery: the heart itself is not incised. As a consequence mortality rates in the hands of experienced cardiac surgeons are quite low when compared to those expected in other types of heart surgery and range from 0.5–4 percent in most series. Major problems, apart from operative death, are infarction precipitated by the surgery itself and postoperative occlusion of the grafted vessels. The latter occurs at a rate of 10–20 percent in the first year following operation.

There seems to be no doubt that coronary bypass surgery is a tremendous advance in the therapy of coronary artery disease, yet the procedure is the source of great controversy among doctors. The issue is whether every patient with coronary artery disease should be operated on once the diagnosis has been made. Many surgeons say yes and offer the operation prophylactically even to asymptomatic patients picked up by routine stress testing; most internists and cardiologists disagree. There is no question that coronary bypass relieves the pain of angina. Thus there is essential agreement that intractable and incapacitating angina which is not responsive to drug therapy is an indication for surgery providing angiography shows a correctable lesion. The question at issue is whether life is prolonged by operation in all forms of coronary artery disease. If so all patients should be operated once the diagnosis is established. Present evidence strongly suggests that if the patient has obstruction in the left main coronary artery (with or without disease in other vessels), survival is enhanced by the grafting procedure. This is much less certain when the blockade is in other vessels. A large cooperative study carried out by the Veterans Administration failed to show prolongation of life in patients treated surgically compared to those treated medically when left main stem disease was not present, but these conclusions have been widely questioned on technical grounds. Additional experience will be required to settle this very difficult issue.

Given this background, my own feelings (which are subject to change as new information is acquired) are as follows: *First,* coronary bypass is the best form of treatment for some patients with coronary artery disease, but surgery is not indicated in all subjects with angina. *Second,* a potential candidate for bypass must have a reasonable life expectancy apart from the presence of coronary artery disease; thus very elderly patients or those with major complications such as severe congestive heart failure or another life-threatening illness (e.g., cancer) should not be operated. *Third,* all patients with significant pain from angina should receive coronary angiograms to determine the nature of the lesions present. *Fourth,* coronary bypass should be carried out in all patients whose normal function is significantly impaired by severe angina despite optimal drug therapy. *Fifth,* surgery should be offered to all symptomatic patients with left main coronary lesions. *Sixth,* asymptomatic subjects (even with left main stem disease)[7] and those with drug responsive angina

[7] When a blood vessel is occluded, it is possible to develop *collateral circulation,* meaning that smaller secondary vessels running parallel to the occluded primary channel carry the blood past the obstruction (a sort of natural bypass). Collateral circulation develops much less efficiently in the heart than in other tissues but can occur when occlusion develops gradually. This accounts for the fact that a coronary artery can be completely occluded in the absence of a heart attack.

who do not have left main stem disease should not be operated routinely. These recommendations are considered prudent and consonant with current data on the effectiveness of bypass surgery. No patient should be hurried into surgery at the first sign of pain; on the other hand, when indicated, operation should not be inordinately delayed.[8] Any person with a question about the necessity for surgery should obtain a second opinion from a cardiologist.

HEART FAILURE

Failure of the heart as a pump can occur because of intrinsic disease of the heart muscle or because the work demands placed upon the myocardium are greater than its capacity to respond. The two most common conditions damaging cardiac muscle directly are *coronary artery disease* (with or without infarction) and the *cardiomyopathies. Cardiomyopathy* is a general term encompassing a variety of conditions that selectively affect the heart muscle. Viruses, alcohol, vitamin deficiencies and diabetes are the significant etiologic entities. Failure of a previously normal myocardium can be caused by increased work due either to *volume* or *pressure* overloads. The most common causes for *volume overload* are leaky valves or abnormal openings between heart chambers. To illustrate the pathophysiology, the effect of a leaky aortic valve can be considered. In the normal heart about 60 milliliters of blood are ejected with each heartbeat. If the aortic valve is incompetent, 20 milliliters of that blood may pass backward through the inadequately closing valve. Under these circumstances the heart will have to pump 80 or more milliliters of blood each beat to assure that 60 milliliters reach the tissues. With severe disease as much blood may leak backward as is ejected forward; thus half or more of heart energy is expended in futile pumping activity. *Pressure loads* are due either to a narrowed valve or systemic high blood pressure. If the aortic valve is stenotic, for example, blood can pass through the valve, but normal volume flow is achieved only at the expense of a great increase in left ventricular pressure and contractile force—in energy terms a

[8] I once had Dr. Thomas N. James, Chairman of the Department of Internal Medicine at the University of Alabama School of Medicine in Birmingham and a distinguished cardiologist, discuss coronary bypass surgery on my television program. At the end of the program, having considered the pros and cons, I asked him what he would do if he had significant angina and left main stem disease. His answer: "I'd see my friendly surgeon."

costly proposition. Similarly increased blood pressure requires greater contraction of the ventricle to force the aortic valve open for the ejection of blood. With both volume and pressure lesions, the heart enlarges in an attempt to meet the demands placed upon it. When that enlargement and the consequent increase in contractile strength is no longer able to compensate for the increased work load, heart failure is said to be present.

When the heart fails as a pump, the symptoms may be due either to a fall in cardiac output (*forward failure*) or, more commonly, to a pooling of blood in the lungs (*backward failure*). The former is most often seen when heart failure occurs rapidly (as following a myocardial infarction) and if severe results in falling blood pressure or frank shock. In the common forms of heart failure, left ventricular function is lost first, followed by sequential failure of the left atrium and the two right-sided chambers. In left heart failure the blood returning from the lungs cannot be adequately pumped forward and backs up in the pulmonary vessels, creating pulmonary congestion. The primary symptom is shortness of breath, produced by stiffness of the blood-engorged lung and occasionally by actual fluid formation in the air space (*pulmonary edema*). Early in the course, shortness of breath occurs only with exertion or exercise. Later it is present whenever the patient reclines, and finally it occurs even at rest. Eventually the increased pressure of the blood in the vessels of the lung causes the right side of the heart to fail, an event signaled by the development of fluid retention in the body.[9] The mechanism by which heart failure causes edema is too complicated to discuss here; suffice to say that fluid retention and edema are due to avid reabsorption of salt and water by the kidneys. The more salt that is ingested, the more edematous the patient becomes. In the end, it is not just the legs that are swollen; the abdominal cavity and pleural spaces also become filled with fluid.

The presence of heart failure is confirmed by X-ray of the

[9] The usual sequence in heart failure is for the left ventricle to fail, resulting in congestion of the lungs, following which the right ventricle fails. However, it is possible to have right-sided failure without involvement of the left ventricle. Such a syndrome can be produced by infarction of the right ventricle, stenosis of the pulmonic valve or a primary elevation of the pressure in blood vessels of the lungs. The latter may occur as a consequence of pulmonary emphysema and other lung diseases, or occur spontaneously for unknown reason (*primary pulmonary hypertension*). Right-sided heart failure due to disease in the lung is called *cor pulmonale* (pulmonary heart).

chest showing cardiac enlargement and congestion of the lungs with blood. In certain situations the diagnosis requires direct demonstration of abnormally elevated pressure in the ventricular chambers. This can be done by passing a special catheter (*the Swan-Ganz catheter*) into the heart (a sort of bedside mini-cardiac catheterization).

Treatment involves multiple approaches. Ideally the causal condition is removed. This is usually possible with high blood pressure and occasionally possible with abnormal heart valves that can be replaced surgically. Atherosclerosis and primary muscle disease are usually irreversible, limiting therapy to relief of symptoms. The *first* line of treatment for heart failure is the drug *digitalis*. Known since antiquity, digitalis has a unique capacity to increase the strength of contraction of the failing heart. It is a powerful drug and must be used carefully under supervision by the physician; in excess it can cause nausea, vomiting, distorted vision (with objects appearing green or yellow) and, most important, abnormal heart rhythms that are potentially extremely serious.[10] The *second* therapeutic principle is to limit salt intake in the diet. Edema formation and lung congestion are clearly reduced by rigid salt restriction (no free salt added during cooking or at table; avoidance of salt-containing foods). The *third* approach is to give diuretic drugs which enhance the production of urine by blocking the reabsorption of sodium chloride in the kidneys. If the patient faithfully adheres to these three measures, heart failure can usually be treated effectively for long periods of time. Fulminant exacerbation of the symptoms of failure, called *acute pulmonary edema*, requires ventilatory assistance with a respirator and oxygen therapy in addition to digitalis and diuretics.

ARRHYTHMIAS

Abnormal heart rhythms (*arrhythmias; dysrhythmias*) are of two general types. In the first the heart rate is too slow (*brachycardia* or *bradycardia*) while in the second it is too rapid (*tachycardia*). Tachycardias, in addition, are also often irregular

---

[10] Digitalis has been used illegitimately in many ways. In the past persons wishing to avoid the military draft induced irregular rhythms in themselves by taking large doses of the drug—an exceedingly dangerous proposition. It was also included in the infamous "rainbow pills" given by certain charlatans to produce weight loss. Digitalis did decrease food intake by making recipients queasy and causing vomiting. Unfortunately it also killed a few.

(tachyarrhythmias). Bradycardias are usually due to atherosclerotic damage to the sinoatrial (sinus) node, or to interruption of some portion of the conducting pathway leading from the node to the ventricular muscle. The term *sick sinus syndrome* is often used for the former while the latter is called *heart block*. Tachycardias may originate from an abnormal trigger zone (that supersedes the normal conduction mechanism) located in either the atria or the ventricles. Occasionally multiple irritable sites exist. While arrhythmias usually indicate the presence of heart disease they can also be due to *drugs* (e.g., digitalis), *chemical disorders of the blood* (particularly deficiency or excess of potassium) or *noncardiac illnesses* (such as thyrotoxicosis, which causes atrial fibrillation in a significant number of patients). One form of tachycardia, *paroxysmal atrial tachycardia* (PAT), occurs in young persons and is apparently not a sign of cardiac disease. Often attacks of PAT can be halted by holding the breath, pressing the eyeballs or submerging the face in cold water, all of which initiate activity of the vagal nerve that slows the heart. *Ventricular arrhythmias* are far more dangerous than those arising in the atrium and require aggressive therapy. The symptoms produced by these abnormalities include palpitations (a fluttering sensation in the chest), dizziness and loss of consciousness. As already noted, ventricular tachycardias, particularly ventricular fibrillation, can cause sudden death. Diagnosis of the type of arrhythmia present is made from the electrocardiogram.

Serious brachycardia requires treatment with an electrical *pacemaker*. Temporary pacemakers (inserted into the heart via a catheter introduced through a peripheral vein) are used if a reversible lesion is thought to be present, but often permanent instrumentation is required. For permanent pacing tiny wires are implanted directly into the heart and connected to a battery-powered generator that is usually placed beneath the skin immediately below the collarbone in the anterior chest. The life span of the batteries varies but may extend up to 3 years before replacement is needed. Generators are of two types. *Fixed-rate pacemakers* fire at a preset rate regardless of the patient's own intrinsic heart rate. Much more frequently used is a *demand pacer* which generates an impulse only when the patient's heart rate falls below a certain predetermined level (say 60 beats a minute). In general the units function exceedingly well, although initial failure in placement of the wire or breakage of the electrode may require a second surgical procedure. Pacemaker function can be checked by long distance telephone using a home adaptor that transmits impulses to a central advisory facility.

Tachyarrhythmias are treated with drugs. The indications are so varied and the number of drugs so large that no attempt will be made to describe their use. The primary agents are digitalis, quinidine, procainamide and propranolol. In emergency situations with ventricular tachycardia, intravenous lidocaine is the drug of choice. All act to delay conduction of electrical impulses or to suppress the excitability of the heart muscle, including trigger zones. As a group the drugs are very potent and dangerous if taken in excessive amounts. They must be used with considerable care.

SPECIFIC DISEASES AFFECTING THE HEART AND BLOOD VESSELS

The number of diseases that affect the heart are too great for detailed discussion. In addition to the primary cardiac disorders many noncardiac illnesses involve the heart secondarily. For example, malignant tumors metastasize to the myocardium not infrequently. In this section brief specific comments will be made regarding atherosclerosis, hypertension, valvular heart disease, congenital heart disease and aneurysms of the aorta.

ATHEROSCLEROSIS

It has already been pointed out that atherosclerosis is the cause of ischemic heart disease and of strokes. The same process operating in peripheral vessels can cause impaired blood flow to any organ or tissue. The atherosclerotic lesion is a deposit of cholesterol and fat in the blood vessel wall that eventually builds up to such a degree that significant blockade or occlusion of blood flow results.[11] The cause of atherosclerosis is not known, but it is clear that the process begins very early

[11] The two major lipids associated with atherosclerosis are *cholesterol* and *triglyceride* (fat). Both are carried in plasma bound to proteins called lipoproteins. Cholesterol is transported in *low density* (LDL) and *high density* (HDL) *lipoprotein molecules*. It turns out that LDL cholesterol is dangerous from the standpoint of producing atherosclerosis while certain types of HDL cholesterol may be protective. This story is still developing. Triglyceride is carried in *very low density lipoprotein* (VLDL) particles and *chylomicrons*. Only the former is thought to be harmful when elevated.

in life, particularly in men. (Women seem to be partially protected by their hormonal makeup until after the menopause.)
The most widely held theory is that the disease is somehow
related to abnormal cholesterol metabolism. This follows from
the observation that if one has a very high cholesterol concentration in the blood, heart attacks occur much more frequently
and at an earlier age than in persons with normal cholesterol
levels. In the disease called *familial hypercholesterolemia*, for
example, cholesterol concentrations in the blood reach 1000
milligrams per 100 milliliters or higher (normal upper limits,
250 milligrams per 100 milliliters), and affected children often
die of heart attacks below the age of 10. Recently it was possible
to autopsy a fetus known to have the disease, and early atherosclerotic changes were found, indicating initiation of blood
vessel disease prior to birth. The major problem with the cholesterol theory is that most patients with heart attacks have
normal cholesterol levels in the blood. However, many
investigators believe that the so-called normal values are far too
high in all Western countries, largely because the fat content of
the diet is elevated by heavy protein intake. Since it is recognized that atherosclerosis is influenced by many other factors
(such as the level of the blood pressure) it is considered that
those who have difficulty are selected out by a combination of
risk factors operating against the background of relative hypercholesterolemia present in the population as a whole. Thus,
two persons may have a cholesterol of 250 milligrams per 100
milliliters, but one is overweight, hypertensive and a smoker,
while the other is devoid of risk factors. The former would
develop accelerated atherosclerosis while the latter would not.

The current theory regarding the role of cholesterol in the
development of atherosclerosis can be elaborated by describing
the now widely held "unitary hypothesis" of atherosclerosis.
According to this formulation, tiny holes or defects develop in
the *endothelium* or lining surface of the arteries which allow
circulating platelets (for a description of blood platelets and
their function, see chapter 14) to adhere to underlying tissues.
These adherent platelets release substances that stimulate
growth of muscle cells in the *media* (middle wall) of the artery
and cause them to enter the *intima* (inner wall). The proliferat-
ing muscle cells then trap LDL cholesterol molecules which
are stored at the site and cannot be digested or broken down.

Eventually the muscle cells repair the endothelial hole, but only after cholesterol has been deposited. The higher the plasma cholesterol at the time of the damage, the more is laid down in the arterial wall. This accounts for the fact that patients with hypercholesterolemia develop atherosclerosis earlier than persons with normal or low cholesterol. As the process is repeated an occluding lesion composed of cholesterol and scar tissue (*atheroma*) is formed. What causes the endothelial holes to develop is not known, but it is suspected that smoking, high blood pressure and stress hormones play a role. Drugs that inhibit platelet function such as aspirin, dipyridamole and sulfinpyrazone are currently undergoing trials to see if they will interrupt the atherogenic process. Preliminary results (in men but not women) show encouraging trends.

HYPERTENSION

High blood pressure predisposes to heart failure, kidney failure and stroke. The common form of the disease is called *essential hypertension,* meaning that the cause is unknown. In a small minority of cases, high blood pressure is due to narrowing of the major artery delivering blood to the kidney (*renal artery stenosis*) or overproduction of salt-retaining hormones by the adrenal gland, particularly the hormone aldosterone (*aldosteronism*). A rare but very interesting tumor causing hypertension is *pheochromocytoma.* Classically it produces a syndrome consisting of episodic high blood pressure coupled with sweating and a fast heart rate. Symptoms are due to the release of the hormones epinephrine and norepinephrine into the bloodstream. Patients with pheochromocytoma commonly have an elevated blood sugar during hypertensive episodes.

High blood pressure presents itself in one of three ways, called *labile, benign* and *malignant. Labile hypertension* means that the blood pressure is elevated only intermittently, usually in association with stress. *Benign hypertension* indicates persistent modest to severe elevation of the blood pressure. It is benign only in the sense that it usually causes symptoms after being present for many years; the name is a misnomer and in fact benign hypertension is a life-shortening disease. *Malignant (accelerated) hypertension* is a rapidly developing, extreme elevation of the blood pressure that kills the patient in weeks to months if untreated. It may develop in a patient who previously had the "benign" form of the disease. A characteristic sign is the development of hemorrhages in the retina of the eye and papilledema (swelling of the optic disc).

Hypertension is usually considered to be present when the blood pressure is greater than 140/90,[12] although slightly higher values may be normal in older persons. Once it has been established that hypertension is present, screening tests are usually run to rule out the rare nonessential causes. These include tests of kidney function, intravenous pyelograms (X-rays of the kidneys), measurement of urinary sodium, potassium and metanephrine content (elevated in pheochromocytoma) and occasionally evaluation of a hormone called *renin* (which may give a clue to the presence of adrenal causes of hypertension). Nonessential hypertension is always suspected when high blood pressure appears in the very young or the elderly.

It is widely believed that expansion of the body fluid volume plays a key role in causing high blood pressure. Therefore, the first principle of therapy is to reduce plasma volume. This is done by diminishing salt intake and giving diuretic drugs (usually one of the class of diuretics called *thiazides*). Since these drugs cause potassium loss in the urine, potassium salts ordinarily have to be given during therapy. If the blood pressure cannot be controlled by diuretics and salt restriction, *propranolol* is usually added. Resistant cases require addition of a third agent such as *hydralazine, methyldopa, clonidine* or *guanethidine.* Benign hypertension can be treated successfully in almost every case with these drugs, and it is absolutely clear that lowering the blood pressure diminishes the appearance of late complications. All of the drugs have significant side effects so that regular examination by the physician is mandatory. Malignant hypertension is a medical emergency. Treatment requires hospitalization and administration of antihypertensive drugs intravenously or intramuscularly rather than by mouth.

VALVULAR HEART DISEASE

It has already been mentioned that the four valves of the heart may become narrowed, obstructing blood flow into or out

[12] When the blood pressure is measured, the appearance of a sound in the stethoscope as the mercury column of the sphygmomanometer falls marks the level of the *systolic* pressure. Disappearance of the sound identifies the *diastolic* pressure. The blood pressure is always recorded as a ratio of the systolic to diastolic (higher to lower) pressures.

of a heart chamber, or incompetent such that back leaks occur. Valvular heart disease may be either *congenital* or *acquired*. The most common cause of acquired change is *rheumatic fever*. Rheumatic fever is a peculiar disease which occurs as a result of infection with the *Streptococcus,* usually a sore throat. After a latent period of 2–4 weeks (during which time the streptococcal infection has cleared), the patient develops fever and arthritis in many joints of the body. The arthritis is migratory, meaning that it moves from joint to joint. Frequently a rash is present and at times abnormal involuntary movements (chorea) appear. Most important, there are signs of inflammation in the heart ranging from a fast rate with murmurs[13] to full-blown heart failure. The attack may clear without heart damage but very often produces permanent valve deformities. The disease is thought to be due to an immune response to constituents in the bacterial cell wall and surrounding capsule: antistreptococcal antibodies are formed that (for reasons which are not clear) preferentially attack the heart muscle and valves, joints and skin. Acute rheumatic fever can be prevented by early treatment of streptococcal infections with penicillin. While only about 0.3 percent of untreated patients get rheumatic fever, the disease is so devastating that every streptococcal infection should be adequately treated. Because recurrent attacks are possible (and even more devastating), all patients who have once had rheumatic fever should receive prophylactic injections of a long-acting penicillin preparation (benzathine penicillin) once a month to prevent recurrent streptococcal infection.

Two other infectious diseases cause permanent valve damage. *Syphilis* attacks the aortic valve almost exclusively and produces incompetency. *Endocarditis* is a direct bacterial infection of the valves which exists in two forms. In both forms bacteria reach the valves via the bloodstream. *Acute bacterial endocarditis* involves previously normal valves and is most often seen with young people who inject illicit drugs intrave-

[13] When one listens to the heart with the stethoscope, ordinarily two sounds are heard, delineating ventricular contraction. The first heart sound is made by the closing of the mitral and tricuspid valves as the ventricles contract. The second sound is due to closure of the aortic and pulmonic valves after contraction is complete. Normally the intervals between sounds are clear. Murmurs are blowing or rumbling noises heard between heartbeats and are due to abnormal blood flow through stenotic or insufficient valves.

nously. Staphylococcus and pneumococcus are the organisms most frequently involved, but other bacteria, funguses and yeasts can likewise cause the illness. *Subacute bacterial endo-carditis* is a disease caused by the implantation of bacteria on valves damaged congenitally or by rheumatic fever. The usual bacteria involved are streptococcal species. Not infrequently the illness begins following dental manipulations with bacteria entering the bloodstream from the mouth. Untreated, valve infections can lead to death from heart failure over short periods of time. The diagnosis of endocarditis is always assumed when a new heart murmur is found in a patient with fever who has positive cultures for bacteria in the blood. The infection can usually be cured with prolonged (6 weeks) intravenous antibiotic therapy using very high concentrations of two drugs in combination (most often penicillin and streptomycin).

In the past heart failure due to valvular heart disease could only be treated medically. In recent years surgical replacement of hopelessly damaged valves has been undertaken with increasing frequency. Several types of prosthetic valves are available and the type chosen depends on the preference of the surgeon. The procedure requires open heart surgery with support of the circulation by an extracorporeal oxygenating system (artificial heart). More than one valve may be replaced in a single operation. Mortality rates are quite high (15–30 percent depending on the preoperative condition of the patient), but the alternative is death from unrelenting heart failure. Postoperative complications include infection at the site of valve replacement, mechanical dysfunction of the valve, clot formation on the valve with embolization to other parts of the body and abnormal destruction of blood cells (hemolytic anemia).

CONGENITAL HEART DISEASE

Congenital heart disease can involve any part of the heart. The defects are due to abnormal development of the circulatory system during embryogenesis. The cause is generally not known although occasionally congenital heart abnormalities are part of recognized genetic diseases such as *Turner's syndrome* or *mongolism* (see chapter 4). *Rubella* (German measles) infection of the mother early in pregnancy is known to cause congenital heart lesions in a high percentage of cases. The recognized abnormalities are too numerous to catalog here, but openings between the atria and ventricles (*atrial* and *ventricular septal defects*) are the most common lesions. Under certain circumstances venous blood passes through the septal defect and out into the peripheral circulation without passing through the lungs. Such babies have *cyanosis* and are commonly called "blue babies." The most frequent abnormality causing cyanotic heart disease is *tetralogy of Fallot*, where a large ventricular septal defect is accompanied by stenosis of the pulmonary artery. Because flow into the pulmonary artery is obstructed, non-oxygenated blood passes through the septal defect into the left side of the heart and from there into the arterial circulation.

Extreme cardiac lesions cause death *in utero* (prior to birth) or early in infancy while septal defects and other milder abnormalities are compatible with survival into adult life. The treatment of congenital heart disease is surgical correction. The achievements of modern pediatric cardiac surgeons are simply superb. Complete repairs are frequently successfully carried out in infants weighing only a few pounds.

ANEURYSMS OF THE AORTA

Aneurysms of the aorta (the main arterial trunk leaving the heart) are fusiform or balloonlike swellings of the vessel due to weakness of the wall structure. They may be located either in the chest or abdomen. The most common cause is *arteriosclerosis* with *syphilis* being the second most frequent etiology. Symptoms are due to pressure on surrounding structures and pain of a variety of types is the usual complaint. The danger is that the aneurysms eventually rupture causing death from internal hemorrhage. Diagnosis is suggested by discovery of a mass on X-ray and confirmed by arteriography of the aorta. Occasionally the aneurysm can be felt on physical examination of the abdomen.

In *dissecting aneurysm of the aorta*, a tear develops in the lining of the aorta and blood dissects into the wall of the vessel. The dissection is accompanied by excruciating pain in the chest, back or abdomen followed by shock. Death occurs, as in fusiform aneurysms, because of rupture with hemorrhage. The rupture is usually into the pericardial sac surrounding the heart or the left chest cavity. Almost all patients with dissection have high blood pressure but usually an underlying disease is present. One congenital disease, *Marfan's syndrome*, is associated with dissection in a high percentage of cases. Patients with the Marfan syndrome are extremely tall and slender with a eunuchoid appearance to the body: the arm span is greater than the height, and the length of the body from pelvis to feet is greater than from pelvis to head, a physical appearance characteristic of eunuchs castrated before the age of puberty. Classically the lens of the eye is also dislocated.

Treatment of both types of aneurysms is surgical with the diseased segment being replaced by an artificial graft.

PREVENTION OF HEART DISEASE

Despite the fact that the treatment of heart disease has improved dramatically over the last 25 years, with rare exceptions treatment is never curative. It follows that prevention represents the only hope for diminishing its impact. At present there is little that can be done to prevent congenital heart disease (although certainly every woman should be immunized against rubella) or the viral cardiomyopathies. On the other hand, rheumatic heart disease can be drastically reduced by adequate treatment of streptococcal disease and the provision of penicillin prophylaxis for all those who have had rheumatic fever. Similarly valvular disease due to syphilis is completely preventable, and control of high blood pressure ought to avert the appearance of hypertensive heart failure in almost every case.

The single biggest problem is atherosclerotic heart disease, but even here much can be done. The known risk factors for developing coronary artery disease and myocardial infarction are *hyperlipidemia* (hypercholesterolemia and hypertriglyceridemia), *hypertension, cigarette smoking, obesity, sedentary life-style, emotional stress, diabetes* and a *strong family history of atherosclerosis*. The first three appear to be most important. The chances of dying from heart disease increase 5 times or more when risk factors are present in combination. If one wishes to reduce the chances of developing heart disease, here are the rules:

1. *Modify the diet.* An antiatherogenic diet is designed to lower the plasma cholesterol by diminishing cholesterol intake and increasing the content of polyunsaturated fat. Basically,

as pointed out in chapter 2, this means eliminating eggs, bacon and cheeses; drinking skim milk or buttermilk in place of whole milk; substituting unsaturated margarine for butter; replacing lard with corn or safflower oil for cooking and salad dressings; diminishing meat and increasing fish and poultry intake. If cholesterol and triglyceride concentrations in the blood are pathologically elevated, drug therapy will also be required (cholestyramine or nicotinic acid for hypercholesterolemia, clofibrate for hypertriglyceridemia).[14] The importance of lowering the plasma cholesterol is indicated by the fact that heart attacks occur 3–4 times less frequently (below the age of 55) when cholesterol concentrations in plasma are below 220 milligrams per 100 milliliters than when the values are above 260 milligrams per 100 milliliters.

2. *Treat hypertension.* Every person above the age of 40 should have a blood pressure check yearly and be aggressively treated for any significant elevation.

3. *Don't smoke.* Period!

4. *Normalize body weight.* Excess weight increases the work load placed on the heart because the fat tissue itself must be supplied with blood and because oxygen demands in the muscles carrying the extra weight also increase. Obesity likewise predisposes to development of diabetes and hypertension, two other significant risk factors.

5. *Exercise regularly.* Exercise should be *dynamic* (moving) rather than *static* (isometric). Examples of the former include walking, bicycling, swimming and jogging. Weight lifting and other static exercises may actually be detrimental, at least in persons with heart disease. Dynamic exercise should be carried out at a sufficient level to increase the heart and respiratory rates. Evidence suggests that a proper exercise program decreases oxygen demand in the heart and increases exercise tolerance both objectively and subjectively even in patients with known coronary artery disease. Excessive exercise is not required. Despite the long-distance jogging craze sweeping the country, there is no evidence that running several miles a day is more effective in

---

[14] There is tremendous excitement about a new experimental drug called *compactin*. While therapeutic trials are only beginning, it appears to dramatically lower plasma cholesterol levels.

preventing cardiac deaths than brisk walking or jogging for shorter distances. Every person over 40 should have a stress test before embarking on an exercise program if the previous life-style has been sedentary.

6. *Avoid emotional stress.* Probably this is easier said than done, but it seems clear that overly tense, stress-ridden individuals have higher rates of myocardial infarction than their more tranquil counterparts.

Obviously if diabetes is present, this should be treated. Nothing can be done about a strong family tendency to develop heart attacks, but the worse the genes, the more aggressive should be the attempt to eliminate other risk factors.

The most encouraging thing about these recommendations is that they appear to work. Deaths from heart attacks have been steadily declining in the United States in the last few years, roughly paralleling the period when prophylactic measures first began to be widely promulgated. The number of cardiac deaths dropped below 1 million per year for the first time in 1975 and in 1977 was down to 959,000 despite an increase in the total population. In view of these figures it seems reasonable to suggest global adoption of the prophylactic measures, especially since a drastic change in life-style is not required.

7

Diseases of the Lungs

It has already been noted (chapter 2) that the energy necessary to sustain life comes from the oxidation of ingested food, a process in which oxygen (O_2) is consumed and carbon dioxide (CO_2) and water are produced. The provision of oxygen for energy-generating chemical reactions and the removal of the end product, carbon dioxide, is the primary function of the lungs, which in simple terms can be considered as an air exchange system between blood and the external atmosphere. The volumes of air handled in the respiratory process are very large. Normally a person breathes about 15 times a minute at rest, each breath representing a volume of approximately 500 milliliters (half a liter); at this rate around 11,000 liters are exchanged each day. During strenuous exercise the ventilatory rate can become twentyfold greater. This enormous capacity means that in the absence of disease, oxygen needs of the body can always be met by the lungs.[1] With pulmonary disease, on the other hand, impairment of lung function may result in diminished oxygenation of blood (*hypoxemia*) or elevated concentrations of carbon dioxide (*hypercapnia*) or both, disturbances that produce a spectrum of symptoms up to and including respiratory failure and death.

---

[1] During maximal exercise it is the capacity of the heart to pump oxygen-laden blood to the tissues that limits the level of exertion, not the capacity of the lungs to deliver oxygen to the blood.

STRUCTURE AND FUNCTION OF THE LUNGS

The lungs are contained in the chest cavity. They lie lateral to and surround the heart and *mediastinal structures*[2] from which they are separated by a double-layered membrane called the *pleura*. The right lung has three major lobes (upper, middle and lower) while the left has only two (upper and lower). Air passes through the nose and throat into the *trachea* which then divides into right and left *main stem bronchi* (singular, *bronchus*)[3] which pass into the right and left lungs respectively. The bronchi are semirigid tubes whose structure is sustained by rings of cartilage. The main stem bronchi branch into increasingly smaller divisions in treelike fashion; the smallest divisions, called *bronchioles*, end in the air sacs or *alveoli* which represent the gas exchange sites. The air sacs are surrounded by the delicate pulmonary capillaries which receive deoxygenated venous blood pumped into the lungs from the right side of the heart. These fragile capillaries are so small that only one or two red blood cells can make the passage through them at one time. The barrier imposed between blood and oxygen by the alveolar and capillary walls is extremely thin— approximately 1 micrometer (about .00004 of an inch)—and as a consequence both O_2 and CO_2 pass through extremely rapidly. The process of gas movement is called *diffusion* and the driving force is a pressure gradient; e.g., if oxygen is present in the alveolus at a pressure of 100 millimeters of mercury and the oxygen pressure in capillary blood is only 40 millimeters of mercury, oxygen will diffuse rapidly to the point of lower tension.[4] The combined surface area of the alveoli is enormous,

[2] *Mediastinum* refers to the central portion of the chest cavity. It is delineated laterally by the lungs, posteriorly by the vertebral column and anteriorly by the sternum and chest wall. It contains the heart, the great blood vessels leading to and from the heart, the esophagus, the trachea and a variety of nerves and lymph vessels.

[3] No gas exchange goes on in the bronchi. For this reason air contained in the mouth, throat, trachea and bronchi is called *dead space* air. In an ordinary breath of 500 milliliters, about 150 milliliters remains in the dead space while 350 milliliters reaches the alveoli for transfer of oxygen and carbon dioxide. Shallow respiration is less effective than deep respiration because most of the air remains in the dead space.

[4] A fundamental property of gases is their tendency to expand. As a consequence all gases exert pressure, which can be considered a measure of the "push" of the gas against any barrier tending to confine it. The greater the concentration of a gas in a fixed volume, the greater will be its pressure. Gas pressures are measured in millimeters of mercury.

about 100 square meters. To put this figure in perspective, the surface area of the entire body of a 6-foot, 180-pound man is only about 2 square meters.

Air moves into the lungs through the bronchial tree in response to a negative (vacuumlike) pressure generated by contraction of the *diaphragm*—the large sheetlike muscle that attaches to the ribs and separates the chest and abdominal cavities—and the muscles that move the rib cage outward. With each inspiration the diaphragm lowers and the rib cage expands increasing the volume of the chest cavity. The lungs, being very elastic, expand in response to the negative pressure, and air flows in to fill the vacuum. At the end of inspiration, the diaphragm moves upward and the chest wall collapses, reversing the pressure gradient and forcing air outside the body.

The rate of ventilation is controlled by many factors acting in concert. The most sensitive control mechanism is the CO_2 concentration of arterial blood acting on the respiratory center in the brain stem. Ordinarily if the CO_2 content of blood rises, respiratory rate quickens and vice versa. The second most potent stimulus to ventilation is low oxygen content of blood, recognized by special receptors (*chemoreceptors*) located in the carotid arteries (the large neck vessels that carry blood from the aorta to the brain). The respiratory rate is also quickened by too much acid in the blood (see chapter 11) and by nervousness, sexual excitement, anxiety and fear. Hyperventilation due to the latter emotions does not occur because the body needs oxygen but is simply a reflex response. Presumably such reflexes developed in the distant past because experience taught that these emotions were frequently followed by intense activity (fighting, fleeing, intercourse, etc.) that would require increased oxygen intake.

GENERAL PATTERNS OF LUNG DISEASE

While many diseases affect the lungs, the disordered functions that result fall into several general categories. It is common, therefore, for physicians to speak of *obstructive* and *restrictive ventilatory defects, abnormalities of diffusion, ventilation-perfusion disorders, disturbances of ventilatory regulation* and *vascular disease* of the lung. Often a single disease causes difficulty by several of these mechanisms. The terms

150 MODERN MEDICINE

refer to generalized abnormalities that affect the lungs as a whole. In addition *localized disease* may occur. With localized disease the patient may be very ill without disturbing overall function of the lung.

OBSTRUCTIVE DISEASE

Obstructive disease means that there is impairment of air flow through the bronchial tree. In its pure form gas exchange mechanisms in the alveoli are normal, but air does not reach the exchange sites in adequate amounts. Obstruction may be *intraluminal* (inside the air passage) or due to disease in the bronchial wall. Aspiration of foreign material such as food[5] or pharyngeal secretions (a common problem postoperatively or after stroke) is a frequent cause of intraluminal obstruction, but *tumors* growing in the bronchus and abnormal production of mucus secondary to *chronic bronchitis* may also produce the syndrome. Acute intermittent obstructive disease is the hallmark of *asthma*, a condition in which bronchial musculature contracts abnormally, narrowing the bronchial channel and obstructing air flow. In *pulmonary emphysema*, destruction of surrounding lung parenchyma allows the bronchioles to collapse during expiration, blocking exit of air from the alveoli. Finally, *external compression* from enlarged lymph nodes or tumors can occlude the bronchus. If air flow is completely blocked, that portion of the lung distal to the obstruction collapses as air is resorbed from the alveoli, a condition that is called *atelectasis* (the collapse is analogous to what is seen when an air-filled balloon develops a slow leak; eventually the walls of the balloon become completely juxtaposed).

RESTRICTIVE DISEASE

In restrictive pulmonary disease expansion of the lung is impaired either because of alteration in the lung tissue itself or

---

[5] About 4,000 persons a year die because of aspiration of food. The most common offender is incompletely chewed meat, but many other materials, including peanut butter, have caused fatalities. The syndrome is characterized by the victim suddenly rising from the chair, grasping the throat and collapsing, unable to breathe or speak (the "cafe coronary"). Immediate intervention is required if the life is to be saved. The rescuer should stand behind the patient, place the arms around the body with the fist in the upper central abdomen and suddenly compress the arms with an upward thrust such that pressure in the chest cavity abruptly rises. The maneuver should be repeated if the obstructing material does not pop out the first time.

because of disease in the pleura, chest wall or skeleton. In contrast to obstructive disease, there is no block to air flow through the bronchial tree. The most common cause is *diffuse interstitial fibrosis* [6] which causes loss of elasticity and stiffness of the lung such that it does not expand well during inspiration. Fibrosis may be seen following *infection,* in association with certain *drugs,*[7] as a consequence of *allergy,* as a manifestation of *collagen diseases* (e.g., scleroderma or rheumatoid arthritis), as a result of *X-ray therapy* for cancer of the lung or secondary to the inhalation of certain *atmospheric pollutants* such as silica dust and asbestos fibers. *Sarcoidosis,* a peculiar disease of unknown origin, results in restrictive pulmonary disease associated with lymph node enlargement in the mediastinum, increased size of the salivary glands (which may resemble mumps) and arthritis. *Congestive heart failure* also causes restrictive disease since fluid in the lung tissue results in stiffness and diminished elasticity exactly as does fibrosis. Interestingly, *exposure to high concentrations of oxygen* for prolonged periods can cause edema in the interstitial tissue and the alveolar sacs, resulting in a stiff lung.

Pleural disease causing a restrictive defect is of two types. In *pleural effusion* the collection of a large amount of fluid in the pleural space compresses the lung and prevents its expansion. The most common causes are heart failure, infections, cancer and transfer of fluid from the abdominal cavity in alcoholics who have cirrhosis and ascites. *Pneumothorax* refers to the admission of air to the pleural space. As a consequence the normal vacuum found in the space disappears resulting in collapse of the lung. Pneumothorax may be secondary to a penetrating wound of the chest, puncture of the lung by a broken rib or spontaneous rupture of a swollen bleb in emphysematous disease.

Less common causes of a restrictive abnormality are diseases leading to *weakness* or *paralysis of the chest wall muscles* (poliomyelitis, tetanus, myasthenia gravis, muscular dystrophy) or *deformity of the spine* which prevents expansion of the rib cage.

---

[6] *Interstitial* means in the alveolar wall. *Fibrosis* refers to scar formation.

[7] Perhaps the most potent drug is the herbicide called *paraquat,* used extensively to spray Mexican marihuana fields. It causes the rapid development of lethal pulmonary fibrosis.

IMPAIRMENT OF DIFFUSION

When this defect is present, oxygen transport across the al-veolar-capillary membrane is slowed such that equilibration between alveolus and capillary blood does not occur. Normally blood passing around the air sac in the pulmonary capillary is exposed to air for about ¾ of a second but requires only ¼ of a second to reach an oxygen concentration equal to that in the alveolus; i.e., diffusion is very rapid. With a diffusion barrier equilibration cannot be obtained even in ¾ of a second and hypoxemia ensues. Symptoms are usually first seen with exercise since the rapid heart rate and increased blood flow diminishes contact time in the capillaries to about ⅓ of a second. Any of the diseases producing pulmonary fibrosis, in addition to causing a restrictive defect, can lead to diffusion abnormalities.

VENTILATION-PERFUSION DEFECTS

By this is meant a mismatching of ventilation and blood flow; either blood perfuses (flows through) sections of lung that are not aerated, or properly oxygenated alveoli are not perfused with normal amounts of blood. Such mismatching is probably the most common cause of hypoxemia in pulmonary disease. The process may occur as a consequence of almost any form of lung disorder. A classic example of ventilation-perfusion mismatch would be lobar pneumonia where blood perfuses a lobe in which the alveoli contain no air because the pneumonia has caused them to be filled with inflammatory fluid. The term used for flow of blood through nonaerated lung is *shunting*.

DISORDERS OF VENTILATORY REGULATION

Underventilation (decreased rate or depth of respiration) is usually due to abnormalities outside the lung; the difficulty is in regulatory centers rather than in the lungs themselves. Depression of the respiratory center in the brain stem can be due to *drugs, infections of the central nervous system, trauma* or *stroke*. Some patients with *extreme obesity* have hypoventilation coupled with somnolence (called the *pickwickian syndrome* after the fat boy in Dickens's *Pickwick Papers*). In addition to hypoventilation, disease of the respiratory center may result in *apnea* (complete cessation of respiration) or a peculiar pattern of breathing characterized by alternating periods of hyperventilation and apnea called *Cheyne-Stokes res-piration*. All three responses are prognostically ominous.

VASCULAR DISEASE

By far the most common vascular disease of the lung is *pulmonary embolism*. Occasionally the pulmonary arteries develop a constrictive lesion resulting in *primary pulmonary hypertension* which means high blood pressure of the pulmonary vessels. The cause is unknown. Arterioles in the lungs may be involved in diseases such as *scleroderma, polyarteritis nodosa* and *lupus erythematosus,* the collagen disorders. Pulmonary arterioles can also be obliterated by nonvascular forms of pulmonary disease; for example, advanced *emphysema* is notorious as a destroyer of capillaries.

Vascular disease causes symptoms in one of two major ways. First, partial obstruction to blood flow puts a pressure load on the right side of the heart leading to right ventricular failure. Second, more complete obstruction leads to death of lung tissue by infarction with subsequent scar formation and loss of function.

LOCALIZED DISEASE

The most common serious (but usually reversible) localized pulmonary disease is *pneumonia,* which may be due to bacteria, viruses or fungi. A special form of pneumonia is the *lung abscess,* a pus-filled cavity in lung tissue most often seen in alcoholics. The second most frequent localized destructive lesion is *cancer of the lung.* Cancer may represent primary neoplastic disease developing in pulmonary tissue or spread to the lung from another primary site.

SYMPTOMS OF PULMONARY DISEASE

The primary symptom of pulmonary disease is *shortness of breath;* it is usually due either to oxygen deficiency or to increased work of breathing secondary to airway obstruction or lung stiffness. *Cough* and *sputum production* accompany most lung disorders. *Hemoptysis* (the coughing of blood) is common with pneumonia, tuberculosis, cancer and large pulmonary emboli. When hypoxia is severe *cyanosis* may develop due to the presence of high concentrations of deoxygenated hemoglobin in the blood. *Chest pain* made worse by breathing (*pleurisy*) is frequently present with pneumonia and pulmonary embolism. *Clubbing* of the fingers is a not unusual accompaniment of severe pulmonary disease (although it may occur in other conditions including cyanotic heart disease). Clubbed fingers are widened at the tips and the nails are beak shaped and spongy.

DIAGNOSTIC TECHNIQUES

The first step in diagnosing pulmonary disease (after obtaining the history and carrying out the physical examination) is to take routine X-rays of the chest. This simple procedure provides a presumptive diagnosis in high percentage of cases. However, it is well known that a number of dissimilar disease processes may produce the same X-ray picture. As a consequence specialized diagnostic techniques are frequently required for definitive identification of diseases causing pulmonary symptoms. The common procedures are outlined below.

Tests for Infectious Disease. The lung is a primary site for infection by bacteria, fungi and viruses. If the patient is coughing up sputum, *microscopic examination* and *culture* will usually identify causative bacterial agents and, less efficiently, fungi. Prolonged culture times are required for the latter as well as for the tuberculosis organism. In the absence of sputum production, *skin tests* and *serologic examinations* are carried out. In the former a small amount of material (*antigen*)[8] is injected into the skin of the forearm. A positive reaction (redness and swelling) within a 48-hour period indicates that the individual has been exposed to the organism from which the antigen was derived. A positive test does not prove current infection but only its possibility, since exposure could have been in the past. Serological tests are designed to show the presence of antibodies to an infecting organism. A rising concentration of antibodies usually indicates recent exposure to the agent being

[8] *Antigen* refers to any substance foreign to the body that is capable of eliciting the formation of *antibodies*. In the case of an infectious agent, the antigen is some material derived from the organism itself; e.g., the antigen for the common tuberculin test for tuberculosis is a protein derivative of the tubercle bacillus. Antibodies are specialized proteins produced by the body to protect the individual against invading foreign agents.

tested. Serologic and skin tests are particularly helpful in tuberculosis, fungal and viral infections.

Pulmonary Function Tests. A variety of tests—some simple, others complicated—are now available to evaluate ventilatory function and to identify specific physiological defects. *Spirometry* refers to measurement of the quantity and speed with which air can be expired in a single maximal effort after full inspiration. Normally about 80 percent of the total expired air is released in one second. A value less than 80 percent implies an *obstructive defect*. If total measured gas movement is less than predicted from tables of normal values but 80 percent or more is expired in one second, a *restrictive defect* is identified. Should the total and one-second values both be diminished, a combined *restrictive-obstructive* disease is present.

Blood Gases. The oxygen and carbon dioxide contents of arterial blood are measured directly and reported in terms of pressure in millimeters of mercury. Normally the oxygen tension (pressure) is about 95–100 millimeters of mercury in young persons and falls with age to a lower limit of 85. Oxygen tension in venous blood is usually about 40 millimeters of mercury, reflecting removal of oxygen by the tissues. Carbon dioxide pressure is ordinarily about 40 millimeters of mercury and does not change with age. With full-blown respiratory failure, the oxygen tension (pO_2) of blood is low and CO_2 tension (pCO_2) is high indicating that oxygen uptake and carbon dioxide removal are both impaired. Oxygen and carbon dioxide do not always move in parallel directions: one may be normal while the other is abnormal, or one may be high while the other is low. Two other values are always reported with blood gases. They are *percent oxygen saturation* and *pH*. *Oxygen saturation* refers to the amount of oxygen bound to the hemoglobin molecule in the red blood cell as a percent of maximal capacity. At a pressure of 100 millimeters of mercury, hemoglobin is about 95 percent saturated with oxygen while at 40 millimeters (the value of venous blood) it is only 75 percent saturated. Below 40 millimeters saturation falls very rapidly. The *pH* is a measure of the acidity of blood. Its value falls (blood becomes more acidic) as CO_2 tension rises and decreases as CO_2 tension falls, since carbon dioxide in solution is an acid.

Bronchoscopy. Bronchoscopy is a technique in which a tube is passed directly into the bronchial tree for diagnostic purposes. The modern fiberoptic bronchoscope is flexible and can be passed into the most distal reaches of the bronchial tree for direct visualization of lesions and to obtain tissue for microscopic examination and culture. It is most useful for the diagnosis of tumors and obscure infections.

Lung Scans. Two types of radioactive scans are available. The most useful measures distribution of blood flow in the lung and is helpful in the diagnosis of pulmonary embolism. The second type of scan, utilizing ^{67}gallium, is beneficial in detecting areas of infection or neoplastic growth, particularly in lymph nodes.

Angiograms. Pulmonary angiograms are carried out by the injection of radiopaque dyes in the pulmonary vessels. They are the definitive method for diagnosing pulmonary embolism.

Bronchography. This technique involves the instillation of X-ray absorbing dye directly into the bronchial tree. It is necessary for the diagnosis of the disease called *bronchiectasis* (see page 158).

Biopsies. It has already been mentioned that biopsies for pathologic examination can be obtained through the bronchoscope. Biopsies of the pleura can be taken with a needle during drainage of pleural effusions. Occasionally direct (open) biopsy of the lung may be necessary when the etiology of the pulmonary disease is obscure. Since general anesthesia is required, this technique is usually used only as a last resort. When mediastinal lymph nodes are enlarged, biopsy is obtained by *mediastinoscopy*, a technique in which a bronchoscopelike instrument is inserted into the mediastinum through an incision at the base of the neck.

THE MAJOR DISEASES OF THE LUNG

PNEUMONIA AND OTHER INFECTIONS

Pneumonia ordinarily begins following several days of a cold or upper respiratory infection. With bacterial forms the first symptom is often a shaking chill shortly after which fever, cough and sputum production make their appearance. The sputum may be rust colored or frankly bloody. Sharp pain with inspiration or cough may be experienced on the side of the infection. If X-ray shows an entire lobe to be involved, the diagnosis of *lobar pneumonia* is made. Patchy infiltration in one or more lobes is called *bronchopneumonia*. On examination the patient with either form usually appears quite ill. *Rales* (a crackling sound in the involved area due to fluid in alveolar sacs) are heard on auscultation, and percussion (thumping of the chest) may show dullness rather than the normal resonant sound of air-filled lung. If harsh breath sounds are also present, the lobe is said to be *consolidated*, meaning that air in the alveoli has been completely replaced by fluid. Patients with extensive pneumonia may show cyanosis and hypoxic blood gas values as a consequence of shunting.

Pneumonia can be caused by a variety of bacteria, the most common of which is the *pneumococcus*. A particularly virulent form of bacterial disease is that due to the *staphylococcus;* it is most often seen in adults as a complication of influenza or as a consequence of contaminated intravenous injection in users of illicit drugs. *Legionnaire's* disease is an epidemic form of pneumonia caused by a bacterium called *Legionella pneumophila*. Untreated it has a high mortality rate. Pneumonia is a common problem in *compromised hosts*. These are patients whose immune defense mechanisms are weakened by primary disease or by the addition of drugs given deliberately to suppress the immune response (for example, patients receiving transplanted organs). Under such circumstances it is common to have infection by unusual bacteria, fungi or viruses that do not cause pneumonia in normal persons. (Such infections are called *opportunistic* to emphasize that the microbial agents have taken advantage of a weakened host.)

Lung abscess is an infection which causes localized destruction of lung tissue with cavity formation. The usual clinical clue is expectoration of large amounts of foul-smelling, pus-filled sputum. X-ray confirms the diagnosis by showing a rounded cavity with an air-fluid level. Lung abscess is usually due to aspiration of food or liquids containing mouth bacteria and is most commonly seen in alcoholics, although any unconscious patient is at risk.[9]

Viral pneumonias tend to be less severe than bacterial forms of the disease and are usually self-limited. *Tuberculosis* and

---

[9] Provided the patient has teeth. The mouth organisms that ordinarily cause abscess are not present in edentulous patients.

fungal infections develop more gradually than bacterial and viral illnesses and are characterized by low-grade fever, cough, weight loss and night sweats. Sputum production and hemoptysis are common in advanced cases but may be absent with early disease. Occasionally tuberculosis manifests itself as a pleural effusion in the absence of other symptoms and without obvious infection of the lung tissue proper. *Bronchiectasis* refers to a structural abnormality (dilatation) of the bronchus that predisposes to infection. Symptoms include chronic cough, sputum production and recurrent episodes of pneumonia.

The bacterial and fungal pneumonias can almost always be treated by antibiotics. The number of effective antimicrobials is quite large and as a consequence cannot be described in detail here; suffice to say that the most difficult task in infectious disease is choosing the proper antibiotic. The choice will depend on the organism causing the pneumonia as identified by culture techniques as well as laboratory testing of the sensitivity of the cultured organism to various drugs. The problem of resistance to antibiotics is real and growing and combinations of agents are frequently required to control the infection. No specific treatment is available for viral pneumonias.

ASTHMA

Asthma is an extremely common pulmonary disease, affecting up to 2 percent of the population. It usually begins early in life. Basically the disease causes episodic shortness of breath lasting from minutes to hours. The mechanism is an abnormal contraction of the muscle layer in the pulmonary bronchi producing marked narrowing and impedance to air flow. It is usual for the lining membranes to become swollen (edematous) during an acute attack, and in addition there is overproduction of thick mucus which may plug smaller air channels. A large portion of cases are *allergic* in nature and are precipitated by dust, pollens, molds or other *allergens* (antigens which induce allergic responses). The ingestion of small amounts of aspirin induces severe symptoms in one subset of patients. *Intrinsic asthma* refers to a form of the disease that appears to be independent of allergy. Occasionally asthma is precipitated by *exercise*. A high percentage of patients outgrow their disease by young adulthood although some subjects have lifetime difficulty.

The hallmark of asthma is wheezing respiration which in severe forms is alarming to both patient and doctor. The respiratory rate is rapid and all muscles of respiration strain to enhance air flow. Cough and sputum production are common. With the stethoscope one hears musical wheezing sounds throughout the lungs, especially on expiration. Oxygen levels in the blood are depressed. An unrelenting attack lasting hours to days is called *status asthmaticus;* untreated it leads to death of the patient.

A variety of excellent drugs are available for treatment of asthma. Mild attacks can be aborted by *bronchodilators* taken orally or by inhalation. Ephedrine, isoproterenol, aminophylline and newer agents such as salbutamol and terbutaline are all effective. In patients with recurrent attacks the bronchodilators can also be taken prophylactically. *Cromolyn sodium* is a useful new drug for the prevention of allergic asthma (it is not helpful during the acute attack). After allergic exposure certain specialized cells in the lung (*mast cells*) release chemicals that cause bronchospasm and initiate the asthmatic episode. Cromolyn appears to block or inhibit the release of these mediators. In chronic severe asthma *steroid hormones* are frequently prescribed. The two most common are prednisone, given by mouth, and beclomethasone, given by inhalation. The advantage of the latter is that it has fewer side effects.

Acute, severe attacks of asthma are treated by the intravenous administration of *aminophylline* and *oxygen* given by a positive pressure respirator.

CHRONIC BRONCHITIS AND EMPHYSEMA

Chronic bronchitis and *emphysema* are the two major components of what most physicians call *chronic obstructive pulmonary disease,* a syndrome characterized by persistent cough, progressive shortness of breath (dyspnea), poor exercise tolerance, repeated infections and ultimately death from respiratory failure. Patients with *chronic bronchitis* have cough and sputum production as predominant symptoms while those with *emphysema* (which means abnormal distension of the alveoli) have dyspnea as the primary complaint. In practice both lesions are usually present together. The etiology of the illness varies but the outstanding factor in most cases is smoking. Exposure to dusts, noxious gases, industrial and atmospheric toxins also plays a role. One form of the disease is genetic and is associated with a *deficiency* of α_1-*antitrypsin*. α_1-Antitrypsin appears to inhibit enzymes in the lung capable of destroying alveolar walls. In the absence of the inhibitor, the enzyme activity can be expressed and alveolar damage results.

Diagnosis of chronic obstructive lung disease is made by pulmonary function studies showing obstructive changes and a characteristic X-ray picture. In advanced stages both hypoxia and carbon dioxide retention are severe.

The single most important therapeutic measure (in smokers) is the avoidance of cigarettes. Bronchodilators and, in severe cases, oxygen and steroids are the major forms of therapy. Removal of bronchial secretions by postural drainage techniques is also helpful. In postural drainage the body is placed head down in several defined positions to facilitate drainage from specific bronchial areas, following which sputum is coughed out.

PULMONARY EMBOLISM

The movement of a clot[10] from peripheral veins or the right side of the heart to the lungs may be of minor consequence if the embolus is small or cause death if it is large. The initial symptom is almost always the sudden onset of shortness of breath. Pleuritic chest pain and hemoptysis follow in some patients. A rapid heart rate is invariable and with large clots the blood pressure drops. Death is due to vascular collapse.

Any condition that leads to sluggish blood flow, abnormal coagulability of blood or damage to the lining of blood vessels predisposes to formation of venous clots which are potential emboli. Prolonged bed rest, congestive heart failure, varicose veins, fractures of the hip or legs, the postoperative state, pregnancy (particularly immediately after delivery) and certain forms of cancer are the major offenders. Pulmonary embolism also appears to occur with increased frequency in young women on birth control pills. The diagnosis is suspected whenever shortness of breath occurs against a background of one of the above conditions, particularly if signs of *thrombophlebitis* such as redness, tenderness and edema of a leg are present. (*Note:* The absence of these signs does not rule out embolism

---

[10] Almost all pulmonary embolism is due to blood clots but embolism with air and fat also occurs. The former occurs most often during too rapid ascent by underwater divers while the latter is a consequence of bony fractures causing release of the fatty bone marrow into the bloodstream.

since clot formation may be in the pelvic or abdominal cavities or in the heart chambers rather than in the legs.) Confirmation of embolization may be extremely difficult; lung scans, angiograms and measurements of the by-products of clot formation (*fibrin split products*) are usually required.

Treatment of pulmonary embolism initially involves intravenous administration of *heparin* (a powerful anticoagulant) to inhibit further clot formation. Subsequently the patient is switched to an *oral anticoagulant* which is continued for several months after the acute episode. Anticoagulants are themselves dangerous, and frequent measurement of clotting parameters such as the *prothrombin time* is required throughout therapy. Currently considerable research is being carried out on the possibility of dissolving fresh emboli by the enzymes *streptokinase* and *urokinase*. The results appear promising. Some patients with extensive venous disease of the legs have recurrent pulmonary emboli. In such patients it may be necessary to surgically *ligate the inferior vena cava* to prevent movement of clots from the extremities to the lungs.

CANCER OF THE LUNG

The incidence of cancer of the lung has increased so greatly that the term epidemic has been applied. It is the commonest form of malignancy in males and is also increasing in women. The major etiologic factor is cigarette smoking,[11] but atmospheric pollutants and occupational toxins such as chromates, arsenic, nickel, asbestos, beryllium and radioactive materials also play a role.

The major problem is that early diagnosis is extremely difficult. The initial symptom is often a minor nonproductive cough ("cigarette cough") and even if an X-ray is obtained, at this stage it may be normal. By the time major symptoms such as weight loss, hemoptysis or dyspnea appear, the lesion is usually inoperable.

Few cancers cause as many complications as those of the lung. Since they arise in the bronchus, *pneumonia* behind the obstructing lesion is extremely common (a high percentage of

---

[11] One recent estimate of death rates for lung cancer is 3.4 per 100,000 population in male nonsmokers, 59.3 per 100,000 when 10–20 cigarettes a day are smoked and 217.3 per 100,000 for 40 or more cigarettes daily.

patients consult the physician because of pneumonia and are then found to have cancer). The tumor may spread to involve the *recurrent laryngeal nerve* and paralyze the vocal cord with hoarseness as a result. *Obstruction of the vena cava* may cause localized swelling of the arms or face. Lung cancers *frequently make hormones* ordinarily produced by the pituitary, adrenal and parathyroid glands, thereby causing syndromes that mimic endocrine diseases such as Cushing's syndrome (overactivity of the adrenal gland) or hyperparathyroidism (with marked elevation of the plasma calcium). Enlargement of the breast (*gynecomastia*) is due to female hormone production. *Muscle weakness* to the point of paralysis and *cerebellar dysfunction* with loss of balance are other complications. *Horner's syndrome* is a peculiar constellation of findings including drooping of the eyelid and loss of sweating over the face on the side of the cancer; it is due to entrapment of sympathetic nerves in the neck by the tumor.

Definitive diagnosis requires biopsy of the lesion either by bronchoscopy or mediastinoscopy. If the lesion is localized, surgery is the first line of treatment with removal of a lobe or the whole lung on one side. Inoperable tumors are treated with X-ray and chemotherapeutic drugs. Overall the outlook is grim, 5-year survival being less than 50 percent even with operable solitary nodules and much less for more advanced disease. *The most important therapy is prevention, which means no smoking!*

DIFFUSE IDIOPATHIC INTERSTITIAL PULMONARY FIBROSIS

As noted before interstitial pulmonary fibrosis can occur in a variety of diseases. It can also develop without apparent cause in which case it is called the *Hamman-Rich syndrome*. Beginning in middle age, the symptoms are shortness of breath, particularly on exercise, and nonproductive cough. Late features include cyanosis, clubbing and eventually respiratory failure. A characteristic honeycombed appearance of the lung is seen on X-ray, but diagnosis requires lung biopsy. A trial of treatment with prednisone is usually indicated but response is varied.

OCCUPATIONAL LUNG DISEASE

A variety of inhaled materials cause lung disease. The most common end result is fibrosis and emphysema. Perhaps best known is *pneumoconiosis,* the "black lung" of coal workers, which is due to carbon dust inhalation. Exposure to silica dust causes *silicosis;* asbestos fibers, *asbestosis;* and cotton fibers, *byssinosis.* Pulmonary disease can also be caused by exposure to aluminum particles, tin oxide, barium sulfate, cobalt, tungsten, carbide, titanium and tantalum. While great strides have been made in prevention of environmental and occupational lung diseases, they still occur and additional safeguards are needed.

RESPIRATORY FAILURE

The end stage of pulmonary disease is respiratory failure. The condition is usually said to be present when the oxygen tension of arterial blood falls to 60 millimeters of mercury or less or when the carbon dioxide tension rises above 50 millimeters of mercury. When oxygen tension reaches 40 millimeters of mercury, headache, somnolence and clouding of consciousness occur. At lower levels convulsions, retinal hemorrhages and permanent brain damage are seen. In the late phases shock results. High carbon dioxide concentrations add to the symptoms and markedly elevate the cerebrospinal fluid pressure causing papilledema. Even in the absence of hypoxia, elevated pCO_2 can cause clouding of consciousness, slurred speech, restlessness and a flapping tremor.

Ordinarily respiratory failure develops gradually against a background of chronic pulmonary disease. Sudden worsening of a previously stable patient is usually due to infection (pneumonia or bronchitis). Respiratory failure can also occur in patients with normal lungs after prolonged vascular collapse. Severe trauma, burns and systemic infections are the most frequent causes. The condition is called *shock lung* or, more correctly, the *adult respiratory distress syndrome.* The lungs show interstitial and alveolar edema with patchy atelectasis, so that oxygenation of blood is impaired. In contrast to chronic respiratory failure, carbon dioxide tension in the blood is not elevated but low. The patients breathe rapidly and, for complicated reasons, are able to remove carbon dioxide from the blood but not exchange oxygen. The condition is extremely serious, and the prognosis is poor once the syndrome is fully developed.

VENTILATORY ASSISTANCE AND OXYGEN TOXICITY

When respiratory failure supervenes, oxygen therapy is absolutely required. With mild hypoxemia it can be administered by mask, but with severe failure artificial ventilators are almost always necessary. Called positive pressure respirators, the machines assist normal inspiration if the patient is able to breathe spontaneously; in apneic subjects the lungs are expanded automatically by intermittently forcing oxygen-containing air into the patient's trachea under pressure. Ventilators can be used with masks, but in comatose or apneic subjects an *endotracheal tube* or *tracheostomy* is usually required. Endotracheal tubes are directed into the trachea through the mouth while in tracheostomy a surgical incision is made in the throat for insertion of the airway.

It is not widely recognized outside of medical circles that oxygen is toxic when given in high concentrations. Ordinarily respiration is controlled by the level of carbon dioxide in the blood as mentioned earlier. Some patients with obstructive lung disease and very high pCO_2 levels no longer respond in the normal way to carbon dioxide and have their respiration stimulated by the low oxygen levels present in the blood. If such patients are given oxygen, respirations may slow or cease with loss of consciousness secondary to dramatic rises in CO_2 tension as the hypoxic stimulus is removed. A second major problem is that high concentrations of oxygen given for more than 2 days can *cause* the adult respiratory distress syndrome. Thus one has the paradoxical situation that the treatment of acute respiratory failure, oxygen, can itself produce or worsen the disease. The usual sequence is for a patient with shock lung to require increasingly higher concentrations of oxygen to treat hypoxemia until the point is reached where the oxygen itself induces further damage to the lung and death. For this reason physicians always administer the lowest possible concentration of oxygen sufficient to prevent dangerous hypoxemia. The message is that oxygen therapy is difficult and tricky.

8

Gastrointestinal Diseases

The gastrointestinal tract is a food-transporting conduit open at both ends to the atmosphere. While its winding canal passes through the body, in one sense it is extracorporeal (outside the body), being separated at all times from direct communication with the interior by the intestinal wall and its surrounding membranes. The intestinal wall is permeable, however, and as a consequence nutrients, water and other materials are normally readily absorbed; conversely, a variety of products are secreted or excreted from the body into the intestinal canal. Some of these materials aid the absorptive process while others are waste products. Beginning with the mouth the tract consists (in order) of the *pharynx, esophagus, stomach, small intestine, large intestine (colon), rectum* and *anus.* The small intestine has three divisions: *duodenum, jejunum* and *ileum.* These divisions, while continuous with one another, are anatomically and functionally distinct. The small intestine is the primary site of food absorption in the system. Fat, sugars, most vitamins, iron and calcium are absorbed in the proximal portion. Amino acids tend to be taken up in the middle segment (jejunum) while bile salts and vitamin B_{12} are transported through the ileum. Other substances are absorbed over the entire length of the small intestine. The large intestine is also divided into segments. The pocketlike beginning of the large intestine, located in the right lower quadrant of the abdomen, is called the *cecum;* it is the entry site of the ileum, the terminal portion of the small bowel. The *appendix* is a fingerlike extension of the cecum. The *ascending colon* rises perpendicularly from the cecum to the right upper quadrant of the abdomen where it makes a right-angle turn, becoming the *transverse colon*. In the left upper quadrant another 90-degree turn signals the beginning of the *descending colon*. The latter connects to the *sigmoid colon* (so named because it makes an S-shaped curve in the pelvis). The final portion of the colon is the *rectum,* a sort of storage chamber for formed stool that opens to the exterior through the *anus*. The primary function of the colon is absorption of fluid and electrolytes such that the liquid intestinal contents are transformed into solid stool. The colon is normally heavily populated with bacteria whose function is to break down excreted and nonabsorbed materials. *Bile* and *pancreatic secretions,* necessary for the absorptive processes, pass into the intestinal lumen through the *common bile duct* which enters in the duodenum. At varying intervals the intestine is demarcated by specialized muscular areas called *sphincters;* contraction of the sphincters occludes the lumen of the canal and blocks the passage of food or intestinal contents. The major sphincters are located at the lower end of the esophagus (*lower esophageal sphincter*), in the distal stomach immediately prior to its entry into the duodenum (the *pyloric sphincter*), between the ileum and the cecum (the *ileocecal valve*) and in the rectum (the *internal* and *external rectal sphincters*). The latter allow the individual to prevent defecation at unwanted times.[1]

After food is chewed and swallowed, it is propelled through the gastrointestinal tract by a series of wavelike contractions of the intestinal wall called *peristalsis*.[2] During passage the constituent carbohydrates, fat and protein are broken down by a series of *enzymes* released from the salivary glands, stomach and pancreas or contained in the intestinal wall. As part of the process large amounts of *hydrochloric acid* are produced by the stomach. Absorption of fat requires the presence of *bile*. A high percentage of ingested food is successfully absorbed, but some

---

[1] When bowel control is normal the individual is said to be *continent. Fecal incontinence* means that feces emerge involuntarily as soon as they reach the rectum, a common problem in stroke and injury to the spinal cord. *Urinary incontinence* refers to loss of bladder control.

[2] The audible gurgling noises in the abdomen experienced by everyone from time to time ("my stomach is growling") are due to peristaltic movements propelling gas and fluid through the intestine. The medical term for this phenomenon is so quaint as to be worth mentioning: *borborygmi* (bore-bore-ridge-me).

materials pass through the entire gastrointestinal tract un-changed. Fiber or roughage, currently a subject of great interest because of speculation that it decreases the incidence of cancer of the colon, is the classic example of unabsorbable ingested food.

Until recently the gastrointestinal tract was considered to be a simple organ system carrying out a single function, the diges-tion and absorption of food. Such a view has proven extremely naive since the stomach and intestine have now been shown to carry out a whole series of complex reactions including the secretion of hormones and production of antibodies. With its great length and multiple functions, the gastrointestinal system is susceptible to disease and malfunction at many points. While some of these disorders are trivial, a high percentage are symp-tomatically distressing or potentially life-threatening.

DIAGNOSTIC PROCEDURES

X-ray Examination. The foundation stone of diagnostic pro-cedures for gastrointestinal disease is X-ray examination. The only portion of the gut not susceptible to radiologic probing is the distal sigmoid colon and rectum. Plain films of the abdomen are helpful in the diagnosis of intestinal obstruction and perfo-ration of the intestinal tract, but usually *barium contrast studies* are required. The radiopaque barium clearly outlines the intes-tinal canal and allows identification of ulcers, constricting and obstructing lesions (such as cancer), abnormalities of the bowel wall and the presence of chronic inflammatory disease. Assess-ment of mechanical function is provided by patterns of move-ment of the barium through the tract. Contrast studies are of three types: *upper GI series,* which covers the esophagus, stom-ach and duodenum; *small bowel series,* which evaluates the jejunum and ileum; and *barium enema,* which visualizes the colon, cecum and ileocecal region. In the first two the barium is swallowed while in barium enema the contrast material is introduced through the rectum.[3] Examination is carried out

---

[3] For reasons that are not clear to me, it is widely believed that the barium enema is an uncomfortable or painful procedure. This is not true. It might be considered slightly undignified, but it is not a difficult experience apart from the fact that laxative purging is usually required ahead of time.

both by direct visualization with the fluoroscope and by taking permanent films.

Endoscopy. The term *endoscopy* refers to direct visual examination of the gastrointestinal tract using one of several types of instruments inserted through the mouth or rectum. The most frequent procedure is *sigmoidoscopy* by which the distal colon and rectum (that portion not seen by barium enema) is examined. It is indicated in every case of rectal bleeding. The sigmoidoscope is a simple tubular instrument with a powerful light source. More complex flexible fiberoptic instruments are required for examination of the esophagus, stomach, duodenum and the large bowel beyond the sigmoid colon. Examination of the large intestine is called *colonoscopy.* Utilizing fiberoptic instruments, lesions can be visualized directly and biopsies taken for tissue diagnosis. Endoscopy is particularly helpful in bleeding diseases of the intestinal tract and in the diagnosis of cancer.

Functional Examinations. A number of tests are available to evaluate gastrointestinal function but many are used for research purposes only. An exception is the study of *gastric* (pertaining to the stomach) *acid secretion.* This is done by placing a tube in the stomach and removing gastric contents in the basal state and after maximal stimulation of acid production by *histamine* or *pentagastrin,* two powerful inducers of acid release. If no acid is present after stimulation, the patient is said to have *achlorhydria,* a condition found in atrophy of the stomach lining (atrophic gastritis), pernicious anemia and some cases of cancer of the stomach. Excess acid secretion is seen in the *Zollinger-Ellison syndrome,* a severe form of ulcer disease associated with a tumor of the pancreas. The *D-xylose absorption test* is a measure of carbohydrate absorption and is carried out when a disease causing malabsorption is thought to be present. The *Schilling test* measures the absorption of radioactive vitamin B_{12} and, like the xylose test, is useful in demonstrating the presence of malabsorptive bowel disease. Measurement of the bicarbonate content of duodenal fluid after injection of the hormone *secretin* (the *secretin test*) is a way of assessing adequacy of pancreatic secretion into the intestine. Diarrhea and malabsorption may be caused by overgrowth of bacteria in the small intestine. *Aspiration of intestinal contents* (by suction through a tube placed in the small intestine) for quantitative culture of bacteria is sometimes done under these circumstances.

Stool Examination. A variety of tests are done on the stool. Perhaps the most important is the test for *occult blood* (amounts of blood too small to be visible to the eye). Occult blood is frequently the earliest sign of cancer of the colon. Culture of the stool for bacteria and examination for parasites is routine in diarrheal states. Microscopic examination for pus cells is important in diagnosis of inflammatory disease. Measurement of stool fat is done when malabsorption is suspected.

DISEASES OF THE ESOPHAGUS

Esophageal Reflux and Hiatal Hernia. The reflux (or regurgitation) of acid-containing gastric contents into the lower esophagus produces burning pain in the upper abdomen or beneath the sternum. It is prone to occur following large meals (*heartburn*) and is aggravated by bending over or lying down. Some patients with heartburn have a *hiatal hernia* demonstrated on X-ray. In this condition a portion of the stomach extends abnormally through the diaphragm into the chest cavity. Treatment of reflux involves ingestion of small meals, antacids to neutralize gastric acidity and elevation of the head of the bed at night. In the past hiatal hernias were routinely repaired surgically, but it is now thought that most do not require surgical intervention.

Diffuse Esophageal Spasm and Achalasia. Both these disorders are due to a disturbance of motor (*peristaltic*) function in the esophagus that interferes with the passage of food into the stomach. The symptoms are difficulty in swallowing and pain in the chest after eating. *Diffuse esophageal spasm* is a benign condition while *achalasia (cardiospasm)* is more serious. Barium swallow in esophageal spasm shows absence of peristalsis and bizarre contouring of the lower esophagus. In achalasia the distal ⅔ of the esophagus is markedly narrowed. The esophagus above the spastic (narrowed) section may be dilated, and in severe cases food regurgitates into the mouth on lying down. If this happens at night, aspiration into the lungs may occur. Some patients with esophageal spasm respond to treatment with *nitroglycerin*, but severe cases of spasm and most cases of achalasia require mechanical dilatation of the obstructed segment using balloon or mechanical dilators. In extreme cases *myotomy*, the surgical interruption of the esophageal muscle fibers by longitudinal incision, is required.

Cancer. Cancer of the esophagus is a terrible disease with a dreadful prognosis. The problem is that by the time symptoms are produced, the lesion is usually beyond cure. The primary symptom is difficulty in swallowing, with pain and hemorrhage occurring as late events. Every case of *dysphagia* (difficulty in swallowing) should be considered cancer of the esophagus until proven otherwise. As the disease progresses weight loss and malnutrition advance at rapid rates. Even with surgically approachable lesions, 5-year survival is only 5–7 percent. X-ray is sometimes palliative, shrinking the cancer and allowing the patient to eat for a while longer. Death is usually due to malnutrition, aspiration of esophageal contents into the lungs or hemorrhage.

DISEASES OF THE STOMACH AND DUODENUM

While the stomach and duodenum are anatomically distinct, functionally they operate as a unit and to a large extent are susceptible to the same types of disease. For this reason they will be considered together.

Peptic Ulcer. The most common of the serious diseases of stomach and duodenum is peptic ulcer. Most (about 80 percent) are located in the duodenum, but gastric ulceration also occurs alone or simultaneously with duodenal disease. Ulcers are irregular rounded defects or holes in the *mucosa* (lining surface) of the two organs. The mechanism of ulcer formation is still poorly understood, but increased gastric acid secretion is thought to be the major factor. The term *peptic* is derived from the fact that the erosion of the surface is considered to be at least partially the consequence of the action of a gastric enzyme called *pepsin* which is capable of digesting proteins and, presumably, protein-containing tissues. *Pepsin* is maximally active in strong acid environments. Thus it is thought that excess acid secretion predisposes to ulcer formation by enhancing pepsin activity. It is almost certain that primary changes in the *resis-*

tance of the mucosa to digestion also play a role since some persons without measurably abnormal acid secretion develop ulcers. Three major factors are considered important in determining susceptibility to ulcer disease: stress and anxiety, ingestion of certain drugs and heredity. In a high percentage of cases, an identifiable stressful situation precedes the onset of ulcer symptoms.[4] The only drug believed to be capable of causing ulcers in humans is aspirin, although some physicians feel that alcohol, caffeine, adrenal steroids and other anti-inflammatory agents should not be given to patients with ulcer disease because they influence ulcer formation in experimental animals. There is a strong association between smoking and ulcers; while smoking does not cause ulcers it is thought to impair their healing. Ulcer disease tends to run in families and 40–60 percent of patients have one or more close relatives similarly afflicted.

The cardinal symptom of ulcer is pain in the *epigastrium* (the upper central portion of the abdomen). Classically the pain develops several hours after a meal or during the night and is relieved by eating or taking antacids. It is usually described as burning or gnawing in nature but may be crampy or simply a vague discomfort. A significant minority of patients experience no pain (*silent ulcer*) and are identified only when they develop a complication of the disease. Occasionally persons with gastric ulcer have pain worsened by food intake. Diagnosis in suspected cases is made by upper GI series or endoscopy.

There are three major complications of ulcer disease. The first is *hemorrhage* due to erosion of blood vessels in the base of the ulcer. If the leakage of blood is small but persistent, the only sign may be the gradual development of anemia. On the other hand, if an artery is eroded the patient will vomit large amounts of blood and is at risk for exsanguination. Major hemorrhage is more common with gastric than duodenal ulcers and tends to occur in older patients. The second complication is *rupture* of the ulcer through the wall of the stomach or duodenum. If the rupture is into another organ (usually the pan-

---

[4] There probably is no such thing as an "ulcer personality" despite the common stereotype that the high-strung, hard-driving business executive is primarily at risk. Ulcer disease occurs in athletes, clerks, bus drivers and every other occupation (stress is no respecter of position). Women appear to have a much lower incidence of ulcer than men, at least before the menopause. It is postulated that female hormones somehow exert a protective effect.

creas) the term *penetration* is used while rupture into the peritoneal cavity is called *perforation*. The primary symptom of penetration is the development of back pain. Perforation is signaled by the sudden onset of agonizing abdominal pain followed by rigidity and tenderness of the abdominal wall. Shock may result. Diagnosis is confirmed by an upright film of the abdomen showing free air under the diaphragm (intestinal gas that has escaped through the perforation). The third complication is *obstruction* of the gastric outlet. The obstruction is due to swelling and scar formation at the site of the ulcer and manifests itself by the appearance of recurrent vomiting. By X-ray the stomach is dilated, and the barium meal is retained for long periods without passage into the duodenum.

The primary aim of treatment for ulcer is the neutralization of stomach acidity. In the past bland diets rich in milk were prescribed, given as frequent small feedings. Such therapy is now considered to be contraindicated since milk actually stimulates acid release. Ulcer patients should eat a regular diet supplemented with large amounts of antacids given 1 and 3 hours after the meal and before bedtime. Liquid antacids containing aluminum and magnesium hydroxides are favored over tablets. Bicarbonate of soda is not good therapy. Using antacids about 80 percent of ulcers will heal in 6 weeks. Drugs capable of blocking acid secretion are also useful. The *parietal cell* (which makes acid in the stomach) is stimulated by the *vagus nerve* (cholinergic stimulation) and by the hormones *histamine* and *gastrin.* Cholinergic effects can be blocked by drugs similar to *atropine* (anticholinergics) while histamine activity can be inhibited by *cimetidine,* a powerful new agent that works by interfering with the attachment of histamine to its receptor on the parietal cell. No inhibitor of gastrin is available. Cimetidine is currently widely used in the treatment of ulcer, occasionally as the sole therapy but more often in combination with antacids or anticholinergics.

Major bleeding from a peptic ulcer is a medical emergency. Fluids and blood are transfused rapidly to sustain the circulation, and gastric contents are aspirated by a large bore tube introduced into the stomach. Ice-cold saline solution is then perfused through the tube to stimulate contraction of the bleeding vessels. Iced saline *lavage* (washing) is repeated until bleeding slows after which endoscopy is undertaken to localize and identify the lesion. This is important since a number of diseases other than ulcer can cause gastrointestinal hemorrhage and may require different treatment. If endoscopy does not reveal the site of bleeding, angiography of the celiac vessels (which supply blood to the stomach and duodenum) is usually carried out. In the majority of cases bleeding can be controlled by aspiration and lavage, but persistent hemorrhage requires emergency surgery.

In addition to hemorrhage, surgery is indicated for perforated ulcers, gastric outlet obstruction and intractable ulcer symptomatology despite long-term aggressive treatment with antacids and drugs. The most popular surgical procedure for bleeding or intractable symptoms is removal of the *antrum* (lower third) of the stomach and severance of the vagal nerves (*vagotomy*). Antrectomy eliminates gastrin-producing cells while cutting the vagus nerve removes the cholinergic drive to acid secretion. Perforations are usually easily closed by direct suturing. If the patient has had long-standing disease, antrectomy and vagotomy may be done at the time of surgery for the perforation. Postsurgical complications include *recurrent ulcer, diarrhea, weight loss, vomiting* and the *dumping syndrome.* In the dumping syndrome, the patient feels lightheaded, dizzy, flushed and nauseated after a meal. The heart rate is fast and vomiting may occur. Symptoms are usually relieved by lying down for 30 minutes to an hour. It is thought that the problem is caused by rapid emptying of gastric contents into the small intestine as a consequence of removal of the distal stomach. Ingestion of small meals at frequent intervals may be required to prevent symptoms in severe cases.

Surgery is also indicated in the *Zollinger-Ellison syndrome,* an illness in which severe ulcer disease (with a high rate of complications) is coupled with diarrhea and malabsorption of foods. The problem is caused by a tumor of the pancreas that produces the hormone *gastrin* in large amounts, thus stimulating gastric acid overproduction. The diarrhea and malabsorption are thought to be due to inhibition of intestinal enzymes by the excess acid. Diagnosis is confirmed by finding high gastrin concentrations in the blood and elevated basal acid secretion in the stomach that responds only minimally to histamine stimulation (because it is already driven to maximal levels). The Zollinger-Ellison syndrome is part of a condition called *multiple endocrine adenomatosis, type 1* (see chapter 15) in which tumors may develop in the parathyroid, pituitary and adrenal glands as well as the pancreas. These tumors must be looked for in every case of the ZE syndrome. In contrast to the partial gastrectomy carried out with ordinary ulcer, the entire stomach must be removed in this condition.

Acute Erosive Gastritis. Acute erosive gastritis refers to diffuse superficial injury of the gastric mucosa with multiple bleeding points. It is a common cause of upper gastrointestinal hemorrhage. Severe gastritis is most commonly seen after acute alcoholic debauch but can also result from aspirin ingestion. It is a complication of burns, trauma, surgery, severe infection or other forms of major stress, particularly if shock has been present. The usual symptom is vomiting of blood. Differentiation from ulcer and other forms of acute hemorrhage in the upper gastrointestinal tract is based on endoscopic examination showing the characteristic picture of gastritis and the absence of ulcer or other lesions. Treatment is similar to that described for bleeding from peptic ulcer except that the hormone *vasopressin,* which causes constriction of blood vessels, is sometimes given intravenously in addition. Painful but nonbleeding gastritis is treated with antacids.

Cancer. The incidence of cancer of the stomach has decreased dramatically over the last few years. Diagnosis is tricky because the cancer may initially appear to be a simple gastric ulcer. Differentiation usually requires biopsy which should be done in any ulcer of the stomach that has not healed after 6 weeks of aggressive antacid therapy. Biopsy is obtained via endoscopy. The usual type of tumor is an adenocarcinoma,[5] but lymphomas and other forms of neoplasm may also be seen. Treatment is surgical removal of the stomach. Unfortunately the cancer spreads to distant sites early and the prognosis is poor. Tumors of the duodenum are rare but when they occur tend to cause jaundice by blocking the common bile duct.

DISEASES OF THE SMALL BOWEL

Malabsorption Syndromes. As noted before the small intestine is the site of absorption of most foodstuffs. As a conse-

[5] Neoplasms are classified as to cell of origin and type. *Carcinoma* means a malignant tumor arising from epithelial cells; *adenocarcinoma* means that the tumor forms glands.

quence chronic disease of the small bowel tends to produce multiple nutritional deficiencies. The usual symptoms are weight loss, abdominal bloating and the development of bulky, oily stools which float in the toilet bowl. Abnormal feces are due to excessive fat content caused by failure of fat absorption (*steatorrhea*). Increased stool frequency may or may not be present. Anemia is common because of iron, vitamin B_{12} and folic acid deficiencies. Low serum calcium, bone pain and pathologic fractures[6] occur because vitamin D cannot be absorbed. A bleeding tendency with easy bruising of the skin results from defective clotting mechanisms secondary to shortages of vitamin K in the body. Edema may be present as a consequence of protein wastage and a low serum albumin.

Malabsorption can be produced by one of three major mechanisms. First, there may be a *deficiency of pancreatic enzymes* necessary for digestion of food. The usual causes are primary diseases of the pancreas such as chronic pancreatitis, cancer of the pancreas or cystic fibrosis. Second, absorption may be blocked by a *deficiency of bile acids* which are necessary for solubilization and transport of many nutrients. Bile acid deficiency can be due to blockade of the bile duct (by gallstones or cancer) or increased destruction of bile acids by bacterial overgrowth in the small intestine. Third, there may be *primary disease of the small intestine.* The abnormality may be in the intestinal wall or the lymph drainage system through which nutrients pass after absorption. One of the most interesting of the primary intestinal disorders is *nontropical sprue.* The disease is due to a toxic effect of *gluten* (a protein constituent of wheat) on the intestinal mucosa. Normally the mucosal surface is completely covered with myriads of microscopic, fingerlike projections called *villi.* These projections extend into the intestinal lumen and provide a tremendous increase in surface area for absorption of food as compared to what would be available with a flat surface. In sprue the villi become flattened out with damage to the absorptive enzymes and consequent malabsorption. The diagnosis is confirmed by biopsy of the small intestine showing the mucosal changes just described and by improve-

[6] *Pathologic fracture* refers to bone injury in the absence of major trauma. With vitamin D deficiency, plasma calcium and phosphorus levels are low resulting in demineralization of bone (*osteomalacia*). This demineralization weakens bone structure and predisposes to fracture with minor stresses.

ment of symptoms on a gluten-free diet.[7] Malabsorption due to lymphatic obstruction is probably most often due to *intestinal lymphoma*, a form of malignancy involving the intestinal lymph nodes. A second cause of lymphatic obstruction is *Whipple's disease*, a rare disorder in which malabsorption and diarrhea are associated with arthritis, fever, increased skin pigmentation and enlargement of lymph nodes throughout the body. The disease appears to be due to bacteria in the intestinal wall (type uncertain) and responds to antibiotics.

Regional Enteritis (Crohn's Disease). Regional enteritis is one of two devastating intestinal illnesses commonly called *inflammatory bowel disease*. It involves both the small intestine and the colon. *Ulcerative colitis*, the second of the two diseases, usually does not affect the small bowel. The cause of regional enteritis is unknown. It is a disease of children and young adults. The primary symptom is *cramping abdominal pain*, especially in the right lower quadrant of the abdomen. *Diarrhea* is almost always present. *Nausea, vomiting, low-grade fever* and *weight loss* are common. Late complications include *perforation of the bowel, intestinal obstruction* and *fistula formation*.[8] The fistulas often open to the outside of the body (most often near the rectum) and drain pus or fecal material. The disease is associated with many *extra-intestinal manifestations* including arthritis of peripheral joints or spine, inflammation of the iris in the eyes, clubbing of the fingers, gallbladder and kidney stones. Diagnosis is made by a characteristic X-ray picture on small bowel series or barium enema.

Treatment is usually carried out with *prednisone*, a synthetic adrenal steroid, often in combination with *sulfasalazine*, a salicylate and sulfa-containing compound. With acute attacks the patient is hospitalized and taken off oral food to provide bowel rest. Nutrition is maintained by total parenteral alimentation (see chapter 2). Surgery is often required to remove obstructing segments of diseased bowel, resect fistulas, drain abscesses or

---

[7] Recently some forms of *nontropical sprue* have been reported in the United States that are apparently not due to gluten sensitivity. *Tropical sprue* is a form of malabsorption occurring in tropical areas of the world, sometimes in epidemic form. The syndrome disappears on moving to temperate zones and in many cases reverses spontaneously even in those who do not change environments. The cause is not known.

[8] *Fistulas* are abnormal channels running between organs or other body structures that are not ordinarily connected. In this case the fistula extends from the inflamed intestine to the exterior of the body.

repair perforations. Because of the chronic nature of the disease and the severe physical and psychological problems it generates, dealing with regional enteritis is one of the most difficult tasks in medicine.

Vascular Disease of the Small Bowel. Atherosclerosis may affect the blood vessels supplying the small intestine as it does other parts of the body. Abdominal pain occurring 15–30 minutes after eating (*abdominal angina*) is the primary symptom. During digestion the intestine needs increased blood flow but cannot receive it due to narrowed vessels; the result is ischemia and pain. Sudden worsening of the pain followed by loss of bowel sounds and the appearance of shock suggests the possibility of infarction of the bowel. The only treatment for acute infarction is surgical resection of the dead segment. Occasionally bypass grafts are successful in restoring the blood supply in patients with chronic disease who have not yet infarcted.

Tumors. Malignant tumors of the small intestine are relatively rare. They cause weight loss, bleeding and mechanical intestinal obstruction. An interesting small bowel neoplasm is the *carcinoid tumor.* The tumor commonly spreads to the liver where it produces attacks of flushing of the skin over the upper chest and head. Vivid color changes ranging from red to purple are followed by pallor during the acute attack. Episodes are often associated with wheezing respiration and explosive diarrhea. The clinical picture is due to chemicals released into the bloodstream by the tumor.

DISEASES OF THE COLON

Cancer of the Colon. Cancer of the colon is a common disease and the second leading cause of death from malignancy in the United States. Patients with *polyps of the colon* [9] are at particularly high risk for development of cancer. Colonic cancers may be located at any site in the colon from cecum to rectum. The symptoms are usually vague and nonspecific at first. The initial sign may be *unexplained weight loss* or discovery of an *anemia*

---

[9] *Polyps* are fleshy projections of the mucosal lining that extend into the lumen of the colon. They may be flat or on a stalk and range in size from 1–10 centimeters in diameter. Their incidence in the general population has been estimated at 5–15 percent.

on routine laboratory examination. The anemia is due to *blood loss in the stool,* an almost invariable accompaniment of colonic cancer. The bleeding is often occult with lesions in the right (ascending) colon but may be bright red with left-sided tumors. A *change in bowel habits* may occur; constipation, constipation alternating with diarrhea and diminution in the size of the stool are common patterns. *Pain* in the abdomen is rare in rectal or distal sigmoid lesions but may be present in other locations. Workup for carcinoma of the colon is indicated whenever any of the above signs appear. Rectal carcinomas can usually be identified by digital examination through the anus, but lesions higher up require sigmoidoscopy, barium enema or colonoscopy.

Treatment of localized lesions is surgical resection. Usually about half the colon is removed. If rectal carcinoma is present a permanent colostomy is required for bowel evacuation after surgery.[10] With early diagnosis (localized disease) the chance of surgical cure is excellent. Unfortunately no good treatment is available when the tumor metastasizes to liver and other sites. There is great interest currently in screening techniques that might enhance early diagnosis. The best procedure would probably be to test for occult blood in the stool at regular intervals in all subjects over 40. Commercially prepared home testing kits are currently undergoing trial. *Carcinoembryonic antigen* (CEA), an antigen in blood originally thought to be diagnostic for the disease, is now known to occur in conditions other than cancer of the colon and is therefore not a good screening test. However, its continued presence after surgery (or its return after a period of normalization) is probably a good indication of metastatic spread of the tumor.

Ulcerative Colitis. Ulcerative colitis is an ulcerating disease of the mucosa and submucosal tissues of the colon. The major symptoms are *bloody diarrhea, weight loss, fever* and *abdominal pain.* The diarrhea can be mild or very severe. An extreme exacerbation of the illness, fatal in a significant proportion of

---

[10] *Colostomy* refers to implantation of the remaining colon through an opening in the abdominal wall. Understandably patients dread this. However, modern techniques have tremendously increased the acceptability of the procedure. Many patients are able to "train" themselves such that extrusion of feces occurs only once or twice a day at predictable intervals, allowing them to dispense with colostomy bags during most of the day. One would never *choose* to have a colostomy, but it is possible to live a normal life despite its presence.

cases, is called *toxic megacolon.* The patient has extremely high fever and shows signs of dehydration. The heart rate is rapid and the abdomen is tender and distended. The colon is markedly dilated and filled with air (hence, *mega*colon—giant colon). Without therapy death occurs due to perforation of the bowel, peritonitis and bacterial infection of the bloodstream.

Like regional enteritis, ulcerative colitis is associated with a host of extra-intestinal complications. *Anemia, fistula formation* and *arthritis* of the spine and other joints are frequent. *Liver disease* resembling hepatitis or even cirrhosis is not uncommon. Inflammation of the internal tissues of the eye (*uveitis*) may be present in up to 10 percent of patients. Ulcerative colitis (in contrast to Crohn's disease) also predisposes to development of *cancer of the colon;* in long-standing disease up to 20 percent of patients develop malignant degeneration. Why ulcerative colitis should be premalignant is not known. Diagnosis of malignancy is extremely difficult because the leading signs of cancer of the large bowel, weight loss and blood in the stool, are seen in ulcerative colitis itself.

Ulcerative colitis should be suspected whenever chronic bloody diarrhea develops in a young person. Sigmoidoscopy shows a characteristic appearance of the mucosa, and barium enema ordinarily readily confirms the diagnosis. Initially bacterial dysenteries, amebiasis and Crohn's disease have to be considered as alternative diagnostic possibilities, but differentiation is usually possible.

The primary modes of treatment are *prednisone* and *sulfasalazine* together with bowel rest and intravenous alimentation during acute exacerbations. At times an immunosuppressive agent, *azathioprine,* is added to the treatment regimen.[11] Surgical removal of the colon (*colectomy*) is required for toxic megacolon, perforation or severe hemorrhage. Occasionally the physician may decide that the colon should be removed because the patient is deteriorating on medical management. Whether total colectomy should be done as prophylaxis for cancer remains an unsettled issue.

Diverticulosis and Diverticulitis. Diverticula are saclike out-

---

[11] The cause of ulcerative colitis and regional enteritis is unknown, but there is some evidence suggesting that an immune component is operative; i.e., that the disease is due to antibodies directed against the patient's own tissues. Azathioprine and prednisone suppress the immune response.

pouchings of the wall of the colon containing a lumen that opens into the colonic canal. If the diverticula are asymptomatic the patient is said to have *diverticulosis*. With inflammation the term *diverticulitis* is used. Inflammation probably begins in a given diverticulum because undigested food residues and bacteria become trapped in the sac, distending the wall and allowing invasion by the bacteria. Symptoms are *lower abdominal pain,* usually on the left, *abdominal tenderness, fever* and *constipation.* The pain is often made worse by defecation. *Perforation* with peritonitis or abscess formation is a serious complication. Diagnosis is made by barium enema, but this should not be done in the acute phase of diverticulitis for fear of inducing perforation.

Treatment of diverticulitis consists of antibiotics in the acute phase. Surgery is ordinarily indicated only to drain abscesses or remove an obstructing inflammatory mass although resection is sometimes recommended with repetitive episodes in the same involved segment. In the nonactive phases it is now thought helpful to increase the fiber content of the diet.[12] This can be done simply by eating bran cereals or using bulk laxatives.

Irritable Colon (Spastic Colon). Irritable colon, an extremely common syndrome, is characterized by *lower abdominal pain* which is relieved by defecation, *alternating periods of constipation* and *diarrhea* and *abnormal stool characteristics.* Usually during acute episodes the feces is of small caliber and often very firm or hard. Pelletlike stools are also seen; less commonly a pasty consistency is present. At times the stool is covered with mucus. Other symptoms include frequent headaches, abdominal bloating and excessive flatulence (passage of intestinal gas through the rectum). The illness is most common in women during young adult life to middle age. It is thought by most investigators to be due to anxiety neurosis: the symptoms are psychosomatic. Examination shows no signs of serious organic disease although excess mucus formation and spasm of the colon are seen on sigmoidoscopy during acute attacks. Spasm may also be seen on barium enema. No specific treatment is available, but most patients respond to reassurance after

[12] In the past patients with diverticulosis were treated with low-residue diets. The history of medicine is replete with examples of initial therapy that subsequently proved incorrect. The wise physician considers all therapies tentative and subject to change as new research provides better information.

workup has shown the absence of cancer or other serious disease. Tranquilizers, antispasmodic drugs and bulk laxatives are often helpful in relieving symptoms.

Vascular Disease of the Colon (Ischemic Colitis). Atherosclerosis may affect the blood vessels supplying the colon exactly as described for the small intestine. It is ordinarily a disease of older persons. The usual symptoms are abdominal pain and rectal bleeding. Partial occlusions may produce only minor complaints, but complete obstruction of a major vessel is not infrequent leading to a fulminant picture of pain, explosive hemorrhagic diarrhea, shock and death. Infarction of the colon can also occur in the absence of complete obstruction if shock or dehydration is present. Arteriography is required for diagnosis. (Barium enema should not be done because of the possibility of perforating the ischemic area.) With infarction the only hope for survival is surgical resection of the involved area. Overall, prognosis is poor in the fulminant forms of the illness.

Acute Inflammatory Disease of the Colon. Acute inflammation of the colon produces diarrhea with or without abdominal pain. The usual causes are bacteria, parasites, viruses and drugs. Fever is common with bacterial diarrheas such as those produced by *Shigella* and *Salmonella* (bacillary dysentery), and examination of the stool usually shows the presence of pus. A similar picture may be produced by *amebic dysentery* but not by the *viruses* that cause most short-term diarrhea. *Parasitic worms* are less commonly a cause of diarrhea than ameba. In recent years it has been recognized that severe inflammatory disease of the colon can be produced by *antibiotics*. Clindamycin and lincomycin are the most common offenders, but ampicillin and tetracycline can also serve to produce the illness. Symptoms may vary from mild diarrhea to *pseudomembranous colitis*, a syndrome characterized by high fever, abdominal pain and bloody diarrhea that must be differentiated from ulcerative colitis.

Since diarrhea with or without bleeding can be produced by many illnesses, the appearance of these symptoms requires multiple approaches to reach the correct diagnosis. Microscopic examination of the stool, culture and sigmoidoscopy are the first lines of attack when acute inflammation is suspected, but ultimately barium enema and other tests are required since the chronic inflammatory syndromes and vascular disease may mimic acute inflammatory illnesses.

Hemorrhoids. Hemorrhoids are dilated veins around the anus. They may be either *internal* or *external.* The cause is not known. Since hemorrhoids often accompany pregnancy and cirrhosis of the liver (where pressure in the abdominal portal vein is elevated), the major theory is that they are a type of varicose vein, produced by a backing up of blood secondary to increased pressure in the abdomen from any cause (including straining at stool). The usual symptoms are pain and rectal bleeding. The latter may be severe enough to produce severe anemia. A sudden increase in pain accompanied by a bluish swelling is due to *thrombosis* of the hemorrhoid. Symptoms can often be controlled by sitting in a warm tub of water, using stool softeners or bulk laxatives (to minimize straining) and application of ointments or suppositories containing local anesthetics and astringents. Bed rest for a day or two will often abort an acute attack. Severe disease requires surgical excision of the hemorrhoidal tissue.[13]

Appendicitis. The appendix is a fingerlike projection of the cecum whose function is uncertain. It appears to be peculiarly susceptible to inflammation, probably because obstruction of the lumen with fecal material is frequent, leading to development of infection behind the block (although many appendices show no obstruction when examined at surgery). The symptoms are *abdominal pain,* usually located in the right lower quadrant of the abdomen, *nausea, vomiting* and *abdominal tenderness. Perforation* of the appendix may cause generalized peritonitis with abdominal distension and rigidity or, more commonly, may lead to abscess formation in the area of rupture. Signs of abscess include fever and a palpable mass in the lower abdomen. Appendicitis, although usually a disease of the young, may occur in the elderly. Because pain and tenderness are less apparent in older persons, perforation often occurs before the patient realizes a serious illness is present.

No specific laboratory test is available to confirm the diagnosis. If the clinical picture is suspicious, operation is required.[14]

[13] Many other forms of treatment are in use, including injection of a sclerosing solution to induce clot formation, freezing with liquid nitrogen and ligation of the hemorrhoids with a rubber band (!).

[14] The term *exploratory laparotomy* is used when the abdomen is entered for diagnostic purposes.

INTESTINAL OBSTRUCTION

Intestinal obstruction refers to impairment of the progression of intestinal contents through the bowel canal. Obstruction may be *mechanical* or *adynamic.* The former refers to physical blockade of the lumen. The usual causes are *postsurgical adhesions, cancer* and a twisting of the bowel which is called *volvulus.* The obstruction may be in the small intestine or the colon. The symptoms are cramping abdominal pain, vomiting, failure to pass stool and abdominal distension. With small bowel obstruction the onset is more acute and the pain sequences more frequent than when obstruction is in the colon. Abdominal distension and a fecal appearance (and smell) of the vomitus usually means colonic obstruction. *Adynamic obstruction (paralytic ileus)* occurs in a variety of clinical conditions. It refers to a general paralysis of the bowel wall with dilatation of the lumen and failure of movement of intestinal contents as a consequence. The condition is extremely common after abdominal surgery, with peritonitis, as a result of vascular occlusion and ischemia of the bowel and with disturbances of blood chemistry such as a deficiency of potassium.

Diagnosis of intestinal obstruction is made on the basis of the clinical picture and characteristic X-ray findings on plain films of the abdomen. If mechanical obstruction is present, barium studies will localize the lesion. Paralytic ileus is treated by removal of intestinal fluids and gas by suction through a gastric or small-bowel tube until the primary disease can be treated. Mechanical obstruction requires surgery to relieve the physical blockade.

9

Diseases of the
Gallbladder and Pancreas

The gallbladder and pancreas are intimately involved in the digestion and absorption of food; in this sense they can be considered appendages of the gastrointestinal tract. The *gallbladder* is part of the *biliary tract*, the bile delivery system of the body. The system originates in the liver with a branching network of small bile ducts called *bile canaliculi*. The architecture of the liver places these ducts in juxtaposition to the regularly arranged cords of primary liver cells (*hepatocytes*) that carry out the multiple biochemical functions of that organ. Bile is formed by transfer of various materials from the hepatocytes into the bile canaliculi. The latter merge into increasingly larger vessels which finally leave the liver as the single major *bile duct*. The gallbladder is located just beneath the liver and is connected to the bile duct by the *cystic duct*. Basically the arrangement is like a "Y," the cystic duct forming one upper arm and the bile duct the other. The stem of the Y is called the *common bile duct;* it empties into the duodenum. A sphincter guards the opening of the common bile duct into the intestine. If the sphincter is open bile flows directly from liver to intestinal canal. If it is closed bile backs up through the cystic duct into the gallbladder which can be considered simply as a storage reservoir (it normally holds 30–50 milliliters of bile). Following a meal, when bile is needed for absorption, the sphincter opens, the gallbladder contracts and bile flows into the small intestine.

Bile is a water solution of *bile acids* (breakdown products of cholesterol), *phospholipids* (phosphorus-containing fat molecules), *cholesterol, salts* (sodium chloride and sodium bicarbonate) and *bilirubin* (the breakdown product of hemoglobin). In addition a variety of other organic materials (including *drugs* and *hormones*) pass into the bile for excretion into the intestine. Fundamentally bile has two roles: enhancing absorption of foods and excretion of waste products. The absorptive function is mediated by the bile acids. Fat is not soluble in water and therefore cannot be transported through the intestinal wall; it can be made soluble by the bile acids which act as intestinal detergents.[1]

The *pancreas* is situated in the posterior abdomen with its head located adjacent to the duodenum and its tail extending beneath the stomach to reach the spleen in the left upper quadrant of the abdominal cavity. It is a complex organ that has two distinctive functions: *exocrine* and *endocrine. Exocrine* activity refers to the synthesis and release of enzymes which digest food in the intestine. These enzymes pass through the *pancreatic duct* which ordinarily empties into the common bile duct but may occasionally enter the intestine directly. The primary enzymes are *amylase* (digestion of starches), *lipase* (digestion of fats) and *proteases* (digestion of proteins).[2] The proteases are secreted as inactive precursor molecules which become activated by an intestinal enzyme called enterokinase. *Endocrine function* refers to the secretion of hormones into the bloodstream for regulation of body fuel and energy metabolism at other tissue sites. Pancreatic hormones are responsible for storage of food energy following absorption of a meal and mobilization of energy stores between meals or during a fast. The

[1] Bile acids (like other detergents) have the peculiar chemical property that one end of the molecule is soluble in water (it is *hydrophilic*) while the other end is soluble in fat but not water (it is *hydrophobic*). In the intestine the fat-soluble portion of the bile acid is inserted into (between) fatty-acid molecules derived from dietary fat leaving the water-soluble portion of the molecule extending from the surface of the bile acid-fatty acid complex. In this way a small water-soluble particle (called a *micelle*) is formed allowing intestinal transport to take place. In the absence of bile acids, fat absorption does not occur and steatorrhea results (see chapter 8).

[2] Pancreatic juice contains a variety of other enzymes which break down nucleic acids and minor food components, but clinically these are of lesser importance.

hormones are manufactured in specialized areas of the pancreas called the *islets of Langerhans*. The two major hormones are *insulin* and *glucagon*. *Insulin* is the primary hormone of *anabolism* (energy storage); it lowers the blood sugar and promotes the formation of glycogen (the storage form of glucose in liver and muscle), fat and protein. *Glucagon* is the primary hormone of *catabolism* (energy breakdown); it raises the blood sugar directly by promoting breakdown of stored glycogen and indirectly by mobilizing amino acids from protein stores for conversion to glucose in the liver. A third hormone, *somatostatin*, is also made in the islets. Its function appears to be modulation (inhibition) of insulin and glucagon release, but there is great interest in the possibility that it may also directly diminish appetite and food absorption.[3]

DIAGNOSTIC PROCEDURES

A number of the diagnostic procedures previously described for other organ systems are applicable in the diagnosis of diseases of the biliary tract and pancreas. These include plain X-ray films of the abdomen, upper GI series, sonography and CAT scanning of the abdominal cavity. Techniques unique to the evaluation of the gallbladder, bile ducts and pancreas are *cholecystography, cholangiography, endoscopic retrograde cholangiopancreatography (ERCP)* and certain *assay procedures for enzymes and hormones.*

Cholecystography and Cholangiography. These radiographic procedures are used for the diagnosis of gallstones and biliary tract obstruction. The most common test is the oral *cholecystogram*. The technique is quite simple. A radiopaque dye is administered in tablet form the evening before the test, and the next day X-rays of the gallbladder are obtained. The test may show a normal gallbladder, gallstones in a functioning gallbladder or a nonfunctioning (nonvisualized) organ. Often a fatty meal is administered at the time films are made to stimulate gallbladder contraction and thus better visualize small stones. The oral cholecystogram does not allow good visualization of

[3] Should this prove to be true, it is conceivable that somatostatin deficiency might play a role in the genesis of obesity. While studies examining this possibility are in progress, for the present such a role for the hormone remains speculative.

the hepatic bile ducts and cannot be done in patients who do not absorb the dye-containing tablets by mouth. In these circumstances *intravenous cholangiography* is carried out with the dye being given by vein. Occasionally it is important to determine whether obstruction to bile flow is inside or outside the liver in a patient whose gallbladder fails to visualize by either oral or intravenous tests. This is done by *percutaneous transhepatic cholangiography,* a technique in which a needle is introduced into the liver through the skin in an attempt to locate a dilated bile duct into which dye can be injected directly into the biliary tree. Failure to find a dilated bile duct implies that jaundice is due to primary disease of the hepatocytes and not to obstruction of the bile ducts.

Endoscopic Retrograde Cholangiopancreatography. In this relatively new technique, an endoscope is passed into the duodenum and a small tube is introduced into the opening of the common bile duct. Injection of contrast dye causes retrograde filling of the pancreatic and biliary duct systems. The technique is particularly useful in the diagnosis of gallstones, benign strictures and obstructing tumors of the biliary tree. It may also be helpful in identifying cancer of the pancreas.

Enzyme Assays. The plasma concentration of the enzyme called *alkaline phosphatase* is elevated in obstructive disease of the biliary tract whether the obstruction is in the bile duct proper or in intrahepatic bile canaliculi.[4] *Serum glutamic oxaloacetic transaminase* (SGOT) and *lactic dehydrogenase,* enzymes from the liver, may also be increased in common duct obstruction. *Amylase* and *lipase* levels in the blood are always measured when pancreatitis is suspected. Elevations strongly suggest presence of that disease.

Hormone Assays. The pancreas is frequently a site of tumor development, and if the site of origin is the islets of Langerhans, abnormal hormone production often results. Diagnosis in suspected cases can be confirmed by assay for hormones in plasma. Most commonly produced are *gastrin, insulin, glucagon, somatostatin* and *vasoactive intestinal polypeptide.* The clinical syndromes produced by these tumors are described below.

---

[4] Alkaline phosphatase is made in bone as well as in bile ducts. The enzyme is, therefore, elevated in some forms of bone disease, occasionally requiring differentiation of the hepatic and bone forms.

DISEASE OF THE GALLBLADDER AND BILIARY TRACT

GALLSTONES (CHOLELITHIASIS)

Gallstones are a common medical problem. Ten percent of men and twenty percent of women between the ages of 55 and 65 have the disease.[5] They may occur spontaneously or develop in association with other illnesses. Obesity, cirrhosis of the liver, regional ileitis, diabetes mellitus, hemolytic anemias and drugs which lower plasma cholesterol are considered to predispose to their development. The most common type of stone consists primarily of cholesterol crystals (*cholesterol stones*), but up to a fourth are made up predominantly of bilirubin and its derivatives (*pigment stones*). The mechanisms whereby stones form are not known with precision, but it is accepted that the final event is precipitation of the formative crystals (cholesterol or bilirubin) either because the bile has become supersaturated or because its solubility characteristics have been altered such that normal levels of cholesterol or bilirubin cannot be maintained in solution.

Gallstones may be totally *silent* (producing no symptoms), cause *painless jaundice* (when a stone becomes impacted in the bile duct thereby obstructing bile flow and allowing bilirubin to accumulate in the blood) or result in the syndrome of *acute cholecystitis* (when the cystic duct is obstructed by a stone).

ACUTE CHOLECYSTITIS

The preeminent symptom of acute cholecystitis is *biliary colic*, severe right upper quadrant abdominal pain that often radiates to the top of the right shoulder or beneath the right shoulder blade. The pain is usually steady but may be intermittent or even crampy. *Nausea* and *vomiting* are essentially always present and with severe disease *fever* and *chills* may be noted. Occasionally the disorder manifests itself by much milder symptoms such as simple epigastric discomfort relieved by vomiting. On physical examination there is *tenderness* to

---

[5] Women of the Pima Indian tribe of Arizona have the world's highest incidence of gallstones. Above the age of 25, 70 percent of the female population is afflicted. The Pimas also have an incredibly high prevalence of diabetes mellitus.

palpation in the right upper quadrant of the abdomen, and occasionally the distended gallbladder can be felt through the abdominal wall. The patient may be mildly *jaundiced*. Laboratory examination shows an elevated white blood cell count, usually mild to moderate increase in the plasma bilirubin concentration and abnormal liver function tests, particularly elevation of liver enzymes in the blood. Diagnosis is confirmed by demonstration of gallstones by oral cholecystography or intravenous cholangiography.

Most attacks of acute cholecystitis end spontaneously. As a consequence conservative treatment is indicated initially: analgesics, intravenous fluids and occasionally antibiotics. Progression of toxicity with worsening fever, jaundice and pain requires surgical intervention in about a fourth of the cases to avoid abscess formation or perforation of the gallbladder with severe peritonitis. In general, however, the surgeon prefers to operate when the patient has recovered from the acute episode if this is at all possible.

Removal of the gallbladder (*cholecystectomy*) probably should be undertaken in any patient with proven gallstones who has ever had an attack of biliary colic or painless jaundice.[6] Most physicians do not believe that asymptomatic stones are an indication for surgery, although there is wide agreement that diabetic patients should be operated on prophylactically because they tolerate acute cholecystitis extremely poorly. In an acutely ill patient with impending rupture of the gallbladder, the surgeon may elect to simply drain the gallbladder (*cholecystostomy*), a much shorter operation than removal, and do definitive surgery electively at a later date. Complications of gallbladder surgery are relatively few; the most common is postoperative *stricture* (scarring) of the bile duct causing obstructive jaundice. Fistula formation may also result. Repair of bile duct damage is possible, but the surgery is difficult.

In recent years it has been demonstrated that cholesterol gallstones can be dissolved in some patients by the long-term oral

---

[6] Removal of the gallbladder, like removal of the appendix, appears to have no deleterious side effects. Occasionally patients continue to have the same symptoms or develop new complaints postoperatively (*postcholecystectomy syndrome*). These are not thought to be due to removal of the gallbladder. In most cases the explanation is that gallstones, though present, were not the cause of the symptoms experienced by the patient before surgery. In a few patients the symptoms are due to postsurgical stricture of the bile duct.

administration of a bile acid called *chenodeoxycholic acid,* provided that gallbladder function is normal. Whether this form of treatment will prove to be of widespread benefit is not yet clear. My own prejudice is that it will not.

OTHER DISEASES

The biliary tract is subject to diseases other than gallstones and cholecystitis, but they are extremely rare. *Cancer of the gallbladder and bile ducts* occurs in elderly patients. The usual symptoms are weight loss, jaundice and right upper quadrant pain with or without a palpable mass. Occasionally the gallbladder is the site of infection with *Salmonella typhosa,* the organism that causes typhoid fever. Such patients are usually asymptomatic but are dangerous as carriers of the disease, contaminating food and water by bacteria passing into the stool via the bile.[7] *Tuberculosis, syphilis* and *fungal infections* of the gallbladder can occur as can infestation with *parasitic worms,* but all are medical oddities. *Gallstone ileus* refers to small bowel intestinal obstruction due to lodging of a large gallstone in the terminal ileum after expulsion from the bile duct.

PANCREATIC DISEASES

ACUTE PANCREATITIS

Acute pancreatitis is by far the most common disease of the pancreas. The condition usually is seen in *alcoholics* but may occur in association with *obstruction of the biliary tract, blunt trauma* to the abdomen, *uremia* (kidney failure), *hyperparathyroidism* (overactivity of the parathyroid glands), *hypertriglyceridemia* (the elevation of plasma fat content), *mumps* and other viral conditions and *drugs.* Pancreatic inflammation as a result of trauma or viral infection is understandable, but the mechanism in other conditions is uncertain. One theory is that *reflux of bile* into the pancreatic ducts somehow initiates the process. Reflux is understandable when a stone blocks the common bile duct below entry of the pancreatic duct but is more difficult to explain in other conditions. It is possible that in some cases it results from *spasm of the sphincter of Oddi* (which prevents

---

[7] "Typhoid Mary," an itinerant female cook who herself was never ill, was the most famous of typhoid carriers. She infected many subjects between the years of 1900 and 1907 in the United States. Typhoid fever is now a rare disease in this country.

entry of bile into the intestine) with subsequent backflow into the ducts. Fatty acids released from plasma triglycerides as a consequence of pancreatic lipase activity are considered to be the toxic agent in hypertriglyceridemia and possibly other forms of pancreatitis. However, none of the theories is completely satisfactory.

The outstanding symptom of acute pancreatitis is *upper abdominal pain,* which radiates through to the back and is relieved by sitting up, flexing the trunk or assumption of the crawling position. *Nausea* and *vomiting* are common accompaniments. *Sweating* and *vascular collapse* with rapid heartbeat and low or immeasurable blood pressures are usual in severe disease as a consequence of hemorrhage into the pancreas or the trapping of large amounts of plasma-derived fluid in the inflamed pancreatic bed. Complications of acute pancreatitis include *gastrointestinal bleeding, ascites* (fluid in the abdominal cavity) and *kidney failure.* Mortality rates are high, varying from 5 to 10 percent with mild symptoms to 80 percent in severe hemorrhagic disease.

Diagnosis is made when the above symptoms are found to be accompanied by elevation of the pancreatic enzymes *amylase* and *lipase* in blood. Plasma *calcium* is usually also low, but this may occur in a number of other conditions and is not diagnostic.

Treatment consists of continuous gastrointestinal suction by gastric tube and the avoidance of food intake to prevent intestinal stimulation of pancreatic secretions.[8] In addition large amounts of fluids must be administered intravenously to restore the circulation (whole blood may be required in hemorrhagic pancreatitis). With high fever, infection of the necrotic pancreatic tissue bed must be assumed to be present and antibiotics administered. Calcium infusions are necessary in those cases where plasma levels become sufficiently low to cause symptoms.

CHRONIC PANCREATITIS

Chronic pancreatitis is a disease found almost exclusively in alcoholics. It may begin as an attack of acute pancreatitis fol-

[8] While the mechanism of induction of pancreatitis remains elusive, it is clear that release of digestive enzymes into the pancreatic tissue is responsible for most of the damage that occurs (the enzymes attack the pancreas like they do food in the intestine). If food is eaten, nondamaged portions of the pancreas release greater quantities of enzymes worsening the pancreatitis.

lowed by multiple relapses over the years or may appear insidiously with mild episodes of pain insufficient to require medical consultation. Some patients never have pain. The repeated episodes of inflammation lead to progressive destruction of pancreatic tissue and scar formation. When a critical mass of tissue is destroyed functional symptoms appear. The earliest sign is usually *steatorrhea;* the bulky, greasy stools (see chapter 8) are due to failure of fat absorption as a consequence of a deficiency of pancreatic lipase secretion into the intestinal canal. Protein absorption is also impaired and *weight loss* may be profound. With advanced disease, destruction of islets results in insulin deficiency and a secondary form of *diabetes* may result.

The diagnosis of chronic pancreatitis is usually suggested by the presence of recurrent abdominal pain and steatorrhea in a chronic alcoholic. With each episode of inflammation, calcium salts precipitate in the pancreas; if X-rays of the abdomen reveal a linear, patchy calcification in the area occupied by the pancreas, the diagnosis is confirmed. Unfortunately not all patients exhibit this sign. In such cases measurement of stool fat and evaluation of the secretory response and chemical makeup of pancreatic juices, obtained by duodenal intubation following stimulation with the enzymes *secretin* or *cholecystokinin,* may confirm pancreatic insufficiency. *Cholecystokinin levels* in the blood can be measured in some hospitals; the values tend to be high in many cases of chronic pancreatitis.

Treatment requires cessation of alcohol intake and oral administration of pancreatic enzymes derived from animals. In general steatorrhea can be well controlled by the exogenous enzymes. Recent evidence suggests that cimetidine, the powerful inhibitor of gastric acid secretion used in the treatment of peptic ulcer, enhances the effectiveness of the digestive enzymes when given in combination with them. No treatment is as good as prevention, however, and all patients who have experienced an episode of pancreatitis should be advised not to drink alcohol.[9]

---

[9] It is a remarkable experience to watch patients with chronic pancreatitis and cirrhosis of the liver continue to drink, slowly (or rapidly) killing themselves despite all exhortations to quit. The same phenomenon is seen in smokers, the obese and users of illicit drugs. Why the need to continue these activities overrides rational response to the presence (or potential presence) of serious illness has never been fully explained, but it is assumed to represent some powerful subconscious drive. Such drives are

PANCREATIC PSEUDOCYST[10]

Pseudocysts are fluid-filled masses in the pancreas that develop as a complication of acute pancreatitis. They usually manifest their presence by aching distress in the abdomen coupled with the presence of a mass detectable by palpation on physical examination or demonstrable by upper GI series. Sonography (echocardiography) is now the most accurate means of diagnosis, but the lesion can also be identified by CAT scan. The cysts may rupture spontaneously and empty their fluid contents into the abdomen, chest, mediastinum or neck, a complication that can be life-threatening. Treatment consists of surgical drainage, usually by anastomosing the cyst wall to an adjacent segment of the small bowel such that drainage occurs into the intestine.

CANCER OF THE PANCREAS

Malignant disease of the pancreas appears to be increasing in frequency in the United States. It accounts for about a fifth as many deaths as cancer of the colon. Chronic pancreatitis seems to predispose to its development, but most patients have no history of previous pancreatic disease. The usual symptoms are *unexplained weight loss* and *abdominal pain*. Like the distress of acute pancreatitis, the pain radiates through to the back (especially in the supine position) and is relieved by bending forward in the sitting position. *Jaundice* due to obstruction of the bile duct is usual at some time in the course but may be late in developing if the tumor is located in the body or tail of the pancreas as opposed to the head (which is adjacent to the entry of the bile duct into the duodenum). For reasons that are not clear, patients with cancer of the pancreas appear to have a *sense of impending death* (or at least an awareness of very serious illness) even before diagnosis is made, a phenomenon that is not seen with other forms of abdominal neoplasm. With bile duct obstruction the patient may complain of *itching* due to elevation of bile acid concentrations in the blood. Complete

---

usually psychologic in origin, but the possibility has to be kept open that an as yet undiscovered chemical imbalance exists. (Presumably any such biochemical abnormality would express itself in the central nervous system.)

[10] A true cyst has an intact membranous wall or capsule. The pancreatic lesion looks like a cyst because it has a hollow cavity, but its "wall" is made up by whatever type of tissue surrounds the damaged area—hence *pseudocyst*.

obstruction results in the appearance of *light or clay-colored stools* since bile pigments (responsible for the normal brown color of feces) do not reach the intestine. Enlargement of the liver (*hepatomegaly*) almost always means that the tumor has metastasized to that organ.

Diagnosis in the early stages is difficult. Upper GI series, sonography and endoscopic retrograde cholangiopancreatography are often required. The only treatment is radical surgical resection (*Whipple procedure*) but the results are miserable. X-ray therapy and chemotherapy are not useful. In general carcinoma of the pancreas must be considered a fatal illness.

CYSTIC FIBROSIS

Cystic fibrosis, one of the commonest of the genetic diseases, has a primary focus in the pancreas and *steatorrhea* is the primary symptom. As a consequence of malabsorption, growth and development are impaired. *Pulmonary disease* is also a feature of the disease, manifested by chronic bronchitis, bronchiectasis, pulmonary emphysema and repeated episodes of bronchopneumonia. Occasionally *cirrhosis of the liver* occurs as a complication.

The cause of cystic fibrosis has not been ascertained, but mucous glands throughout the gastrointestinal tract and lungs are known to produce a thick, abnormal mucus that may contribute to the clinical picture by blocking small ducts in the pancreas as well as terminal bronchioles in the lungs. Diagnosis is made from the characteristic clinical picture and the demonstration of abnormally high concentrations of sodium chloride in sweat. Why the sweat glands secrete elevated concentrations of salt is not known. Sweat chloride concentration is a good screening test in children but is less helpful in adults who may normally have concentrations equivalent to those seen in cystic fibrosis.

Treatment consists of the administration of pancreatic hormones as in other forms of pancreatic malabsorption together with the fat-soluble vitamins A, D and K. Aggressive pulmonary hygiene including postural drainage, inhalation of wetting agents, thumping of the chest to loosen mucus and therapeutic coughing are mandatory. Antibiotics are used only during episodes of acute pulmonary infections and not prophylactically. With the use of these measures, life expectancy has increased significantly for children with the disease. Death usually results from pneumonia.

ENDOCRINE DISEASE OF THE PANCREAS

By far the most common endocrine disease of the pancreas is *diabetes mellitus*. The elevated blood sugar and other metabolic abnormalities that characterize diabetes are due to disease of the islets of Langerhans, which results in insulin deficiency and glucagon excess in blood. Diabetes is discussed in chapter 15. All other forms of endocrine disease arising in the pancreas are due to development of hormone-producing tumors which may be benign but are often malignant. These tumors, while quite rare, are now being recognized with increasing frequency due to the availability of much more accurate assays for hormones in blood. They may occur alone or in association with *adenomas* (glandular tumors) of other endocrine glands (*multiple endocrine adenoma syndrome*).

Insulinoma. Insulinomas are tumors of the beta cells of the islets of Langerhans. They secrete insulin at inappropriate times or in inappropriate concentrations and as a consequence cause *hypoglycemia*. The lowering of the blood sugar may be very profound resulting in convulsions or loss of consciousness. Diagnosis is made by demonstration of abnormal insulin concentrations at a time of spontaneous symptomatic hypoglycemia or during a fast deliberately undertaken to induce hypoglycemia. In a normal person the plasma insulin becomes unmeasurable after 24–72 hours of fasting as the blood sugar decreases to below normal (but asymptomatic) levels. The normal fall in insulin does not occur in insulinoma despite the fact that symptomatic hypoglycemia may be produced.[11] Treatment is surgical removal of the tumor.

Ulcerogenic Islet Cell Tumor (Gastrinoma). Gastrinoma is the cause of the Zollinger-Ellison syndrome. Intractable ulcer disease is caused from high gastric acidity induced by secretion of the hormone *gastrin* by the tumor. Hemorrhage and perfora-

---

[11] The diagnosis of an insulin-secreting tumor is not secure even if hyperinsulinism is demonstrated. The problem of *factitious hypoglycemia*, meaning that patients deliberately induce hypoglycemia in themselves by surreptitiously injecting insulin or taking oral hypoglycemic drugs ordinarily used in the treatment of diabetes, is a very common one. The self-induction of disease is apparently done for psychiatric reasons. The problem is most often seen in medical or paramedical personnel but is not limited to this group.

tion of ulcers are common. Diarrhea and steatorrhea are associated features. Treatment is total removal of the stomach, not removal of the gastrin-producing tumor.[12]

Diarrheogenic Islet Cell Tumor. This tumor causes explosive watery diarrhea accompanied by low potassium levels in blood. The syndrome is sometimes called *pancreatic cholera,* reflecting the fact that the severe diarrhea resembles the infectious diarrhea caused by the cholera organism elsewhere in the world. For reasons that are uncertain, acid concentrations in the stomach are low. Elevated plasma levels of calcium and glucose are seen in some patients. The hormone produced by these tumors has been the subject of disagreement, but most investigators now consider *vasoactive intestinal polypeptide* to be the cause of symptoms. Treatment is surgical removal of the primary lesion.

Glucagonoma. Glucagonoma, as the name implies, is a tumor of the glucagon-producing alpha cell of the pancreatic islet. It results in a syndrome characterized by a migratory, scaly, crusting skin rash and elevated blood sugar. Weight loss and anemia are common and arthritis may be present. Most of the tumors are malignant and rapidly metastasizing, making treatment difficult.

Somatostatinoma. The rarest of the islet tumors, somatostatinoma, has been associated with hyperglycemia, anemia, steatorrhea and gallbladder disease.

Mixed Tumors. Some pancreatic islet tumors simultaneously produce more than one hormone: the same tumor may produce insulin, gastrin, serotonin and ACTH (adrenocorticotrophic hormone). As a consequence, one tumor may cause symptoms suggesting primary disease in several endocrine glands. Differentiating these possibilities is an extremely difficult proposition.

---

[12] In theory the disease should be cured by removal of the gastrinoma. In practice this does not turn out to be the case, probably because the tumors have already metastasized at the time surgery is undertaken such that complete removal of gastrin-producing tissue is impossible.

10

Diseases of the Liver

The liver, the largest solid organ in the body, is located in the right upper quadrant of the abdomen, nestled against the diaphragm just under the lower border of the rib cage. Anatomically it is divided into a large right lobe (with subdivisions called the quadrate and caudate lobes) and a smaller left lobe. Ordinarily the liver cannot be felt on physical examination and becomes palpable only if it is enlarged or if it is pushed below the rib border by overexpansion of the lungs as occurs with pulmonary emphysema. The blood supply of the liver is unique. In most organs blood arrives via artery and leaves through the veins. The liver, by contrast, receives only about 30% of its total blood flow from the hepatic artery. The remainder arrives via the portal vein which carries venous blood from the intestine and spleen. This arrangement means that almost all absorbed nutrients pass to the liver before entering the general circulation,[1] allowing it to play a critical role in the control of fuel metabolism in the body. Venous blood leaving the liver reaches the inferior vena cava via the hepatic veins.

The liver is not only the largest solid organ, biochemically it is the most complex, carrying out multiple hundreds of enzymatic reactions necessary for the proper functioning of all other tissues. Some of these functions can be assumed by other or-

[1] The exception is dietary fat, which, it will be recalled (chapter 2), is absorbed into intestinal lymph, reaching the general circulation via the thoracic duct. Fat thus passes to the liver in arterial rather than portal venous blood.

gans in the case of extensive liver disease but others cannot. Nonreplaceable functions which become manifest in severe liver disease include the production of glucose during fasting, the synthesis of albumin (the major protein of plasma), the manufacture of clotting proteins, the disposal of bilirubin (the breakdown product of hemoglobin), the detoxification of endogenous metabolic products and the metabolism of drugs. Impairment or loss of these functions may lead to *low levels of glucose in the blood* (with convulsions and loss of consciousness), *depression of the albumin concentration in plasma* (with generalized edema and the accumulation of fluid in the abdomen and chest),[2] *spontaneous bleeding* (in the skin, gastrointestinal tract and other parts of the body), *jaundice* (the yellow discoloration of skin due to bilirubin accumulation in plasma), *drug toxicity* (on dosage schedules handled by a normal person without difficulty) and *hepatic coma* (due to the inability to dispose of toxins generated within the body and gastrointestinal tract). These findings are not specific to any one form of liver disease but represent the common parameters of extensive liver damage however produced.

DIAGNOSTIC PROCEDURES

Liver Function Tests. A variety of biochemical tests are available to evaluate liver function. Routine screening tests (obtained on almost every patient who has blood drawn during a physical examination) include plasma bilirubin, alkaline phosphatase and transaminase activities. *Bilirubin,* as noted, is the breakdown product of hemoglobin responsible for jaundice. *Alkaline phosphatase* is an enzyme whose concentration in blood goes up whenever there is obstruction in the biliary tract. That obstruction may be extrahepatic, as with a gallstone in the bile

---

[2] Albumin is primarily responsible for the effective osmotic pressure of the blood. Osmotic pressure refers to the attraction or holding power of a molecule in solution for its solvent (in the body the solvent is water) when the molecule cannot pass through a semipermeable membrane (in this case the blood vessel wall) while the solvent can. As albumin concentration decreases, plasma-effective osmotic pressure (*oncotic pressure*) falls, allowing fluid to leave the plasma compartment and enter the interstitial space that surrounds cells. The kidney recognizes that the plasma volume is diminished and avidly retains salt and water in an attempt to compensate (replace the lost fluid). However, because the albumin is low the fluid retained by the kidney also passes out into the already expanded interstitial compartment. The end result is pitting edema of the soft tissue and, in some cases, accumulation of large amounts of fluid in abdominal and chest cavities.

duct, or intrahepatic due to inflammation in the liver. As noted before in chapter 9, alkaline phosphatase levels also rise in certain forms of bone disease, requiring that the liver and bone enzymes be differentiated under some circumstances. *Transaminase* levels are a sensitive indicator of hepatic inflammation (particularly hepatitis) but are nonspecific since inflammation or damage to other tissues also cause the enzyme to rise. *Leucine aminopeptidase* and *5'-nucleotidase* are enzymes that are more specific for liver damage but more difficult to assay. They are ordered only in difficult cases. Tests of clotting function are regularly carried out. The two most common are called the *prothrombin time* and *partial thromboplastin time*. A markedly prolonged prothrombin time which does not return to normal on administration of vitamin K[3] is indicative of extensive liver disease. Many physicians believe that the degree of prothrombin abnormality is the best indicator of overall prognosis in liver disease: mild liver disease does not cause deficiency of clotting factors sufficient to make the test abnormal. *Blood ammonia levels* may also be measured but are usually reserved for patients with impending hepatic coma.

Liver Scans. Several types of isotopic scans are available for visualization of the liver. With the commonly used radioactive colloidal gold or sulfur colloid scans abscesses or tumors show up as filling defects: the uptake of isotope by normal tissue surrounding diseased areas makes the latter appear as "holes." With [67]gallium scans the inflammatory or neoplastic (tumor) mass preferentially takes up radioactivity relative to normal tissues thus appearing as a hot spot. Scans are useful in identifying large lesions but may be negative if the abnormality is smaller than 2–3 centimeters in diameter. Cirrhosis of the liver, which markedly distorts liver architecture, often gives false positive scans suggesting the presence of tumor. Since hepatic cancer frequently develops in patients with cirrhosis, the gallium scan is the test usually ordered in known cirrhotic subjects.

Needle Biopsy of the Liver. Needle biopsy is done through the skin (*percutaneously*) using only local anesthesia. A slender core of tissue moves up the needle shaft as it passes into the

[3] Vitamin K is necessary for the synthesis of prothrombin and clotting factors VII, IX and X. Coagulation defects due to deficiency of these factors can be the consequence of a failure to absorb vitamin K (as in intestinal malabsorption) or inability of the liver to carry out clotting factor synthesis. If one administers vitamin K by injection and prothrombin time normalizes, a deficiency of the vitamin can be assumed. Failure to normalize after vitamin K means intrinsic liver disease is present.

liver substance and is removed for microscopic examination. With generalized hepatic disease a diagnosis can almost always be made by such biopsies; with localized disease the technique is less successful since the involved area may be missed. It is helpful in identifying viral or drug-induced hepatitis, cirrhosis, disseminated metastatic cancer, lymphoma and infiltrative diseases like sarcoidosis or tuberculosis. The procedure is quite safe although occasionally complications such as bleeding, pneumothorax or perforation of the gallbladder occur when the needle tip (which is not under direct visualization) encounters a structure other than liver.

Peritoneoscopy. In this technique a tubular instrument is passed through a small incision in the abdomen for direct visualization of the liver and other abdominal viscera. Its tremendous advantage is that biopsy can be taken under direct visualization and localized lesions may be identified. There is almost no hazard and little discomfort. It is an extremely helpful procedure in difficult diagnostic problems.

Immunologic Tests. It is now possible to detect the presence of hepatitis B virus antigen and antibodies to the B virus by immunologic assays. Such assays are regularly ordered in patients with hepatitis or suspected hepatitis. Hepatitis B virus causes that form of hepatitis transmitted by blood transfusion and blood banks now test all blood for B antibodies before allowing it to be transfused. Tests for hepatitis A virus are not yet routinely available in hospital laboratories. Antibodies to mitochondria are often found in biliary cirrhosis while antibodies to nuclei and smooth muscle are signs of chronic active hepatitis. A test called the LE (*lupus erythematosus*) cell test, ordinarily a sign of the collagen disease of that name (see chapter 13) may be positive in chronic active hepatitis. Measurement of alpha-fetoprotein may be helpful in the diagnosis of hepatic cancer.

HEPATITIS

VIRAL HEPATITIS

Viral hepatitis is the most common of the liver diseases. Two of the viruses causing the illness have been identified and partially characterized: *hepatitis viruses A and B*. It is certain that

other viruses also cause the syndrome since patients with classic hepatitis have been carefully studied without finding evidence of either A or B virus. In the past the terms *infectious
hepatitis* and *serum hepatitis* were often used to describe the
illnesses caused by the A and B viruses respectively. It is now
recognized that distinction between the two cannot be made on
clinical grounds, although the A virus usually has a shorter incubation time and tends to be transferred by infected feces
while the B virus has a longer incubation time and is more often
transmitted by blood transfusion or use of needles contaminated with virus. The latter is an extremely common problem
among users of illicit drugs who often share a community needle. The incidence of B infection is increasing relative to A, and
in a significant percentage of cases there is no history of injections or transfusions. It is now known that hepatitis B virus is
secreted in tears, oral and vaginal secretions, semen, urine and
feces, rendering transmission to intimate contacts by the oral
route not only possible but likely.[4]

The symptoms of viral hepatitis fall into two phases: *preicteric* and *icteric* (icteric means jaundiced). The preicteric phase
usually lasts 1 to 2 weeks and is characterized by *loss of appetite, nausea, vomiting* and *fatigue. Headache, cough, symptoms
of a cold* and *sore throat* may be present. *Joint* and *muscle
pains* are common. *Fever* is characteristic, but rarely goes above
102°F. Occasionally a *skin rash* is noted. When *jaundice* appears the generalized symptoms usually improve.[5] With severe
infections the *stools become light colored* and the *urine turns
dark* as excretion of bile pigments into the bile is impaired by
inflammatory obstruction of bile canaliculi; this obstruction
causes regurgitation of pigments into the urine, giving a brown
color. On physical examination, in addition to jaundice, one
usually finds the liver to be enlarged and tender. There may be
a generalized increase in lymph node size, and in a minority of
patients the spleen is enlarged and palpable.

Diagnosis is made on the basis of the characteristic clinical
presentation coupled with the demonstration of abnormal liver
function tests. The first test to become abnormal is the *trans-*

---

[4] Some authorities now classify hepatitis as one of the venereal diseases since it can
clearly be transmitted by intimate physical contact. However, the vast majority of cases
are not transmitted sexually.

[5] Some patients never develop jaundice. They are said to have *nonicteric* hepatitis.

aminase level in blood. The *hepatitis B surface antigen* (equivalent to virus)[6] is positive in the preicteric and early icteric phases when B virus is the causal agent. *Antibody* to the hepatitis B surface antigen usually becomes positive only in the convalescent phase of the illness. A positive test for B antigen means active disease or a carrier state while a positive antibody test means previous exposure to the virus. *Liver biopsy* is probably indicated only if there is a question about diagnosis.

The prognosis for complete recovery is excellent in viral hepatitis. Mild disease does not even require hospitalization. However, a few patients develop a fulminant form of the illness called *massive hepatic necrosis* and die in hepatic failure. Worrisome signs include marked prolongation of the prothrombin time, elevation of the bilirubin above 20 milligrams per 100 milliliters of plasma (normal, less than 1), significant lowering of the plasma albumin and the presence of hypoglycemia. There is no specific treatment for hepatitis. Adrenal steroids in high doses are usually given to patients with massive necrosis, but their benefit is questionable. While the vast majority of patients with hepatitis recover completely, a few with type B disease develop a late complication called *chronic active hepatitis*.

It is possible to prevent the appearance of clinical hepatitis by administration of *immune serum globulin* (gamma globulin). Its major effectiveness is in hepatitis A, although large doses are often given to subjects (particularly medical personnel) known to have been exposed to B virus. Prophylaxis is given only to intimate contacts of patients with sporadic hepatitis; i.e., gamma globulin would be offered to family members of a proven case but not, for example, to classmates of a student with the disease.

DRUG-INDUCED HEPATITIS

A number of drugs cause a clinical picture indistinguishable on clinical grounds from viral hepatitis. The reaction is called *idiosyncratic*, meaning that it strikes unpredictably and that

[6] The B virus is thought to consist of an inner *core* and outer *coat* or *surface*. Viral proteins (antigens) may be derived from either the surface or core, and antibodies may develop to each. The core antigen has been found in liver but does not reach the blood in contrast to surface antigen. Other viral-associated proteins include the *e* antigen and an enzyme called *DNA polymerase*, both of which appear to correlate better with the infectivity of blood than the B surface antigen.

most patients given the drug do not develop the problem. An outstanding cause of this type of injury is the anesthetic agent, *halothane.* Toxicity usually occurs in patients who have been exposed to halothane on a previous occasion. Other drugs causing hepatitislike injury are *phenytoin,* an anticonvulsant drug commonly used in the treatment of epilepsy, *methyldopa* and *chlorthiazide,* both of which are used in the treatment of high blood pressure and *isoniazide,* the most effective drug in the treatment of tuberculosis. Some drugs produce a picture more compatible with obstructive jaundice than hepatitis. These drugs, called *cholestatic agents,* include *methyl testosterone* (a form of the male sex hormone), *oral contraceptive agents, sulfonylureas* (the oral blood-sugar-lowering drugs used in the treatment of diabetes), certain tranquilizers such as *chlorpromazine,* and *methimazole,* a drug used in the treatment of hyperthyroidism. While the liver injury associated with drugs is usually reversible, some apparently cause permanent damage, including cirrhosis.

TOXIC HEPATITIS

Organic solvents, the prototype of which is *carbon tetrachloride,* cause hepatic damage in all patients given heavy enough exposure: the effect is *dose related* and not idiosyncratic. As little as 4 milliliters of carbon tetrachloride may be fatal when ingested. It may also cause damage by inhalation. A common scenario predisposing to inhalation toxicity is the use of a carbon-tetrachloride-containing solvent to clean rugs or furniture in a nonventilated room. Industrial chemicals such as *trichlorethylene, yellow phosphorus, arsenic* and *ethylene glycol* are other toxic agents that may damage the liver. *Ethylene glycol* and *diethylene glycol,* common constituents of permanent commercial antifreeze mixtures, are often ingested by alcoholics when they cannot obtain alcohol. Many of these agents damage the kidney and other organs in addition to the liver. An interesting form of toxic hepatitis is due to the ingestion of certain species of *poisonous mushrooms.*

CHRONIC ACTIVE HEPATITIS

Chronic active hepatitis is a disease characterized by longstanding inflammation of the liver accompanied by cell death and scar formation. A high percentage of cases result in cirrhosis and death in liver failure. Chronic active hepatitis should be distinguished from *chronic persistent hepatitis*. The latter term refers to a condition, usually seen following a classical acute episode of viral hepatitis, where the clinical picture of fatigue, anorexia, enlargement of the liver and abnormal liver functions continue for 4 to 8 months before finally disappearing. Biopsy is usually required to distinguish between the two. Differentiation is important since chronic persistent hepatitis, in contrast to chronic active hepatitis, is not a progressive disease and does not lead to cirrhosis; recovery is eventually complete.

Chronic active hepatitis can be caused by a variety of agents, some quite common and others extremely rare. About 30 percent of the cases begin with what appears to be typical viral hepatitis. Often the patients appear to recover, only to develop signs of progressive liver disease over the next 1 to 3 years. The blood of such patients is persistently positive for the hepatitis B surface antigen, and it is assumed that they have ongoing active viral infection in the liver. The onset of symptoms in other patients is insidious, and there is no history suggestive of previous viral illness. Some of these patients have hepatitis B antigen circulating while the remainder do not. Most such patients fall into a diagnostic category called *lupoid hepatitis.* Other causes include viruses that usually do not cause hepatitis, drugs, a condition of abnormal copper storage in the body called Wilson's disease and a genetic disease, α-1 antitrypsin deficiency. The latter has already been mentioned as a cause of pulmonary emphysema (chapter 7). Patients with constant hepatitis B infection tend to be men in the 30–50 year age range while those with lupoid hepatitis are most often young women (15–25 years of age). All forms of chronic active hepatitis result in the gradual onset of *fatigue, malaise* and *jaundice. Fever* may be present intermittently. Patients with lupoid hepatitis are distinguished by the presence of *menstrual abnormalities, joint pains* or *frank arthritis, pleural* and *pericardial pain* (with or without effusions), *skin rashes* (including acne), *positive LE cell tests* and high levels of *antinuclear, antimitochondrial* and *smooth muscle antibodies.* In short the syndrome resembles the collagen disease called *lupus erythematosus* with the exception that liver disease predominates (hence, *lupoid*-resembling lupus). Patients with lupoid hepatitis have a high incidence of associated autoimmune diseases, including ulcerative colitis.

The course of chronic active hepatitis is variable. Some patients with disease due to hepatitis B apparently remit without progression to cirrhosis. Others have a rapidly progressive downhill course resulting in early death, while yet a third group exhibits a pattern characterized by remissions and exacerbations of symptoms ending finally in cirrhosis of the liver. It should be noted that the cirrhosis resulting from chronic active hepatitis is called *postnecrotic cirrhosis* and has nothing to do with the ordinary alcoholic (*Laennec's*) cirrhosis. (See below.)

Chronic active hepatitis appears to respond to treatment with *prednisolone* [7] with interruption of the downhill course and (at times) complete remission. In patients not responding to steroids *azathioprine*, another immunosuppressive agent, is often added to the therapeutic regimen. (Azathioprine is always used in conjunction with prednisone. It is ineffective when given alone.)

CIRRHOSIS OF THE LIVER

Cirrhosis of the liver is a general term describing diffuse liver disease characterized by destruction of primary liver cells and extensive scar formation in the supportive tissues. Surviving liver cells are stimulated to multiply, resulting in a nodular appearance of the organ. The normal, regularly arranged architecture is replaced by an irregular pattern of extensive scars separating regenerating patches of new liver cells. The scars constrict the portal vessels and block blood flow through the liver causing a rise in pressure through the portal system (*portal hypertension*). All symptoms can be accounted for either by destruction of hepatic cells or portal hypertension. Several types of cirrhosis are recognized: *Laennec's cirrhosis, postnecrotic cirrhosis, biliary cirrhosis* and *cardiac cirrhosis*. Certain features are common to all forms but each also has distinctive clinical or pathologic manifestations. Laennec's and postnecrotic cirrhosis account for the vast majority of cases.

---

[7] *Prednisone* and *prednisolone* are synthetic steroid hormones which have slightly different properties and are much more potent, milligram for milligram, than the naturally occurring hormone, *hydrocortisone*. They presumably function in chronic active hepatitis to suppress the autoantibodies that are thought to play a role in the inflammatory process. Since prednisone has to be converted to prednisolone in the liver to become active, the latter drug is preferred by many physicians in severe liver disease because of the possibility that the activation process might be impaired.

LAENNEC'S CIRRHOSIS
(ALCOHOLIC OR PORTAL CIRRHOSIS)

Laennec's cirrhosis is the most common form of cirrhosis in the United States. It is a disease that occurs almost exclusively in alcoholics. Earlier studies suggested that the effect of alcohol was indirect, causing malnutrition which then damaged the liver, but it is now clear that alcohol itself is the primary toxin. This is not to imply that malnutrition does not play a role, only that it is not necessary.[8] Ordinarily large intakes of alcohol for prolonged periods are required. The estimate is that 50 percent of persons drinking a pint of whiskey a day will develop cirrhosis over a 25-year period. In the early stages of the disease, the only finding may be an *enlarged liver* with mildly abnormal liver function tests detected by chemical examination of the blood. As the disease progresses the patient develops *weakness, fatigue, jaundice* and *abdominal swelling* due to the accumulation of fluid in the abdominal cavity (*ascites*). Ascites develops because increased pressure in the portal system and low plasma albumin concentrations combine to cause leakage of fluid from surface vessels in the liver and portal vein branches into the abdomen. Since blood flow through the liver is impaired, return of venous blood from the intestines to the heart must occur through alternate (*collateral*) pathways. As a consequence, the patient with cirrhosis develops dilated veins in several characteristic sites, each representing part of the alternative venous return system. These include veins over the abdomen, particularly around the umbilicus, hemorrhoidal veins and, most important, fragile channels on the inner surface of the esophagus (*esophageal varices*). The latter are highly susceptible to spontaneous bleeding and frequently lead to death of the patient.[9]

A large number of physical findings accompany the cirrhotic state in addition to jaundice and ascites. Delicate, dilated blood capillaries appear over the upper chest and face (*spider an-*

---

[8] Chronic alcoholics are usually malnourished because their caloric intake is essentially limited to alcohol, which is a carbohydrate energy source devoid of protein and vitamins.

[9] Patients with cirrhosis have a high incidence of duodenal ulcers which are often symptomatically silent until they bleed. The point is that upper gastrointestinal hemorrhage is not always due to bleeding varices.

giomas).[10] *Weakness* of leg muscles, *ankle edema, gynecomastia* (enlargement of the breast in males), *clubbing* of the fingers, redness of the palms of the hands (*palmar erythema*), *enlargement of the parotid glands* (resembling mumps) and palpable *distension of the spleen* are common features. In the late phases *purpura* (bleeding into the skin) may be noted. *Testicular atrophy* is frequent in men.

Laboratory examination shows disturbances in a variety of liver function tests, including elevation of the plasma bilirubin, increased liver enzymes, lowered plasma albumin and abnormal clotting functions. Anemia is essentially invariable and is due to folic acid deficiency, often complicated by blood loss. Electrolyte abnormalities are frequent, including lowered blood levels of potassium, magnesium, calcium and sodium, but these are primarily due to alcoholism and not cirrhosis *per se*.

The diagnosis of cirrhosis is usually clear from the clinical picture and should be suspected in any alcoholic patient with enlargement of the liver and abnormal liver function tests. Definitive diagnosis requires liver biopsy.[11]

The course of Laennec's cirrhosis is variable. If the disease is diagnosed early and the patient abstains from alcohol, the outlook is quite good. However, most patients will not (or cannot) stop drinking and as a consequence 60 percent die within 5 years of diagnosis.[12] Death most commonly results from *mas-*

---

[10] The capillary branches radiate from a central point and resemble the legs of a spider. Characteristically compression of the central point with a pencil tip or pinhead occludes flow in the radiating branches.

[11] The earliest stage of alcoholic liver disease shows *fat infiltration* on microscopic examination. Subsequently, inflammatory cells are seen as liver cells die, a phase called *alcoholic hepatitis*. Finally, the characteristic *scarring* appears and the liver begins to shrink in size, becomes firm or hard in consistency and develops a nodular surface in place of the normally smooth external capsule. The nodules in Laennec's cirrhosis are smaller and more uniform (finely nodular) than those in postnecrotic cirrhosis which tend to be larger and more irregular (coarsely nodular).

[12] The monetary and human costs of alcohol-related problems in society are astounding. A partial list of these problems includes absenteeism from work, disintegration of families, trauma to self and others (a high percentage of traffic deaths and private plane crashes, falls and personal violence occur under the influence of alcohol), cirrhosis of the liver, beri-beri, alcoholic convulsions, delirium tremens, the Wernicke-Korsakoff syndrome (deterioration of the central nervous system), alcohol-induced hypoglycemia, hypertriglyceridemia, neuropathy with muscle paralysis, gastritis with upper GI bleeding, myopathy (death of muscle cells) with myoglobinuria (leakage of muscle constituents that damage the kidney), impotence, infertility, feminization with gynecomastia in men, anemia and increased susceptibility to infection, particularly aspiration pneumonia.

sive upper gastrointestinal bleeding, usually from esophageal varices. Other major mechanisms include *hepatic coma* (see page 210) and *kidney failure.* The latter complication, called the *hepato-renal syndrome,* is a peculiar form of renal disease seen in hepatic failure of any cause. Despite intensive study, its cause remains an enigma.

Treatment, apart from withdrawal of alcohol, consists of the administration of a *nutritious diet* supplemented with *vitamins* and *limitation of salt* if edema and ascites are present. *Diuretics* are usually given in addition. If ascites is massive enough to interfere with eating and breathing, small amounts of fluid may be removed by a needle inserted in the abdominal wall (*paracentesis*). Recurrent ascites is often treated by placement of a *LeVeen shunt* (named after the originator of the technique). In this procedure a tube is placed in the abdominal cavity and brought through the chest wall (beneath the skin) to the neck where it is inserted into a jugular vein. The ascites is thereby brought back into the systemic circulation and the excess fluid excreted in the urine. Bleeding esophageal varices are treated by infusion of a hormone called *vasopressin* (which diminishes portal venous pressure) and placement of a *Sengstaken-Blakemore tube.* This tube has an inflatable balloon around it which can be blown up, compressing the esophageal veins to stop the bleeding. Surgery to relieve portal hypertension and prevent recurrent bleeding from varices involves anastomosis of the portal vein to the inferior vena cava, thus bypassing the block in the liver (*portacaval shunt*). Mortality rates from the procedure are high, and it is only recommended when the outlook without surgery appears hopeless.

POSTNECROTIC CIRRHOSIS

This form of cirrhosis is not associated with alcoholism but represents the end stage of chronic active hepatitis. The disease should be suspected in any young person or nonalcoholic with a clinical picture suggesting cirrhosis. It is thought that jaundice is more severe early in postnecrotic cirrhosis than is the case with alcoholic liver disease, but this is by no means invariable. Clinically patients may present with upper gastrointestinal bleeding, ascites or signs of portal hypertension exactly as in the Laennec form. Laboratory findings are also similar, although plasma gamma globulin levels tend to be higher in postnecrotic cirrhosis. Diagnosis is made by liver biopsy. Overall the prognosis is poor, and death within 5 years of the appearance of clinical signs is usual. Liver transplantation may provide some hope in the future, but at present the procedure is still in the developmental stage.

BILIARY CIRRHOSIS

Biliary cirrhosis is much less common than the two previous forms of the disease. It can occur whenever there is long-standing obstruction in the biliary tract. *Primary biliary cirrhosis* tends to be a disease of middle-aged women and is associated with intrahepatic obstruction to bile flow. The cause is unknown. *Secondary biliary cirrhosis* is due to obstruction of the bile duct by gallstones, tumors or strictures following gallbladder surgery. A fulminant form of the disease in infants is due to a congenital defect in development of the biliary tree. Clinically patients first develop signs of *obstructive jaundice* with marked itching due to elevation of bile acids in the blood. The stools become light colored as jaundice increases, and steatorrhea may be present. The plasma cholesterol becomes markedly elevated and deposits of cholesterol (*xanthomas*) appear over bony prominences and in tendons. Subsequently ascites and portal hypertension appear.

As expected with obstruction to bile flow, laboratory examination shows marked elevation of alkaline phosphatase in association with the rise in plasma bilirubin. Bile acids in the blood are increased, but these are rarely measured. A peculiar lipoprotein (*lipoprotein X*) is characteristically present. It appears in the blood in all forms of biliary obstruction. Diagnosis is made, as in other forms of cirrhosis, by liver biopsy.

Treatment is unsatisfactory except in the secondary forms where extrahepatic obstruction can be surgically relieved. Itching may be relieved by cholestyramine, a resin that binds bile acids in the intestine and can be taken by mouth. Survival beyond 10 years is unusual.

CARDIAC CIRRHOSIS

Cardiac cirrhosis is the consequence of chronic congestion of the liver secondary to long-standing heart disease. The usual etiology is rheumatic heart disease with deformity of the mitral or tricuspid valves. Constrictive pericarditis and cor pulmonale (see chapter 5) are other causes. The hepatic congestion is caused by a block in return of venous blood to the heart. Somehow the pressure of excess blood in the liver initiates a scarring process. Cardiac cirrhosis is quite rare, and the clinical consequences are much milder than in other types of the scarring liver disease. Treatment requires reversal of the heart abnormality. Cardiac surgery is necessary in the case of rheumatic valvular disease or constrictive pericarditis.

HEPATIC COMA
(HEPATIC ENCEPHALOPATHY)

Hepatic coma is the name given to the central nervous system dysfunction that accompanies end-stage liver disease. It may result from acute disease, such as massive hepatic necrosis in viral hepatitis, or as a consequence of gradual liver failure, as occurs in the various forms of cirrhosis. The clinical picture is quite characteristic. The earliest sign is a *failure of memory* or *reasoning capacity*. Patients are unable to make simple calculations such as serial subtractions or additions of small numbers. *Disorientation* as to time, place and person often appears next. *Bizarre behavior* such as drinking from a urinal or shouting incoherently is occasionally seen. As the disease progresses *stupor* and finally *coma* supervene. A classic finding on examination is the presence of a *flapping tremor*, technically called *asterixis*. With the arms extended the hands drop and then extend upward again in repetitive fashion. In extreme forms the arms and head may also be involved in the flapping movements. The breath exhibits a musky, somewhat pungent odor called *fetor hepaticus*. Once smelled it will never be forgotten. Hyperactive reflexes and other abnormal neurological signs complete the picture. The electroencephalogram shows a typical pattern of slow waves that supports a diagnosis of hepatic coma.[13]

The cause of hepatic coma is not known with certainty although elevation of blood ammonia (NH_3) levels is thought to

---

[13] Alcoholics with cirrhosis may be confused and lose consciousness for many reasons besides hepatic coma. The physician always has to rule out trauma to the head from falls, hypoglycemia, ingestion of toxic substances, bleeding into the brain, acute Wernicke-Korsakoff syndrome, simple alcohol intoxication and delirium tremens.

play a central role. Ammonia, generated in the body (particularly by the kidney) and absorbed from the gastrointestinal tract where it is produced by bacteria acting on ingested protein, is ordinarily detoxified in the liver. With hepatic cell damage this process is impaired. Moreover, the high portal vein pressure shunts blood from the intestine away from the liver through collateral channels, thus allowing its entry into the general circulation. The key role of ammonia is emphasized by the fact that hepatic coma is often precipitated by bleeding into the intestine or the ingestion of large amounts of protein. Both blood and dietary proteins lead to increased production of NH_3 by intestinal bacteria. Certain drugs also predispose to development of encephalopathy; opiates, sedatives and powerful diuretics are notorious in this regard and should be avoided.

Treatment involves limitation of protein intake, the use of laxatives and enemas to clear the colon of potential sources of NH_3 and administration of *neomycin* (a nonabsorbable antibiotic) to diminish the concentration of NH_3-forming bacteria in the gut. *Lactulose,* a synthetic sugar, also appears to be helpful by decreasing ammonia absorption. These measures, combined with aggressive attention to supportive parameters such as the administration of IV fluids, often allow reversal of hepatic coma, particularly if the episode was induced by bleeding, drugs or increased protein intake. Encephalopathy due to loss of liver cells alone may be irreversible.

TUMORS OF THE LIVER

Two types of cancer are found in the liver: *primary* and *metastatic. Primary cancers* are most often malignancies of the hepatic cell (*hepatocellular carcinoma; hepatoma*), but tumors of the bile ducts (*cholangiocellular carcinoma*) also occur. While hepatic cell tumors may develop in patients who have never had liver disease, the vast majority occur in patients with underlying *cirrhosis* (especially the postnecrotic form) or *hemochromatosis.* The latter is a disease characterized by the abnormal storage of iron in multiple tissues of the body, including the liver. The abnormal iron deposits cause a bronze coloration of the skin, diabetes mellitus, testicular atrophy in men, arthritis, heart failure and cirrhosis of the liver.[14] Hepatomas usually herald their presence by *increasing size of the liver* coupled with *weight loss, fever* and occasionally *pain in the right upper quadrant.* On physical examination a separate *mass* may be felt in the liver, and rarely auscultation with the stethoscope reveals the presence of a rubbing sound (*friction rub*). *Anemia* is common and the tumor may cause *hypoglycemia* or *hypercalcemia.* The finding of elevated blood levels of a protein called *alpha-fetoprotein* is strongly suggestive of primary hepatoma. Diagnosis is confirmed by liver scan, peritoneoscopy and liver biopsy.

Metastatic cancers of the liver usually arise in the gastrointestinal tract and spread to the liver via the portal vein. Primary tumors in other sites, including the lung, breast and prostate also reach the liver. Symptoms are usually those of the primary tumor, with metastasis heralded by the presence of an enlarging liver.

There is no effective treatment for primary cancer of the liver; metastatic lesions can be treated only if the primary tumor is susceptible to chemotherapy.

OTHER DISEASES

The liver is vulnerable to a variety of other diseases, most of which are quite rare relative to those discussed before. *Pyogenic abscesses* (pus-filled cavities due to bacterial infection) are usually secondary to rupture of the appendix or infection secondary to obstruction of the bile duct. *Amebic abscess* is ordinarily seen in travelers returning from tropical countries (it is not necessary to have amebic dysentery prior to developing liver abscess). Both types of abscess cause fever, chills, sweating, weight loss, right upper quadrant pain which may radiate to the shoulder, enlargement of the liver and abnormal liver function tests. A pleural effusion on the right side is not un-

---

[14] The cause of hemochromatosis appears to be a genetically determined abnormal rate of absorption of iron from the diet. Many years of increased absorption are required before symptoms appear. The disease is much less common in women than men, presumably because of the protective effect of regular menstrual periods which cause loss of significant amounts of iron in the menstrual blood. This loss, which protects against iron storage disease, also makes normal women vulnerable to iron deficiency anemia (see chapter 14).

usual. Diagnosis is made by liver scan or ultrasound. Treatment involves surgical drainage, antibiotics or antiamebic drugs.

The liver may be enlarged by infiltration with *leukemia* or *lymphomas* (e.g., Hodgkin's disease). Systemic illnesses such as *sarcoidosis* and *amyloidosis* also involve the liver. The former, already mentioned in the chapter on lung disease, is a disease of unknown etiology characterized by disseminated patches of inflammation (*granulomas*) in lungs, liver, lymph nodes and other parts of the body. *Amyloidosis* is a condition which may occur spontaneously or be secondary to chronic inflammatory diseases (e.g., ulcerative colitis, rheumatoid arthritis, tuberculosis). Symptoms are due to the deposition of a peculiar protein (*amyloid*) in the liver and other organs.

The *hepatic porphyrias* are a series of conditions in which the porphyrins, precursors of the hemoglobin molecule, are overproduced and released into the bloodstream. The most severe forms, called *acute intermittent porphyria* and *variegate porphyria*, are characterized by excruciating abdominal pain, involvement of the nerves (sometimes sufficient to cause paralysis), urine which turns dark on exposure to sunlight and sometimes a blistering skin rash. *Porphyria cutanea tarda*, a variant seen in alcoholics, has a skin rash made worse by exposure to light as the primary symptom. All forms of porphyria are inherited diseases causing abnormalities in the enzymes controlling the conversion of porphyrins and porphyrin precursors to heme, the oxygen-binding component of hemoglobin.

Reye's syndrome is an illness (presumably virus induced) of children up to age 15. The symptoms are recurrent vomiting, stupor, seizures and coma. The liver is enlarged and massively infiltrated with fat. Death usually occurs within a few days after onset. The mechanisms of liver and brain damage remain obscure.

11

Diseases of the Urinary Tract

The urinary tract consists of two *kidneys,* two *ureters,* the *bladder* and the *urethra.* The ureters are long tubelike structures connecting each kidney to the bladder while the urethra is the conduit for urine flow from bladder to the external environment. The male urethra passes through the penis and thus is considerably longer than its female counterpart which travels only a short distance before opening just above the vaginal vault. This anatomical relationship is important in the increased prevalence of bladder infections in women. The male urethra passes through the prostate gland,[1] an accessory organ of male reproduction, as it leaves the bladder on its way to the penis. Enlargement of the prostate, a common affliction in older men, constricts the urethra and obstructs urine flow. Because of these close anatomical relationships, the lower excretory system is often called the *genitourinary tract.* The kidneys carry out the primary chemical duties of the excretory system while the ureters, bladder and urethra have only mechanical ("plumbing") and storage functions. The entire excretory system is *retroperitoneal,* meaning that it lies posteriorly in the body, separated from the abdominal organs by the peritoneal membrane that

---

[1] The prostate produces fluids for transport of sperm in the semen. Sperm are made in the testes, passing through a tubular system (epididymus, vas deferens, seminal vesicles and ejaculatory ducts) to enter the urethra at the time of orgasmic ejaculation. Prostatic fluids enter the urethra as it passes through the gland (via the prostatic ducts). It is this fluid that accounts for continued ejaculation at orgasm in men who have been sterilized by *vasectomy* (surgical interruption of the vas deferens).

lines the abdominal cavity proper. This accounts for the fact that kidney pain is felt primarily in the back and that the surgical approach to the kidneys is usually from the posterior flank.[2]

The microstructure of the kidney can be described as follows. Blood passes in through the renal artery which breaks up into increasingly smaller branches that end in a tuft of threadlike capillaries surrounded by a membrane that forms the beginning of the *renal tubule*. The capillary structure and its surrounding capsule are called the *glomerulus;* in shape it looks like a boll of cotton at the end of its stem. Fluid filtering out of the capillaries passes into the funnel-like opening of the tubule for its long journey to the collecting system. Each kidney contains about one million of the glomerular-tubular units (*nephrons*). Multiple tubules converge into one of several *renal papillae* which drain into the central collecting system (the *renal pelvis*). From the pelvis urine passes into the ureters for transport to the bladder. Normally about 100 milliliters of fluid a minute pass from the glomeruli into the tubules (144 liters a day!), but most of this is reabsorbed so that only about 1 or 1.5 liters of urine are produced in a 24-hour period. The glomerular filtrate is essentially identical to plasma except that it contains no cells and normally almost no protein. During passage through the tubule, needed body constituents are reabsorbed leaving the final urine a solution of waste products mixed with excess salts and other chemicals ingested in the diet.

Kidney functions can be divided into four large areas: (1) control of the volume and composition of body fluids; (2) regulation of acid-base balance in the body; (3) excretion of waste products and toxic materials; and (4) the production of hormones. Body fluid volume is normally maintained at a constant level by the coordinated activity of a thirst center located in the brain stem (which signals the need or absence of need for water intake) and the kidneys, which can vary urine volume over a wide range. An important mediator of the volume of urine produced is *antidiuretic hormone* (also called *ADH* or *vasopressin*) which is released by the pituitary gland. If the body needs fluid, antidiuretic hormone is produced and water is avidly reabsorbed by the renal tubule. With water excess ADH release

[2] Externally the position of the kidneys is marked by the junction of the lower ribs with the vertebral column (the *costovertebral angle*).

is inhibited, water reabsorption by the kidney is blunted and urine output becomes large.[3] Normally body fluid composition and volume is maintained within a narrow range, but disease, stressful environmental conditions and powerful drugs used in therapy may overwhelm the kidney's capacity to compensate.[4]

Most lay persons are unfamiliar with the concept of acid-base balance. Normally the body makes strong acids continually from the breakdown of foods and body tissues. Primary protection against these acids is provided by sodium bicarbonate present in the blood. In a process called *buffering*, strong acids (such as phosphoric and sulfuric acids) are converted to a weak acid (carbonic acid) by reaction with bicarbonate (which is a *base*). The carbonic acid can then either be excreted by the kidney or converted to carbon dioxide for expiration by the lungs.[5] The primary role of the kidney in acid-base balance is to maintain plasma bicarbonate levels in the normal range. If too much acid is present in the body, the subject is said to have *acidosis;* if there is too much base the term is *alkalosis.*[6] In

[3] Alcohol is a potent inhibitor of ADH release. Persons who drink large amounts of alcohol urinate excessively partially because fluid intake is high and partially because antidiuretic hormone is inhibited.

[4] Disturbances of body fluids may involve volume or concentration. These fluids are water solutions containing sodium and potassium salts as their major constituents. If the concentration of salts is normal, fluids are said to be *isotonic*. If a water deficit occurs such that salt content in body fluids rises as volume shrinks, the patient is described as *dehydrated* and body fluids are *hypertonic*. (A clinical example is a person working under a hot sun with no access to water.) If the total volume of fluid in the body is less than needed but its composition is normal (i.e., water and salts have been lost proportionately) the subject is said to be *volume depleted*. (Common causes are vomiting, diarrhea or use of diuretic drugs.) If body fluids are present in excess but composition is normal, then *edema* is the descriptive term. (Clinical examples are heart failure and kidney failure.) If salt content of body fluids is diluted by excess water, the patient is said to be *hypotonic* or *water intoxicated*. (Examples include abnormal or inappropriate release of ADH and a form of anxiety neurosis called *pathologic water drinking*.)

[5] An illustration of the buffering reaction, using phosphoric acid as the strong acid, is as follows:

(a) $\quad$ H_3PO_4 $\quad$ + $\quad$ $2NaHCO_3$ $\quad$ $\rightarrow$ $\quad$ Na_2HPO_4 $\quad$ + $\quad$ $2H_2CO_3$
$\quad\quad$ (phosphoric acid) $\quad\quad$ (sodium $\quad\quad\quad\quad$ (sodium $\quad\quad\quad$ (carbonic acid)
$\quad\quad\quad\quad\quad\quad\quad\quad\quad\quad\quad$ bicarbonate) $\quad\quad\quad$ phosphate)

(b) $\quad$ $2H_2CO_3$ $\quad$ $\rightarrow$ $\quad$ $2CO_2$ $\quad$ + $\quad$ $2H_2O$
$\quad\quad$ (carbonic acid) $\quad\quad$ (carbon dioxide) $\quad\quad$ (water)

[6] The acid-base state is assessed by measuring the acidity (hydrogen ion concentration or *pH*) of blood. The pH depends on the ratio of carbonic acid to bicarbonate content ($H_2CO_3:NaHCO_3$), which is normally about $\frac{1}{20}$. If carbonic acid is increased relative to bicarbonate, *acidosis* is present; if bicarbonate is increased relative to carbonic acid, *alkalosis* exists. Carbonic acid content is controlled by the lungs. If carbon

acidosis bicarbonate reabsorption is maximized while in alkalosis the response is a loss of bicarbonate in the urine; the kidneys thus play a protective role in both acidosis and alkalosis.

The body has essentially two ways to dispose of toxic and waste materials. The first is through the intestine (via bile) and the second is through the kidneys. Most water-soluble materials utilize the latter route. As a consequence kidney disease is accompanied by accumulation in the blood of the waste products of body metabolism. The same is true of external materials such as drugs that ordinarily would be removed by excretion in the urine.

Three major hormones are synthesized and released into the bloodstream by the kidney: *erythropoietin, renin* and *1,25-dihydroxycholecalciferol.* Deficiency of *erythropoietin* (which normally stimulates the bone marrow to make red blood cells) is associated with anemia, a common feature of renal (kidney) failure. The hormone may also be produced in excess amounts by cancers of the kidney, resulting in overproduction of red blood cells (*polycythemia*). *Renin* is a hormone that functions in the regulation of blood pressure. Its production is increased when the blood supply to the kidney is impaired and causes the high blood pressure that occurs with disease of the renal arteries. Renin also stimulates the production of *aldosterone,* the major salt-retaining hormone released from the adrenal gland and thereby indirectly regulates salt content in the body. *1,25-dihydroxycholecalciferol* is a metabolite of vitamin D that is necessary for the absorption of calcium and phosphorus from the intestine. The biochemistry of vitamin D is complicated. When taken in the diet it passes first to the liver where it is converted to 25-hydroxycholecalciferol. The latter is then transported to the kidney where the 1,25-derivative is formed. In renal failure, 1,25-dihydroxycholecalciferol formation is decreased, calcium absorption in the gut is impaired and calcium

---

dioxide is breathed off rapidly, carbonic acid content falls because of increased conversion to CO_2 according to equation (b) in footnote 5. Underventilation increases carbonic acid levels. Bicarbonate is under control of the kidneys. Four major types of acid-base disturbance are recognized: *metabolic acidosis* (the accumulation of strong acids, as in kidney failure), *metabolic alkalosis* (the accumulation of bicarbonate, as in the ingestion of sodium bicarbonate), *respiratory acidosis* (the accumulation of CO_2 and thus carbonic acid, because of lung disease) and *respiratory alkalosis* (low CO_2 levels due to hyperventilation, as in anxiety neurosis).

levels in the blood fall. The parathyroid gland then releases parathyroid hormone in an attempt to compensate by mobilizing calcium from bone. This process results in the extensive demineralization of the skeleton that occurs in advanced renal failure.

DIAGNOSTIC TESTS

Urinalysis. The simplest of the diagnostic tests for renal disease is the routine urinalysis. There are several components to the examination. All urines are tested for *protein* and *glucose*, neither of which should be present. The former usually indicates kidney disease, especially of the glomerulus, while the latter suggests diabetes. The *specific gravity* or *osmolality* is a measure of the kidney's ability to concentrate the urine. Dilute urine may be a sign of intrinsic renal disease, absence of antidiuretic hormone or simply excess water intake. The *acidity* (*pH*) is also routinely measured but is not as important as other aspects. Finally, *microscopic examination* is carried out. The presence of white blood cells is indicative of infection in the bladder or kidneys while red blood cells may occur with bladder infections, kidney stones, cancer of the urinary tract (bladder or kidney) or glomerular disease.[7] *Casts* are cylindrical molds of the tubules that appear with protein leakage; they may contain red or white blood cells or have a granular appearance. They usually indicate serious renal disease.

Other tests done on the urine include bacteriological culture when infection is suspected and literally hundreds of chemical measurements for diagnostic purposes: hormones, drugs, electrolytes, etc. In many cases 24-hour collections are required to quantitate the daily output of the tested material.

Renal Function Tests. The two most common tests of renal function are measurement of blood levels of *urea nitrogen* (*BUN*) and *creatinine*. Both of these materials accumulate in the blood as renal function decreases. When elevated the patient is said to have *azotemia*. The BUN (which is derived from protein breakdown) may be influenced by the amount of pro-

---

[7] Red blood cells may appear normally in the urine of menstruating women because of admixture of urine and menstrual discharge.

tein in the diet and other factors while the creatinine is specific for kidney function.[8] Plasma creatinine concentration usually does not rise until significant loss of renal function has occurred. For this reason a test called *creatinine clearance* is often done. In this test the total amount of creatinine in a 24-hour sample of urine is divided by the plasma creatinine concentration as an estimate of the amount of plasma that is filtered (cleared) per minute by the glomerulus (normal value, about 120 milliliters per minute). Since clearance falls before a rise in plasma concentration of creatinine occurs, it is a more sensitive test of renal function.

X-ray Procedures. The most common X-ray procedure for kidney disease is the *intravenous pyelogram.* A radiopaque dye that is excreted by the kidney is injected intravenously and serial films are taken; both structure and function of the kidneys can be estimated by the technique. In *retrograde pyelography,* which is used much less commonly, the dye is injected directly into the ureters through an instrument (*cystoscope*) placed in the bladder. *Arteriography* is done when renal vascular disease or cancer is suspected.

Sonography. Sonography is a useful tool for determining kidney size, identifying renal masses (including cysts) and delineating abscesses.

Cystoscopy. The cystoscope is used for direct visualization of the bladder lining when bleeding into the urinary tract is present. The instrument is similar to the endoscopes described in earlier chapters but is adapted to the small size of the urethra through which it is inserted. Its major diagnostic use is in bladder cancer.

Biopsy. Needle biopsy of the kidneys and prostate are done in order to obtain tissue for diagnostic purposes. The procedure is similar to the technique used for liver biopsy.

Renal Vein Catheterization. When it is suspected that high blood pressure may be due to renal vascular disease, it is sometimes necessary to get venous blood directly from the renal vein

[8] Both tests may be elevated in the absence of renal disease when a patient is severely dehydrated, volume depleted or in shock. This is due to the fact that blood is shunted away from the kidneys to more vital organs (e.g., brain and heart) whenever circulation is impaired. The kidney excretes any creatinine or BUN reaching it, but because of diminished blood flow, the waste materials do not arrive at the glomerulus. Accumulation of BUN and creatinine due to circulatory deficiency is called *prerenal azotemia,* indicating that the problem is not in the kidney itself.

for measurement of renin levels. This is done by passing a catheter through a peripheral vein into the renal vein under fluoroscopic control.

INFECTIONS

Infections of the urinary tract are extremely common, especially in women. Men only rarely develop infections spontaneously. The infecting organisms are almost always bacteria that inhabit the large intestine. Such organisms intermittently contaminate the skin surrounding the anus (*perineum*) at the time of defecation. They can migrate spontaneously to the genital region but more commonly are spread by toilet tissue or genital contact during sexual intercourse.[9] The bacteria enter the bladder through the urethra, which is much closer to the anus in women than in men. Bacteria may also be introduced as a complication of medical instrumentation such as catheterization or cystoscopy. In persons with paralyzed or obstructed bladders requiring constant indwelling bladder catheters, infection is extremely common; experiments have shown that bacteria on the skin around the anus migrate on the catheter almost like it was a highway. Other predisposing factors include pregnancy, obstruction to urine flow (as by prostatic enlargement or postgonococcal scarring of the urethra) and congenital structural abnormalities of the urinary tract in children.

Three types of urinary tract infection are recognized. *Cystitis* refers to infection localized to the bladder. *Pyelonephritis* means that the bacteria have moved from the bladder up the ureters to infect the kidneys. *Nephric or perinephric abscesses* are localized collections of pus in the kidney or immediately adjacent to it. In contrast to cystitis and pyelonephritis, abscesses are usually not due to colon bacteria but are caused by staphylococci and other organisms that arrive by the bloodstream rather than through the ureters.

---

[9] *Honeymoon cystitis,* a loose term frequently used by physicians, refers to the frequent appearance of lower urinary tract infection following initial sexual activity after marriage. In a day where a high percentage of young persons have sexual experience prior to marriage, the "honeymoon" appellation is probably no longer appropriate, though intercourse-related cystitis remains a common problem. It can be largely avoided by carefully washing the perineum and genital areas with soap and water prior to coitus.

Cystitis. Infection of the urinary bladder produces local symptoms without (or with minimal) fever or systemic complaints. *Urinary frequency* is increased, and there is a sense of *urgency* as though urination cannot be prevented (even though volumes are small). A stinging or burning sensation (*dysuria*) is present as the urine is passed, and aching pain may be felt above the pelvic bone immediately after completing the act. The urine may be *bloody* during the acute phases; red and white blood cells are seen on microscopic examination.

Pyelonephritis. Acute pyelonephritis is characterized by *fever, chills, pain in the flanks or back, nausea, vomiting, frequency of urination and dysuria.* On examination pressure or percussion over the costovertebral areas produces or worsens the pain. Diagnosis is made by examination of the urine (which shows many white blood cells and bacteria); confirmation requires a positive urine culture.[10] Patients with pyelonephritis are much sicker than those with cystitis and frequently require hospitalization. *Papillary necrosis* is a dangerous complication of pyelonephritis occurring in persons who have underlying disease of the renal papillae. Patients with diabetes, sickle cell anemia, chronic alcoholism and vascular disease of the kidney appear to be peculiarly susceptible. Papillary necrosis is suspected whenever renal function suddenly deteriorates in a patient with signs of acute pyelonephritis (which by itself does not cause loss of function). The papillae may actually sluff off and be recovered as bits of tissue in the urine.

Nephric and Perinephric Abscesses. Abscesses are heralded by the abrupt onset of *chills, fever* and *unilateral flank tenderness.* Frequency of urination and dysuria are absent. Examination of the urine shows bacteria but no white blood cells. Perinephric abscesses often cause elevation of the diaphragm on the affected side, frequently with a pleural effusion. Sonography is helpful in making the diagnosis.

Treatment. The treatment of cystitis and pyelonephritis is antibiotics chosen on the basis of culture results. Pending report of culture and antibiotic sensitivity (which require 48 hours), a drug known to be effective against colonic bacteria is given. The drug is changed if culture shows the offending or-

---

[10] Most hospitals now do quantitative cultures. If urinary tract infection is present, more than 100,000 organisms will be found per milliliter of urine.

ganism to be resistant. Sulfonamides, tetracycline and ampicillin are frequently used in initial management. Antibiotics are also given for abscesses, but surgical drainage is usually required.

GLOMERULONEPHRITIS

Glomerulonephritis is a general term describing a type of disease in the kidney in which the primary pathologic abnormalities are found in the glomerulus (filtering unit). Acute forms are characterized by *bloody or tea-colored urine,*[11] *edema, high blood pressure* and, in some cases, *heart failure.* The edema may cause swelling or puffiness around the eyes and in the hands as well as in the legs, a distribution that is unusual in edema due to heart failure or cirrhosis. Some patients develop the *nephrotic syndrome* (see page 223). Subacute or chronic forms may be manifested by progressive loss of kidney function without ever passing through a stage of gross hematuria.

Glomerulonephritis can be produced by a variety of mechanisms which usually can be differentiated only by microscopic examination of tissue obtained by needle biopsy. The major types are *poststreptococcal glomerulonephritis, nonstreptococcal immune glomerulonephritis, hereditary nephritis* and the *nephrotic syndrome.*

Poststreptococcal Glomerulonephritis. This form of glomerulonephritis appears 2–3 weeks following an acute streptococcal infection of throat or skin. It is usually a disease of children and young adults. In contrast to rheumatic fever, which can be caused by many subtypes of streptococci, only a few streptococci (*nephritogenic strains*) cause glomerulonephritis. The kidney damage is thought to be due to the formation of antibodies to the streptococcus. These antibodies bind to bacterial antigens, forming what are called *immune complexes.* The immune complexes become trapped in the glomerulus and initiate the inflammatory reaction that causes tissue damage. Recovery

[11] The brown color is due to hemoglobin released by rupture of red blood cells; its normal red color is changed to brown by acid in the urine. If the concentration of the urine and its acidity is such that red cells do not lyse or hemoglobin is not altered, the urine will be red. In some patients the urine will remain clear although red blood cells are identified by microscopic examination.

is usually complete, although some adults apparently develop progressive disease leading to a form of chronic glomerulonephritis that eventuates in renal failure. No specific treatment is available; therapeutic efforts focus on controlling edema, hypertension and heart failure until recovery occurs. Adequate treatment of streptococcal infections with penicillin prevents the illness.

Nonstreptococcal Immune Glomerulonephritis. Immune-complex glomerulonephritis also develops in patients who have not had a streptococcal infection. Known causes include *viruses, vaccines, drugs* and *systemic diseases* such as lupus erythematosus and subacute bacterial endocarditis. Many cases appear spontaneously, however, and are thought to be *autoimmune* in origin: for one reason or another antigens from the person's own tissues induce an antibody response resulting in immune-complex formation and glomerulonephritis. Three subgroups are recognized on microscopic examination: *membranous, membrano-proliferative* and *proliferative.* The only importance is that the prognosis (which may include complete recovery) is much better in the membranous form.

A devastating variant of immune glomerulonephritis is *Goodpasture's syndrome.* This disease is not due to immune complexes but to antibodies that directly attack both glomeruli and lung tissue. In addition to glomerulonephritis, the patients have massive pulmonary hemorrhages. The coughing of blood may be severe enough to cause death either by asphyxiation or exsanguination. Treatment is not satisfactory although removal of both kidneys seems to slow pulmonary hemorrhage in some cases. Chronic dialysis is then required to sustain life.

Hereditary Nephritis (Alport's Syndrome). This form of glomerulonephritis is familial and is transmitted as an autosomal dominant trait. The kidney disease may appear in isolation but is often associated with *congenital deafness, cataracts or abnormalities of the cornea and retina.* Males are more seriously affected than females for reasons that are not clear. The disease is progressive and renal failure usually appears before the age of 40.

Nephrotic Syndrome. The nephrotic syndrome is a specific constellation of findings consisting of *massive protein loss in the urine, low plasma albumin concentrations* (due to urinary protein loss), *extensive generalized edema and elevations of the cholesterol content of blood.* It may appear as a phase of any of the glomerulonephritic diseases and in association with a wide variety of other conditions varying from bee stings to diabetes mellitus. A common form of the disease occurring in children is called *lipoid nephrosis.* Its recognition is important because recovery is usual in contrast to other forms. The cause of the nephrotic syndrome is sometimes difficult to ascertain, even with renal biopsy. Prednisone therapy is helpful in lipoid nephrosis and is often tried in other forms as well, although success is less frequent. Other immunosuppressive chemotherapeutic agents are sometimes used in patients who fail to respond to steroids.

OBSTRUCTIVE UROPATHY

Mechanical obstruction to urine flow can occur at any site in the urinary tract. *Urethral obstruction* in men is most commonly due to prostatic enlargement. Urethral strictures (due to venereal disease, congenital abnormalities or surgical procedures) and urethral cancers occur in both sexes. *Obstruction in the ureters* (unilateral or bilateral) can be caused by kidney stones, cancer, congenital narrowing and a peculiar disease called *retroperitoneal fibrosis* in which dense scar formation surrounds and occludes ureters, blood vessels and other structures. The cause of the latter is unknown in most cases, although methysergide, a drug given for migraine headache, produces the illness in some patients. Finally, ureters (unfortunately) are sometimes tied off accidentally during pelvic surgery such as hysterectomy or tubal ligation.

Because pressure builds up behind the obstruction, dilatation of the urinary tract occurs above the block. In urethral obstruction the bladder may be felt extending above the navel.[12] Retrograde transmission of pressure to the kidneys causes them to dilate and enlarge (a condition called *hydronephrosis*). If the pressure is unrelieved, urine production stops.

Diagnosis of obstructive uropathy is made by intravenous and retrograde pyelography coupled with sonography. Treatment

---

[12] The bladder may also be dilated due to loss of its nerve supply in diseases such as multiple sclerosis, diabetes, tabes dorsalis (a form of late syphilis) and spinal cord injury.

obviously requires removal of the obstruction. This is accomplished temporarily by passage of a small urethral or ureteral catheter, but ultimately surgery is usually necessary. Cancerous obstruction often requires a bypass procedure in which the ureters are transected above the block and implanted in the sigmoid colon such that urinary waste products pass out in the stool. Treatment of prostatic obstruction and kidney stones, perhaps the two most common causes of obstructive disease in the urethra and ureters, respectively, is covered in the following sections.

Prostatic Disease. There are three common diseases of the prostate: *benign prostatic hypertrophy, cancer of the prostate* and *prostatitis.* They cause obstructive symptoms in decreasing order of frequency. *Benign prostatic hypertrophy* is a condition of aging; it appears to be due to an accumulation of a male sex hormone (*dihydrotestosterone*) in the prostate. Overgrowth of the gland begins centrally, occluding the urethra and pushing the normal prostatic tissue to the periphery. The primary symptom is difficulty in starting urine flow. Additional problems include decreased projectile force and narrowing of the stream of urine, frequency, involuntary dribbling following completion of the urinary act and a sense of incomplete emptying of the bladder. *Cancer* of the prostate is extremely common in older men, reaching an incidence of up to 60 percent beyond the age of 80. Most of the tumors arise posteriorly where they can be felt as a distinct hard nodule on rectal examination. The cancer may be localized and asymptomatic, grow to cause obstructive symptoms or produce pain by spread to bone, especially in the lower spine. Diagnosis can be made by needle biopsy of the nodule. An additional clue that cancer is present is elevation of the enzyme *acid phosphatase* in blood. The third disease, *prostatitis,* generally affects young men but may also occur in older subjects. It is characterized by high fever, often with chills, painful, frequent urination and a tender prostate on rectal examination.

Prostatitis is treated by antibiotics; if abscess formation occurs, surgical drainage is required. Therapy of prostatic hypertrophy is carried out with a form of surgery called *transurethral resection (TUR).* An instrument is passed through the urethra, and the prostatic mass is cut away without the necessity of external surgical incision. Localized cancer is treated by total surgical prostatectomy after which X-ray therapy is given to the prostatic bed. If the tumor has spread locally or systemically, female hormones (*estrogens*) are administered and the testes are removed (*orchiectomy*). Orchiectomy is designed to prevent testicular release of the male sex hormones that promote tumor growth, and estrogens are given to neutralize the small amount of male hormones produced by the adrenal glands. Painful metastatic areas can often be relieved by additional X-ray treatment. Even with distant metastases prolonged survival is possible.

Kidney Stones. The primary symptom of a kidney stone is severe (often excruciating) *pain* in the back or flank which radiates to the lower abdomen, genital region or inner thigh. The pain tends to be colicky or crampy in nature and may be associated with *hematuria*. Some stones pass spontaneously while others become impacted in the ureters causing obstruction and requiring surgical removal. The most important issue in stone formers is determination of the underlying disorder predisposing to their formation. *Calcium-containing stones* may result from hyperparathyroidism, increased calcium absorption in the gastrointestinal tract or increased excretion of calcium in the urine. Gout causes *uric acid stones* and the rare inherited diseases called cystinuria and primary oxaluria result in *cystine-* and *oxalate-containing stones* respectively. Oxalate stones also occur after intestinal bypass surgery for obesity and in extensive small bowel disease such as regional ileitis. When the primary diseases are treated, stone formation ceases or at least occurs with decreased frequency. Specific forms of therapy will not be discussed, but effective treatment is available in almost every case, regardless of etiology.

RENAL FAILURE

In one sense renal failure can be said to be present whenever tests of kidney function become abnormal (elevation of the BUN or creatinine) even if the patient is asymptomatic. Generally, however, the term is reserved for the clinical picture that results when damage to the kidney becomes severe enough to produce symptoms. The composite clinical picture produced by renal failure is called *uremia*. Renal failure is divided into two categories: *acute* and *chronic. Acute renal failure* refers to the sudden appearance of *oliguria* (decreased urine output) or *anuria* (absent urine output) in a patient who previously did not have kidney disease. If the patient can be kept alive during the period of renal shutdown, recovery will occur. *Chronic renal failure* is the consequence of ongoing destructive disease in the kidney and usually appears in slowly progressive fashion. Occasionally a rapid period of deterioration may mimic acute renal failure.

Acute Renal Failure. The common denominator in the development of acute renal failure (sometimes called *acute tubular necrosis*) is collapse of the circulation. When shock develops for any cause, intense constriction of the blood vessels leading to the kidney causes patchy destruction of cells in the renal tubule effectively converting it into a sieve; fluid filtered at the glomerulus thus "backleaks" into the circulation rather than reaching the ureter for excretion.[13] If the patient can be brought through the illness that caused the shock in the first place and survives the complications of renal failure, repair of the tubules occurs and urine output resumes. The causes of acute renal failure are as numerous as the diseases that cause shock, but the most common precipitating events are *trauma* (particularly with crush injuries), *hemorrhage, surgery, septicemia* (invasion of the bloodstream by bacteria), *incompatible blood transfusions, large-scale burns* and the *ingestion of toxic chemicals or drugs.*

The syndrome is heralded by a fall in urine output;[14] the urine may be clear or bloody. *Loss of appetite, nausea* and *vomiting* are almost invariable. There is fluid retention resulting in *edema* and the *blood pressure rises.* Because of the increased blood pressure and fluid overload, *heart failure* is common. As waste products accumulate in the blood, the patient becomes *confused, somnolent* or even *comatose. Convul-*

---

[13] This is a vastly oversimplified description of the problem; the exact sequence by which anuria is produced is still a matter of debate, but the interpretation given is one acceptable view of the process.

[14] The most important differentiation that has to be made is between *acute renal failure* due to kidney damage and *prerenal azotemia* due to volume depletion or dehydration where oliguria occurs because the kidney absorbs the bulk of filtered fluid in an attempt to repair the fluid deficit. One clue is that the sodium content of the urine is extremely low in prerenal azotemia but not in acute tubular necrosis. Urine output rapidly returns in prerenal states when intravenous fluids are given.

sions are not unusual. The most dangerous chemical abnormality is a *rise in the potassium concentration of the blood* (potassium is normally excreted in the urine). High potassium levels cause cardiac standstill: the heart simply stops beating. During the period of renal failure, patients are *vulnerable to infection* and may die from that complication.

Treatment consists of limiting fluid intake, restriction of dietary protein (since protein is a source of potassium and will also increase the level of the BUN) and prevention of hyperkalemia by administration of potassium-binding agents (*chelators*) by mouth or enema. Infection and heart failure are treated aggressively. If recovery is delayed or potassium levels cannot be controlled, peritoneal or hemodialysis (see page 229) is initiated until the kidneys begin to function again. During recovery urine output is very large for a period of 1 to 3 weeks (the *diuretic phase*). With the availability of dialysis, it is expected that essentially all patients surviving the precipitating event will recover.

Chronic Renal Failure. Chronic renal failure rarely results in anuria. Even in the advanced stages urine flows of 150–500 milliliters a day may be maintained. As in acute renal failure, *fluid retention, hypertension, heart failure* and *altered central nervous system function* are present. The skin has a sallow appearance and in the final days may be covered with powdery white crystals of urea (*uremic frost*) as urea-containing sweat evaporates. *Anemia* is a major problem and is due both to decreased red cell production (because of erythropoietin deficiency) and an increased red cell fragility resulting in the accelerated rates of destruction. One of the most distressing complications is a *bleeding tendency* due to impairment of platelet function. Bruising of the skin, oozing of blood from around the teeth, nosebleeds and hemorrhage into the gastrointestinal tract often result. Persistent *hiccuping* may interfere with rest and eating. Failure to form 1,25-dihydroxycholecalciferol (active vitamin D) results in *dissolution of bone* and predisposes to pathologic fractures. Some patients develop a *peripheral neuropathy* with numbness, tingling and pain in the extremities; muscle weakness or frank paralysis may result. *Pericarditis* (see chapter 6) may cause chest pain, and occasionally bleeding into the pericardial sac produces sudden death. The accumulation of acid waste products causes a *metabolic aci-*

dosis with rapid respiration. *Potassium retention,* as in acute renal failure, is a continual threat.

Patients with chronic renal failure are treated with low-protein diets designed to be of high biologic value; that is, to contain proteins rich in essential amino acids (see chapter 2). An alkalinizing solution (*Shohl's solution*) is often given to combat the acidosis. Antacids are prescribed in an attempt to prevent ulcer formation and to diminish phosphorus absorption (phosphorus levels in the blood rise in uremia). These measures are ancillary to definitive treatment which requires either chronic dialysis or transplantation of a kidney.

Dialysis. In the absence of kidney function, waste products can be removed from the body by exposing blood to solutions that are free of the noxious materials (*dialysis*). Under these circumstances the chemical toxins pass from the solution of high concentration (blood) to that of low concentration (the dialysis fluid). Two techniques are available. In *peritoneal dialysis* a catheter is placed through the abdominal wall, and dialysis fluid is run into the peritoneal cavity. The exchange is between capillaries in the peritoneum and the infused fluid which remains in the abdominal cavity. After equilibration (usually about an hour) the fluid is removed and replaced by a fresh volume. Ordinarily the process is repeated 30–40 times. Peritoneal dialysis is usually used for short-term dialysis. Its major advantage is that no complicated equipment is required. *Hemodialysis* requires use of a dialysis machine (*artificial kidney*). It is required for all long-term dialysis and is preferred by many kidney specialists even for short periods, as in acute renal failure. Basically the technique involves passing blood from the patient through a coil of semipermeable tubing exposed to dialysis fluid. Access to the patient's blood is achieved by surgically grafting a bovine blood vessel between a major artery and vein in the arm to produce a high flow *fistula*. At the time of dialysis the fistula is entered by two needles placed through the skin, one carrying blood to the instrument, the other serving as the return. Treatments are usually carried out 3 times weekly and last for 4 to 8 hours, depending on the instrument used. Dialysis is often done in special centers, but intelligent, highly motivated families can be trained to carry out the procedure at home. Chronic dialysis is remarkably successful, and a high percentage of patients can be treated essentially indefinitely, living a normal life except for the treatment periods. The psychological effects resulting from being dependent on a machine for sustenance of life have been far less than originally predicted.

Transplantation. The ideal form of treatment for chronic renal failure is transplantation of a functioning kidney to replace the nonfunctional organ. Successful transplantation has now been achieved in thousands of patients. Since each person has two kidneys but only one is required to maintain normal body function, living donors can be used in contrast to transplantation of single organs like heart and liver. Often, therefore, the donor of the kidney is a living first-degree relative of the patient (parent or sibling). In cases where a living donor is not available, cadaver kidneys are used. Every attempt is made to procure such organs from accident victims or other persons whose heart and lungs are still functioning with the help of artificial support systems but whose electroencephalogram shows brain death.[15] Following removal kidneys are preserved on special perfusion instruments until transplanted. A nationwide exchange system exists for transfer of kidneys between transplant centers.

The techniques for grafting the foreign kidney into the host are now well worked out and surgery itself is not a problem. The difficulty is that the kidney is foreign to the recipient's body and will be rejected by the host's immune system unless that system is blocked. Several techniques are utilized in an attempt to minimize the rejection process. Tissue typing is now possible and allows selection of a donor whose genetic makeup appears relatively compatible with the recipient.[16] While typing techniques are far from perfect, advances continue to be made. The immune system is suppressed by the administration of prednisone in combination with azathioprine or cyclophosphamide.[17] High doses are used initially and then gradually

[15] The slogan seen on many bumper stickers, "Don't bury kidneys, transplant them" emphasizes the fact that the majority of the population has made no arrangement to donate their useful tissues (corneas, skin, kidneys, etc.) to others in the case of sudden death. It seems to me the right and proper thing to do—somehow comforting (ahead of the event) to know that my death may bring life to someone waiting for that gift.

[16] The technique is somewhat analogous to the typing of blood for transfusion but is much more complicated.

[17] Some centers also infuse antilymphocyte globulins (which can be considered a kind of vaccine against the cells that mediate rejection) while others attempt to deplete the body lymphocyte pool by draining lymph, removing the lymphocytes and reinfusing the lymphocyte-free fluid.

tapered to lower levels. Suppression is required throughout the life of the patient. Despite these techniques a significant number of kidneys are rejected and have to be removed. Some are rejected immediately (*hyperacute rejection*) while other rejections occur days to months later. Long-term survival of the transplanted kidney is about 50 percent using cadaver organs and 60–80 percent with a living, related donor. Rejection of one kidney does not preclude subsequent retransplantation.

Side effects of immunosuppression are not trivial. Infections with organisms that do not ordinarily cause disease (*opportunistic infections*) are common and difficult to treat because the immune defense mechanisms are paralyzed. High-dose steroids stunt growth in children and often produce the signs of Cushing's syndrome (chapter 15). The hair may fall out. There is a small but definite increase in the incidence of cancer, reflecting the fact that the immune system ordinarily protects against tumor formation.

CANCER

Cancer can develop at any site in the urinary tract, but the bladder and kidney are most often involved. The initial symptom is often *painless bleeding* into the urine although kidney tumors may manifest themselves only as an *abdominal mass*. This is particularly true for *nephroblastoma (Wilms' tumor)*, the most common renal cancer in children, which may grow so large as to distend the entire abdomen. *Pain in the flank or back* may accompany the mass. *Hypernephroma,* the most frequent form of renal cancer in the adult, often causes *systemic* as well as local symptoms. These include fever and elevation of the white blood cell count in the absence of signs of infection, hypercalcemia, polycythemia (rather than the anemia which is usual with other cancers) and hypoglycemia. Hypernephromas metastasize to lung, bone, liver and brain. (The relationship between renal carcinoma and chromosomal abnormalities is discussed on page 84.)

Hematuria in the absence of signs and symptoms of cystitis should be considered cancer until proven otherwise. The first step is cystoscopy to rule out bladder cancer. Any suspicious lesion is biopsied. Identification of tumors in the kidney requires multiple approaches including intravenous pyelography, arteriography and sonography. Solitary benign cysts of the kidney may be confused with cancer but usually can be differentiated by the techniques just mentioned coupled with needle aspiration. Since cysts are fluid filled while cancers are solid, recovery of fluid strongly suggests a benign lesion. The fluid is also examined microscopically for tumor cells since a tumor may rarely develop in the wall of a cyst.

Treatment is surgical removal of the involved kidney. Irradiation and chemotherapy are utilized in metastatic disease. A high percentage of children with Wilms' tumor, invariably fatal in the past, can now be salvaged using the chemotherapeutic agents actinomycin D and vincristine after surgery.

OTHER DISEASES

The number of pathological processes affecting the kidney is large. Many *systemic diseases* including hypertension, the collagen-vascular diseases, gout, multiple myeloma, amyloidosis, sickle cell anemia, hepatic failure, sarcoidosis and hyperparathyroidism affect the kidney as part of the clinical picture and can cause renal failure. A variety of *drugs* are direct renal toxins. Gentamicin, a widely used antibiotic and phenacetin, a common ingredient in over-the-counter analgesics advertised for headache and pain relief, are classic examples. *Congenital abnormalities* such as single or horseshoe kidneys are not unusual. In the former case one kidney fails to develop and in the latter the two kidneys are fused at the lower pole. Duplication of ureters is not rare. *Hereditary diseases* are also known. The most common is *polycystic kidney disease* in which giant cysts form in the kidneys, compressing and eventually destroying normal renal tissue. The disease is usually easily recognized because the kidneys enlarge to enormous size. Transmission is by autosomal dominant mode. Associated conditions include cysts of the liver and aneurysms of the blood vessels at the base of the brain which rupture and cause death in 10 percent of cases. *Nephrogenic diabetes insipidus* is a disease in which the kidney tubule is unresponsive to the action of antidiuretic hormone. Concentration of the urine is not possible and urine flows are extremely large. The syndrome is identical to that produced by a deficiency of pituitary antidiuretic hormone (*true diabetes insipidus*), but plasma levels of ADH are high and there is no response to exogenously administered hormone. *Renal tubular acidosis* refers to a group of disorders characterized by the inability of the kidney tubule to excrete acid in the urine. The defect may exist in isolation or be accompanied by leakage into the urine of glucose and amino acids. Primary features are metabolic acidosis, low plasma concentrations of potassium, loss of calcium in the urine and a softening of bone similar to rickets. *Vascular diseases* of the kidney may be of several kinds. Narrowing of the renal artery may be congenital or acquired as a result of atherosclerosis. Renal arteries may also be blocked by emboli arising elsewhere in the body. If the arterial supply is impaired, high blood pressure may result due to overproduction of the hormone renin. Sudden complete occlusion of a renal artery by an embolus causes pain on the affected side, hematuria and fever. If both kidneys are involved pain is bilateral and urine formation ceases. Thrombosis of the renal veins, a complication seen in hypernephroma, congestive heart failure and severe dehydration, causes enlargement of the affected kidney, flank pain, hematuria, protein loss in the urine and occasionally the nephrotic syndrome.

12

Diseases of the
Reproductive System

The reproductive system in males consists of *penis* and *testes* while *vagina, uterus* and *ovaries* constitute the female counterpart. The *breasts* are also considered part of the reproductive system since they develop under the same hormonal influences. Anatomically distinct from the primary sex organs are the endocrine glands that control their development and function: the *hypothalamus, pituitary* and *adrenal glands.* The hormones produced by these glands, which operate in response to intricate biological clocks, program the manifestations of normal sexual development during fetal life, initiate sexual maturation at puberty and sustain germ cell function during the reproductive years. A brief review of the normal sequence will set the stage for understanding abnormal function of the system.

The *genetic sex (chromosomal sex)* of an individual is determined at the time of conception: two X chromosomes define a genetic female while the XY combination results in maleness (see chapter 4). Genetic sex (*genotype*) in turn determines *gonadal sex;* the XX genotype leads to development of ovaries while the XY genotype causes testes to appear. Finally, the gonads determine *phenotypic sex,* the outwardly apparent sex indicated by male or female genitalia and body structure. It is quite remarkable that in the absence of gonads phenotypic development is invariably female whether the genetic sex is male or female. Stated another way, unless testosterone (the male sex hormone)[1] is produced by the primitive testes at a critical point in embryonic life (about the 40th day after conception), the penis and scrotum do not develop, and the newborn child will have a vagina instead even when the chromosomal complement is XY. The reasons for this built-in femaleness (which is also independent of estrogens since it occurs despite removal of the ovaries early in fetal life) are not known. Any process interfering with testosterone synthesis in the male or causing androgen production in the female during embryonic life will result in a discrepancy between genetic and phenotypic sex: a genetic male will have the appearance of a female or a genetic female will appear masculinized. The initiation of testosterone synthesis in the male and estrogen synthesis in the female during fetal development is almost certainly under pituitary control.

Following birth hormonal activity is quiescent until the time of puberty. In the immediate prepubertal period, changes occur in the hypothalamus (the specialized area of the brain that controls pituitary hormone release) and the pituitary gland which result in the accelerated release of *luteinizing hormone (LH)* during sleep; subsequently *follicle-stimulating hormone (FSH)* secretion also increases.[2] Under the influence of these hormones, testes and ovaries begin to grow and to produce their respective male and female sex hormones. Two categories of change result. *First,* the secondary (nonreproductive) sexual characteristics develop: growth of the uterus, breasts, pubic (genital) and axillary (underarm) hair in girls; growth of the penis, pubic, axillary and facial hair in boys. In addition body shape and muscle development differentiate into feminine and masculine patterns. *Second,* the reproductive sequence becomes operative. Sperm formation starts in the testes and ovulation is initiated in the ovary. In the female menstrual periods

---

[1] There are a number of sex hormones produced in the body. Female sex hormones go by the generic name *estrogens* while their male counterparts are called *androgens.* Each sex produces both types of hormones normally, but androgens are produced in greater quantities in males while estrogens are predominant in females.

[2] Luteinizing hormone and follicle-stimulating hormone are called *gonadotropins,* signifying that they control growth and function of the gonads (testes and ovaries). They are secreted in response to a hypothalamic hormone called *LH-RH* (luteinizing hormone-releasing hormone). Adrenal hormones play an ancillary (though important) role in the development of secondary sexual characteristics but not in the growth of ovaries or testes.

begin (*menarche*) and continue (unless interrupted by disease) until menopause.[3]

The maturing testis produces testosterone in specialized cells (*Leydig cells*) that are regulated by the action of LH while sperm are manufactured in the *seminiferous tubules* under the influence of FSH. Hormone production and sperm synthesis are essentially constant in the male. In women the picture is much more complicated with wide swings in hormone production occurring cyclically and repetitively throughout the reproductive phase of life. Each month an egg (*ovum*) is produced and each month the uterus is prepared for implantation of that egg should conception take place. The menstrual cycle is usually about 28 to 30 days in length, but normal women may have regular periods at intervals as short as 25 days or as long as 37 days. The menstrual cycle is divided into two phases by *ovulation* (release of the egg) which occurs approximately at the midpoint of each period; the preovulatory interval is designated the *follicular phase* because during this time the follicle (which contains the egg) matures under the influence of pituitary FSH. Increasing amounts of *estradiol* (the primary ovarian estrogen) are produced during this interval. Ordinarily only one of the multitudinous ovarian follicles develops completely each month. How this selection is accomplished remains a mystery. At the time of ovulation, the mature follicle is positioned at the surface of the ovary and ruptures to the outside, releasing the egg into the mouth of the adjacent fallopian tube which then transports it to the uterus.[4] Ovulation appears to be induced by an abrupt surge in LH and FSH release from the pituitary immediately prior to the event. That portion of the follicle remain-

---

[3] The changes of puberty do not occur simultaneously. In girls the first change is usually breast development which ordinarily starts at about the age of 8 to 10 but may not occur in normal subjects until the early teens. Breast enlargement usually precedes the appearance of pubic hair by a few months, but occasionally the sequence is reversed. Menarche begins, on average, between 12 and 13 years of age. However, it is now thought that attainment of a critical body weight (about 48 kilograms or 106 pounds) is more important than chronological age. The later stages of puberty are accompanied by accelerated growth and development of a female body contour.

In males puberty begins a year or two later than in females; the initial events are an increase in the size of penis, testes and prostate gland. The scrotal skin becomes wrinkled and pigmented, following which pubic and axillary hair appear. Body growth then accelerates (the rate of increase peaking on average about 15½ years), muscles develop, shoulders broaden, the voice deepens and beard and body hair appear. Final sexual development in the male may not be complete until the mid-twenties.

[4] Ovulation is often signaled by a brief episode of abdominal pain (*mittelschmerz*). It is also associated with a rise in body temperature, which is the basis of the rhythm method of planning pregnancies.

ing in the ovary after release of the ovum becomes the *corpus luteum* and directs the second half of the cycle which is called the *luteal phase*. In the luteal phase a second ovarian hormone, *progesterone*, is produced. If pregnancy does not occur, the corpus luteum begins to degenerate after about 8–10 days, estradiol and progesterone secretion fall and, approximately 14 days after ovulation, menstruation ensues. The actual mechanism is a sloughing of the lining of the uterus (*endometrium*) as a consequence of hormone withdrawal.[5] Rupture of small blood vessels accounts for the bleeding.

From this brief description it follows that disturbances in hormone production or action can result in a variety of abnormalities. Manifestations include *anatomic defects; delayed, absent or precocious puberty; amenorrhea* (the absence of menstrual periods); *discordant sexual development* (masculinization in the female, feminization in the male) and *infertility*. In addition, the reproductive system, like all other organ systems, is subject to *infection* and development of *cancer*. Finally, since sexual function is dependent not only on an intact sexual apparatus but also on a healthy psyche, dysfunctional states such as *impotence* and *frigidity* may occur even when no physical disease is present.

Diagnostic Tests

Endocrine Function Tests. The most important type of test done in working up disease of the reproductive system is the measurement of the various hormones involved in regulating ovarian and testicular function. Extremely sensitive radioimmunoassays are now available in most hospitals for the assay of the gonadotropins (*luteinizing hormone, follicle-stimulating hormone*), male (*testosterone, dihydrotestosterone*) and female (*estradiol, estrone*) sex hormones and *prolactin*. The latter hormone is produced by the pituitary gland and is responsible for

[5] During the follicular phase, estradiol causes growth and thickening of the endometrium preparatory to receiving the fertilized egg. In the luteal phase glands in the endometrium increase in size and complexity, and blood vessels proliferate to provide the nourishing function required at fetal implantation. Hormone withdrawal leads to spasm of the endometrial (*spiral*) arteries, causing the lining cells to die and separate from the uterine wall. If conception occurs the corpus luteum is maintained ("rescued") by gonadotropins (*chorionic gonadotropin, HCG*) produced in the placenta. Ovarian hormone production continues and the endometrium remains healthy and intact.

milk production by the breast during pregnancy. It has become very important as a marker of small pituitary tumors that cause milk production and amenorrhea in nonpregnant women. Adrenal and thyroid hormones are also often measured since dysfunction of these glands can affect the reproductive system.

Biopsies. A nonsurgical form of biopsy is the familiar *Papanicolaou smear* for cervical cancer. The cervix and uterus can also be biopsied directly. *Dilatation* and *curettage* (D & C) is a common procedure utilized in abnormal uterine bleeding. The uterus is mechanically dilated and portions of the endometrium are removed for diagnostic purposes. *Testicular* and *ovarian biopsies* are obtained less frequently but are important in certain conditions. A relatively new technique, available only in research centers, is to establish *permanent cultures* (for growth outside the body) of cells taken from biopsies of genital skin. Because reproduction of these cells provides a virtually unlimited source of tissue, it has been possible to identify the specific biochemical defect in a number of disorders of sexual development.

Tests of Infertility. In males the primary test is a *sperm count.* Semen is obtained by masturbation and examined under the microscope. A normal volume of ejaculate is 1 to 4.5 milliliters; each milliliter should contain about 60 million sperm, and at least 60 percent of the total number should be normally shaped and actively moving in the fluid. An important issue in female infertility is whether the fallopian tubes are obstructed. *Hysterosalpingography,* the technique of choice, involves the retrograde injection of a radiopaque dye through the tubes to show that they are open. X-rays of the abdomen reveal whether dye has reached the abdominal cavity. *Culdoscopy* involves direct visualization of tubes, ovaries and uterus by insertion of a viewing instrument through an incision in the posterior wall of the vagina. It is helpful in discerning pathologic changes of the reproductive organs including abnormalities of the fallopian tube.

DISORDERS OF WOMEN

ABNORMAL MENSTRUATION

Absent or diminished menses is an extremely common problem in women. If menstruation has never occurred *primary amenorrhea* is said to be present. If menarche occurs normally but periods subsequently cease, the diagnosis is *secondary amenorrhea.*

Primary Amenorrhea. Primary amenorrhea is generally considered to be present if menses have not appeared by the age of 16. The two most common causes are *gonadal dysgenesis* (the Turner syndrome) and *congenital absence of the vagina.* The former disease, due to absence of one of the two X chromosomes, is discussed in chapter 4. Girls with absence of the vagina usually have only a skin dimple at the normal vaginal site, but a very short, blind-ending vaginal canal is occasionally present. A rudimentary uterus is characteristic, and structural abnormalities of the kidneys are also frequently found. Ovarian function is normal, but menstruation does not occur because of the abnormal uterus and the absent or closed vagina.[6]

The third most common cause of failure to menstruate is *polycystic ovary disease (Stein-Leventhal syndrome),* a condition characterized by amenorrhea,[7] infertility, obesity, hirsutism and enlarged, cyst-filled ovaries. Estrogen production is maintained but the patients do not ovulate; as a consequence the corpus luteum does not develop, progesterone formation does not take place, the endometrium does not mature and menstruation does not occur. The state of persistent estrogenization is called *chronic estrus.* If progesterone is administered, menstrual bleeding promptly ensues. Hirsutism is due to overproduction of the ovarian androgens androstenedione and testosterone. Polycystic ovary disease appears to be due to abnormal function of the hypothalamic-pituitary system. LH levels are high but FSH levels are normal or low, suggesting a miscommunication sequence. Treatment is quite successful in inducing ovulation, menstruation and pregnancy. Acceptable methods include surgical resection of a wedge of ovarian tissue (which for some reason induces ovulation), the administration of gonadotropic hormones or treatment with a drug called *clom-*

[6] A vagina can be constructed surgically. Surprisingly, nonsurgical treatment is also successful. The technique involves applying pressure against the vaginal dimple with a mechanical dilator several times a day.

[7] Polycystic ovary disease can cause either primary or secondary amenorrhea. It may also cause dysfunctional bleeding (see section on abnormal uterine bleeding). Other gynecologic diseases also manifest themselves as more than one syndrome; e.g., pituitary insufficiency may cause primary or secondary amenorrhea depending on whether it develops pre- or postpubertally.

iphene which stimulates release of LH and FSH from the patient's own pituitary.

A fourth common cause of primary amenorrhea and delayed sexual development is *deficiency of pituitary gonadotropins* due to disease in the pituitary gland or the hypothalamus. Pituitary insufficiency can occur spontaneously but may also be produced by brain tumors and other central nervous system diseases. Fifth, a significant percentage of phenotypic females who do not menstruate turn out to be genetic males: they are *pseudohermaphrodites* who have no ovaries (see page 251). Other causes of primary amenorrhea, such as *hypothyroidism*, are occasionally seen but are rare compared to the major entities just described.

Secondary Amenorrhea. The most common cause of secondary amenorrhea during the reproductive period is *pregnancy*, and pathologic entities should never be sought until the patient has a negative pregnancy test. In maturing women amenorrhea normally appears with *menopause*. Pathologic secondary amenorrhea is usually divided into diseases in which *estrogen is still produced* and those with *absent estrogen production*. The most common cause of the former is the previously mentioned *polycystic ovary syndrome;* affected patients may have a few periods around the time of puberty and then cease to menstruate. A second frequent cause is *endometrial sclerosis* (Asherman's syndrome) in which the endometrium becomes scarred (and thus incapable of response to hormones) following dilatation and curettage to remove retained uterine contents after an incomplete spontaneous abortion (miscarriage). The D & C is usually complicated by uterine infection in these patients. Secondary amenorrhea with estrogen production can also be caused by *estrogen-secreting ovarian tumors, extensive liver disease* and *severe obesity.*[8]

If estrogen is absent, the cause of amenorrhea is either an acquired *disorder of the hypothalamic-pituitary system* (in which case LH and FSH levels in plasma will be low) or *pri-*

---

[8] While the bulk of estrogens are directly secreted from the ovary, one hormone, *estrone*, can be produced in peripheral tissues from circulating androgens made in the ovary and adrenal. Adipose tissue is a favored site for this conversion; thus in obesity, overproduction of estrone occurs as a direct result of the excess fat. In liver disease androgens are not taken up normally by the liver and as a consequence are diverted to peripheral tissue where they are available in greater quantities for conversion to estrone.

mary ovarian failure (in which case the LH and FSH levels will be high in an attempt to overcome the defect). Decreased gonadotropin production can be produced by *pituitary insufficiency* (of any cause), *psychogenic stress*,[9] *dieting* (starvation), *malnutrition, severe systemic illnesses, prolactin-secreting pituitary tumors* (see galactorrhea-amenorrhea below) and following *prolonged use of oral contraceptive pills. Androgen-secreting ovarian and adrenal tumors* also cause amenorrhea by suppressing LH and FSH release. The cause of primary ovarian failure *(premature menopause)* is usually indeterminant, although infections and autoantibodies directed against the ovary are involved in some cases.

Painful Menstruation. Some degree of discomfort afflicts most women immediately before and during the early phases of menstruation. This discomfort is thought to be due to contractions in the uterus stimulated by *prostaglandins,* the hormone-like fatty-acid derivatives that play a primary role in initiating uterine contractions at the beginning of labor during pregnancy. Aspirin inhibits the formation of prostaglandins and may ameliorate menstrual cramps if begun the week prior to menses. Abnormally severe menstrual cramps are designated *dysmenorrhea.* Patients with severe pain should be carefully examined for pelvic pathology (such as a uterine tumor) but usually no cause is found. Pain occurring during menses but localized in areas away from the pelvis may be due to *endometriosis,* a peculiar condition in which endometrial tissue is found aberrantly located outside the uterus (in other organs and tissues).

ABNORMAL UTERINE BLEEDING

During the reproductive phase of life the most common cause of abnormal or irregular vaginal bleeding is *spontaneous abortion* or *ectopic pregnancy* (implantation of the fetus in the fallopian tube rather than the uterus). All premenopausal abnormal bleeding should be considered pregnancy related until proven otherwise, even if the patient is unaware that she is pregnant. Postmenopausal bleeding is highly suspicious of

[9] During the German air raids on London in World War II, it was noticed that a significant percentage of the female population ceased menstruating due to stress. In general the stress must be persistent and severe for amenorrhea to be produced. The precipitating problems may be either internal (psychogenic) or external (situational).

cancer of the endometrium (uterus) but may also be due to *cancer of the cervix* or *vagina*. The latter two diseases often manifest themselves as bleeding after sexual intercourse (*postcoital bleeding*). If bleeding occurs at the expected time of menstruation but is heavier or longer than usual, the term *menorrhagia* is used. The cause is usually localized disease in the uterus such as a *fibroid tumor (leiomyoma)* located just under the surface lining or *adenomyosis,* a condition wherein endometrial tissue is abnormally located in the muscular wall of the uterus. Systemic diseases causing *bleeding disorders* (e.g., acute leukemia) may first manifest themselves by vaginal hemorrhage at the time of menstruation or cause bleeding between periods. *Dysfunctional bleeding* refers to irregular or spotty bleeding, often relatively small in amount, occurring in patients who do not ovulate but have chronic estrogen production. Presumably chronic estrogenization results eventually in scattered endometrial sloughing despite the absence of progesterone. The same conditions that cause secondary amenorrhea with chronic estrogenization may also present as the dysfunctional bleeding syndrome.

MENOPAUSE

The menopause, an inevitable event in the life of every woman who does not die prematurely, has both psychologic and physiologic consequences. Psychologically it is a reminder that aging is occurring relentlessly. It is often erroneously interpreted as a sign that physical attractiveness is doomed to disappear and that sexual drive (*libido*) is destined to vanish. During the same period homemakers find their children grown up with little further need for the maternal function around which their life has centered for two decades or more. The result is often a significant depression. In fact neither libido nor attractiveness has anything to do with menopause; freedom from recurrent monthly bleeding (with the constant threat of pregnancy if sterilization has not been carried out) should herald a period of enriching freedom, even as diminished family responsibility opens the door to opportunities for personal growth. In short, properly understood it can be the best of times.

Physiologically the menopause is caused by cessation of ovarian function. As the ovaries shrink in size and cease to make estrogen,[10] LH and FSH levels rise in an attempt to stimulate hormone synthesis. These gonadotropins are probably responsible for the *hot flashes* and *sweating* that bother many women during the initial phases of estrogen withdrawal. There may be some atrophy of the vaginal lining such that lubrication during sexual activity is less than optimal. Thinning of the bones (*osteoporosis*) occurs at an accelerated rate following cessation of menses and may be severe enough to cause spontaneous fractures, particularly collapse of the vertebrae. *Atherosclerosis*, which is less common in premenopausal women than in men, develops at a more rapid rate after menopause.

Whether postmenopausal women should receive estrogen replacement therapy remains a controversial question. Many patients feel better on replacement, and there is suggestive evidence that estrogens slow the rate of development of osteoporosis. On the other hand the evidence is persuasive (to me) that long-term estrogen therapy increases the incidence of cancer of the uterus. (I realize that despite the increased risk most patients given estrogen will never get cancer.) My view is that short-term estrogen therapy is acceptable in patients with severe estrogen withdrawal symptoms, but that it should not be given for more than a few months and certainly not prescribed routinely in every menopausal woman. Mucosal atrophy in the vagina can be treated locally with estrogen-containing creams without the necessity for systemic hormone therapy.

HIRSUTISM AND VIRILIZATION

Hirsutism means the abnormal growth of body hair. Frequently the new hair is distributed in a male pattern with growth occurring on the face, chest, around the nipples or on the extremities. Commonly the pubic hair (*escutcheon*) changes from the classic inverted triangle of the woman (where a straight base extends across the lower abdomen) to the upright triangle of the male (where the pubic hair extends upward toward the navel to form the apex of the triangle.) Hirsutism may occur in isolation or as part of the more serious problem called *virilization* (masculinization). Virilization is often subdivided

---

[10] Estrogen deficiency is relative and not absolute. As previously mentioned the weak estrogen *estrone* can be synthesized from adrenal androgens by peripheral tissues. Women with few menopausal symptoms likely have more efficient peripheral production of estrone than their more symptomatic sisters.

into categories of *defeminization* and *true virilization*. The former includes loss of menses, decrease in breast size and disappearance of female body contours, while the latter consists of enlargement of the clitoris (the *sine qua non* of true virilization), acne, coarsening of the voice, increase in size of shoulder girdle muscles and loss of hair in the frontal region of the head (*male pattern baldness*). The presumption is that both hirsutism and virilization are the consequence of abnormal androgen production in the woman, with hair growth the result of mild excesses and masculinization the response to higher levels of male hormones.

Many cases of simple hirsutism are never explained. Some are familial and are presumed to be genetically determined. Abnormal hair growth may be produced by *drugs* such as phenytoin (an anticonvulsant), steroid (e.g., prednisone) and androgenic (male sex) hormones. *Systemic diseases* such as acute intermittent porphyria, anorexia nervosa and Cushing's syndrome are often associated with hirsutism. *Pregnancy* causes a moderate increase in body hair in some women. The most common cause is *polycystic ovary disease* (which can also cause true virilism). While earlier discussion of this syndrome emphasized persistent estrogen production, the cystic ovary also overproduces testosterone and another androgen called androstenedione to account for the hirsutism and virilization. If virilization is present (and the patient does not have polycystic ovaries) the most likely diagnosis is an *androgen-producing tumor* of the ovary or adrenal gland. Virilization can also be produced very early in life by *congenital adrenal hyperplasia (adrenogenital syndrome)*. This term refers to a group of genetically transmitted diseases in which there are defects in one of several enzymes leading to hydrocortisone production by the adrenal gland. Because of diminished synthesis of hydrocortisone (the most important adrenal hormone), the pituitary gland releases excess ACTH, the adrenal-stimulating hormone, in an attempt to overcome the deficit. This ACTH stimulates androgen production by the adrenal as a side effect, thereby causing virilization.

Diagnosis of the cause of virilization and hirsutism involves measurement of plasma testosterone (and other androgens) and urinary 17-ketosteroids (which are metabolic products of androgen breakdown). A number of complicated functional tests are often required to localize the site of androgen overproduction, including (sometimes) catheterization of the venous drainage of ovaries and adrenals. Tumors are treated by surgical removal while polycystic ovaries are managed as previously described. The adrenogenital syndrome is easily treated by supplying exogenous hydrocortisone or an analogue such as dexamethasone or prednisone. Under these circumstances ACTH release reverts to normal and androgen overproduction ceases.

GALACTORRHEA-AMENORRHEA

Galactorrhea refers to pathologic (nonpregnancy related) production of true milk from the breast. Milk release may occur spontaneously or only be demonstrated by squeezing the breast. Small amounts of clear secretion expressed on pressure are not galactorrhea and have no clinical significance. For practical purposes galactorrhea can be considered to be caused by excess release of the pituitary hormone *prolactin,* although a few cases occur in the absence of measurable increases of the hormone in plasma.[11] Amenorrhea appears to result from a prolactin-induced inhibition of LH-RH release in the hypothalamus, preventing the preovulatory surge of gonadotropins needed for rupture of the ovarian follicle. Infertility is universal in amenorrheic patients. The most common cause of the illness is a *prolactin-secreting pituitary tumor.* The majority of these tumors are so small as to be invisible by routine skull X-rays and hence are called *microadenomas.* Their presence is deduced by multiple thin-section X-rays (*tomograms*) of the sella turcica, the bony cavity which is the anatomic location of the pituitary, and by CAT scanning. Other causes of galactorrhea include *major tranquilizing drugs, tumors and other diseases of the hypothalamus, hypothyroidism, trauma to the chest wall* and possibly withdrawal from *oral contraceptives.* Regular and vigorous *stimulation of the breasts and nipples* is accompanied by increased release of prolactin and may cause galactorrhea in some patients.[12]

---

[11] Even when absolute levels of prolactin are in the normal range, suppression of prolactin concentration (with drugs) causes galactorrhea to disappear. This suggests that all galactorrhea is prolactin dependent.

[12] It is widely believed that the nonpregnant wet nurses described in literature developed the capacity to secrete milk through mechanical stimulation of the breast. Since no systemic study of such patients has ever been carried out, it is possible that successful wet nurses all had prolactin-secreting microadenomas and that breast stimulation only exaggerated an already present galactorrhea. Certainly such asymptomatic microadenomas are common in the general female population (up to 10 percent in pituitaries examined at autopsy).

If galactorrhea is due to drugs, withdrawal reverses the syndrome as does treatment of the causal diseases (e.g., hypothyroidism). Therapy of microadenomas is in a state of flux. Until recently all such tumors were removed by *transsphenoidal hypophysectomy*, a beautiful technique (with low complication rates) in which the pituitary is approached without opening the skull by inserting the resecting instrument (under microscopic control) beneath the upper lip, through the sphenoid sinus into the floor of the sella. Patients receiving the operation are up and about the next day. Prolactin levels fall following successful surgery, but it is becoming increasingly clear that in many patients they do not completely normalize. As a consequence resumption of menstruation and reappearance of fertility may not occur. A new drug called *bromocriptine* lowers prolactin in essentially every case and is more successful in restoring fertility. At present it is not certain that all patients with microadenomas should be operated on, although large tumors (*macroadenomas*) clearly require surgery. Since adenomas may increase in size during pregnancy, it is generally agreed that patients desiring treatment because of infertility should have surgery first, then be treated with bromocriptine. Patients not desiring pregnancy may not require any therapy if it can be demonstrated through careful observation that the microadenoma is not enlarging.

INFERTILITY

Experience has shown that when a couple is unable to have children, the problem lies with the wife about 70 percent of the time and the other 30 percent with the husband. There are three major causes: *anovulation* (failure to ovulate), *mechanical blockade of the fallopian tubes* and *endometrial sclerosis*. The causes of anovulation and endometrial sclerosis have been previously described. Gonorrhea is probably the leading cause of obstructive disease in the tubes, but other pelvic infections, including tuberculosis, can result in obliterative scarring. Rarely, *an abnormality in cervical mucus* (which results in killing of sperm before they reach the egg) appears to interfere with normal conception. About 15 or 20 percent of infertile women (whose husbands have been proved fertile) have no demonstrable cause for their inability to reproduce even after careful study; such patients are classified as having idiopathic infertility.

Workup for infertility includes careful physical examination, hormone assays in plasma, measurement of body temperature to help define the presence or absence of ovulation and hysterosalpingography to rule out tubal obstruction. Anovulatory women are treated either with clomiphene or exogenous human gonadotropins. The former drug effects endogenous release of LH and FSH, thereby inducing ovulation. If pregnancy is successfully achieved there is an increased incidence of multiple births (7 percent twins, 1 percent triplets or more). Gonadotropins are given to those patients who have an inability to produce LH and FSH on their own. The only hope for patients with tubal blockade is surgical reconstruction.[13]

DEVELOPMENTAL ABNORMALITIES

Delayed Onset of Puberty. Delayed onset of puberty may result from many of the dysfunctional states already mentioned in this chapter. The most common cause is a relative or absolute deficiency of gonadotropins due to disease in the hypothalamus or pituitary gland. Stress from other systemic illnesses and emotional factors of a variety of types can selectively inhibit release of LH and FSH. All such cases have low levels of gonadotropins in plasma; if gonadotropins are high failure to develop is due to disease of the ovaries. Puberty (at least development of secondary sexual characteristics) can almost always be induced by hormonal replacement therapy whatever the underlying cause.

Precocious Puberty. Precocious puberty in girls refers to onset of sexual development (including menses) before the age of 8. Maturation of genitalia and appearance of secondary sexual characteristics without reproductive capacity is called *pseudopuberty*. About 80 percent of patients with precocious puberty have no demonstrable underlying disease; the problem is apparently an early setting of the biological clock that controls hypothalamic-pituitary function. Diseases causing premature development include *brain tumors* in the hypothalamic region, *hormone-producing ovarian tumors, adrenal tumors* and, very rarely, *hypothyroidism.* Another rare etiology is *polyostotic fibrous dysplasia of bone (Albright's syndrome)*, a disorder char-

---

[13] Another approach, still experimental, is the removal of an ovum for fertilization by sperm outside of the body. The fertilized egg is then implanted in the uterus. While apparently normal "test-tube babies" have resulted from this procedure, the potential for developmental abnormalities would, on the face, seem high. I believe great caution should be exercised until more experience is obtained.

acterized by multiple bone cysts (leading to fractures after minor trauma), irregular brown spots on the skin (*café au lait* spots) and precocious puberty. The cause of the illness is unknown.

Female Pseudohermaphroditism. The term *pseudohermaphroditism* refers to patients who appear to have both male and female sex characteristics but whose gonads are appropriate to the genetic sex; i.e., female pseudohermaphrodites have ovaries but have become masculinized because of the influence of androgens during uterine life.[14] The most common cause of female pseudohermaphroditism is the previously mentioned *adrenogenital syndrome.* At birth the external genitalia are ambiguous; that is, both male and female features are present. The clitoris is enlarged and the labia have fused to form a rudimentary scrotum, although no testes are present. Occasionally a prostate gland can be felt. The internal female structures (uterus and ovaries) are normal. The children grow rapidly, progressively virilize during early life and do not menstruate at puberty. The excess androgen causes early cessation of bone growth and untreated patients are thus short in stature. The condition can be well controlled by administration of exogenous adrenal steroids if it is recognized early. Reconstructive surgery is sometimes required to remove the enlarged clitoris and refashion the vagina. *Nonadrenal causes* of female pseudohermaphroditism are rare. In the past pregnant women threatening to have a miscarriage were treated with certain hormones that had androgenic side effects. Abortion was often prevented, but a significant proportion of the children were masculinized, leading to abandonment of this form of therapy.

CANCER

The three most common forms of cancer involving the reproductive system in women are *cancer of the cervix, cancer of the uterus* (endometrium) and *cancer of the breast.* The latter is

[14] *True hermaphrodites,* who are rare, have two sets of gonads—separate testes and ovaries or a combined ovotestis. Almost all true hermaphrodites are at least partially masculinized and ⅔ are raised as males. The genitalia can take almost any appearance. Those who appear more feminine have a vaginal canal with an enlarged clitoris resembling a small penis; phenotypic males have a rudimentary vagina (*urogenital sinus*). Almost all subjects have breast enlargement at puberty and about half menstruate. In the more masculine subjects the uterus commonly empties into the urinary tract resulting in monthly bleeding in the urine (the equivalent of the normal menstrual period).

the leading cause of death from malignant disease in women. All three are susceptible to early diagnosis: carcinoma of the cervix by routine Papanicolaou smears; carcinoma of the uterus by dilatation and curettage at the earliest sign of abnormal vaginal bleeding (particularly in the menopause); and carcinoma of the breast by regular manual examination.[15] Unfortunately these simple techniques are frequently ignored and women die needlessly.

The importance of diagnosing breast cancer early is that it rapidly metastasizes to regional lymph nodes in the axilla, neck or chest. From there spread occurs to bone, lungs, liver, brain and many other areas. If a mass is found the next step is usually biopsy although *mammography* (low voltage X-ray examination of the breasts) may be done as an intermediate procedure, particularly in patients with large breasts where palpation is difficult. This technique can usually distinguish between benign and malignant lesions. Mammography is not done routinely as a screening test since the X-rays themselves have a certain (small) risk of inducing cancer. Benign tumors (*fibroadenomas*) and *fibrocystic disease* can sometimes be confused with cancer. In fibrocystic disease multiple nodules and cysts develop in the breasts. The condition usually appears in women who have experienced marked tenderness and engorgement of breast tissue in association with menstrual periods. Because the incidence of cancer is increased by fibrocystic disease, affected women require repeated biopsies as new nodules develop. In severe disease simple mastectomy is sometimes recommended as a prophylactic measure.

Treatment of cervical and endometrial carcinomas varies depending on the state of the disease at the time of diagnosis. Extensive tumor masses are treated by X-ray to the entire pelvic region followed by radium therapy in the upper vagina and cervical areas. Hysterectomy (removal of the uterus) is then carried out. With more localized tumors generalized pelvic irradiation is not necessary prior to surgery and radium-surgical therapy is given. Cancer of the breast traditionally has been treated by radical mastectomy—removal of the breast, lymph

[15] The technique of self-examination of the breast is easily learned and should be regularly performed (monthly, after menstruation) by every woman. Suspicious areas (which oftentimes turn out simply to be glandular tissue) should be checked at once by the physician.

nodes, muscle and soft tissues on the affected side. However, a strong trend toward less radical surgery has now developed; simple mastectomy followed by X-ray therapy is recommended with increasing frequency.[16]

In the past little could be done for metastatic cancer of the breast, but this is no longer true. Many patients can now be given prolonged periods (years) of productive, pain-free life with modern therapy despite spread of the disease to other parts of the body. If the cancer develops premenopausally, it is often dependent on estrogen for growth. In such cases metastases are treated first by castration—surgical removal of the ovaries (*oophorectomy*). About 60 percent of patients have shrinkage of symptomatic metastases following oophorectomy with its resultant fall in estrogen production. Paradoxically, cancers developing after menopause act in exactly opposite fashion, regressing when treated with estrogen. Great advances have been made in chemotherapeutic techniques for carcinoma of the breast. By far the most effective drug is *doxorubicin* which is always used in combination with other cytotoxic (cell-killing) agents. Many physicians administer combination chemotherapy immediately following mastectomy if lymph nodes are positive (adjuvant chemotherapy). Results appear promising. Painful metastases, particularly in bone, are treated with X-ray to the involved area.

A brief word should be said about the psychologic effects of breast cancer. In addition to the multitude of emotions and fears generated by the diagnosis of any cancer, there is the additional burden of losing a breast in a sexually oriented society that often seems to equate physical attractiveness with the dimensions of the female chest. This anxiety is entirely unwarranted since it is now possible to purchase skillfully designed prostheses that completely mask the loss (even in a bathing suit). Moreover, for those who are not satisfied with an external prosthesis, *mammoplasty* is routinely available. In this procedure the plastic surgeon reconstructs the breast with a silicone implant.[17]

---

[16] Details about the evolving status of treatment for cancer of the breast are beyond the scope of this chapter. I want to make clear that some responsible surgeons still believe radical mastectomy to be the treatment of choice in most patients with breast carcinoma.

[17] Hopefully, one of these days both men and women in our society will mature enough to realize that beauty is not exclusively defined by two masses of glands and fat suspended from the pectoral region. One of the most incandescently beautiful women

DISORDERS IN MEN

Reproductive function in the male is much simpler than in the female because there is no requirement to develop an environment conducive to growth and nourishment of the fetus. Absence or dysfunction of the testes has two effects: failure of androgen production and the inability to synthesize sperm, a combination of symptoms that is called *hypogonadism*. The clinical picture produced by hypogonadism depends on the time of its development. In fetal life the result is *male pseudohermaphroditism*. At later stages manifestations include *absent puberty, infertility* and *loss of secondary sexual characteristics*. While hypogonadism makes up the largest category of male reproductive disorders, other conditions are also important. These include *precocious puberty, gynecomastia* and *tumors of the testes*.

HYPOGONADISM
Fetal Hypogonadism. There are two critical periods of testicular testosterone release: during fetal development and at puberty. If the testosterone burst is missing in fetal life, virilization is impaired and the child will be born a *pseudohermaphrodite* (because anatomic development is constituently female in the absence of effective androgen action). There are two major causes of male pseudohermaphroditism. The first is a *failure to synthesize testosterone* because of a defect in one of the five enzymes that are necessary to convert cholesterol to the male hormone. The second is *tissue resistance to the action of testosterone*. Some cases of resistance are due to an absent cellular receptor necessary for the action of testosterone while in others the enzyme that converts testosterone to its active form (*dihydrotestosterone*) is missing. The clinical picture in the various forms of male pseudohermaphroditism ranges from the *Reifenstein syndrome*, characterized by *hypospadias* (opening of the urethra in the base rather than the end of the penis)

I ever knew had neither breast (she had cancer in both), no ovaries, no left kidney, no hair (chemotherapy caused it to drop out so that she had to wear a wig at all times) and a colostomy (because the cancer obstructed her colon). Possessed of a radiant religious faith, she spent the last years of her life (throughout the multiyear fight against her disease) driving for the Red Cross and in many other ways ministering to the sick and wounded of this world. Whenever she came into a room she became the center of attention of both men and women.

and *enlarged breasts,* to the remarkable syndrome called *testicular feminization* in which genetic males appear to be perfect females except that pubic and axillary hair is absent or scanty. In the latter syndrome the breasts are full and feminine, but the vagina is short and blind ending. No uterus or ovaries are present. Since there is no scrotum the testes are located in the abdomen or groin (inguinal) region. Testicular feminization is due to a complete resistance to the action of testosterone; the testes overproduce the hormone in an attempt to overcome the block and plasma levels are higher than those of normal men.[18] Simultaneously testicular estrogen formation is enhanced to account for the complete feminization.

Pubertal Hypogonadism. If androgen formation and action is normal during fetal life but is deficient during the pubertal development phase, anatomic sex is normal but sexual maturation does not occur. Such patients tend to be tall and extremely slender.[19] The body proportions are abnormal and resemble the developmental pattern seen in castrated boys: the length of the outstretched arms is greater than total height, and the legs are disproportionately long such that the span of the upper body is less than half the span from pelvic bone to floor. Such an appearance is called *eunuchoid* (like a eunuch). Beard development does not occur and pubic hair takes a female distribution. Perhaps the most common cause of hypogonadism manifesting itself at puberty is the *Klinefelter syndrome* (see chapter 4), a chromosomal disorder characterized by extremely small, firm testes, gynecomastia, absence of sperm, low testosterone production rates and elevated gonadotropin levels.[20] A second

[18] Patients with testicular feminization are always raised as girls and usually come to the attention of physicians because they do not menstruate. Psychosexual orientation as well as physical appearance is feminine and they should be treated as women. (One patient was the Mother Superior of a Roman Catholic convent.) Explanation of why amenorrhea and infertility are present is a delicate matter and potentially devastating psychologically. The discussion must be handled with sensitivity; in most cases it appears wise to indicate that there is a hormonal disturbance without stating that the patient is a genetic male. The testes have to be removed surgically because their abdominal or inguinal location predisposes to tumor formation.

[19] The *epiphyses,* or growing portions of the long bones, diminish their activity under the influence of the sex hormones at the end of puberty in both sexes (*closing of the epiphyses*). In the absence of sex hormone action, epiphyseal closure is delayed resulting in greater than normal height.

[20] By now the reader will have noticed that whenever ovaries or testes fail to produce normal amounts of estrogen or androgen, the pituitary releases more gonadotropin in an attempt to stimulate production. This type of response is characteristic of the relationship between the pituitary and all the glands under its control (see chapter 15).

major cause is *hypogonadotropic hypogonadism,* a condition in which testes do not mature and testosterone is not produced because LH and FSH are not synthesized or released in adequate amounts by the pituitary gland. The most common form is called *Kallmann's syndrome;* boys with this syndrome have an inability to smell (*anosmia*) and undescended testes in addition to their hypogonadism. A less severe form of hypogonadotropic hypogonadism is the *fertile eunuch syndrome.* These patients have low LH levels but normal FSH production. They can (because of the FSH) produce sperm and reproduce even though they lack signs of virilization. Failure of gonadotropin secretion in a previously normal pituitary may occur spontaneously or be caused by *destructive lesions* such as brain tumors. If the gonadotropic failure occurs very early in life the syndrome of *microphallus* results; the penis in this condition is normal in structure but so small as to be hardly visible (considerably smaller than the female clitoris in many cases). Delayed or absent puberty can also be produced by *direct testicular injury* (and failure of androgen production) occurring before the expected age of maturation. The causes are identical to those listed under adult testicular failure.

Adult Hypogonadism. Testicular failure in the adult can be caused by a variety of diseases. The most common is *mumps orchitis,* a condition in which one or both testes become painful and swollen in the course of infection with the mumps virus. A significant proportion of affected testes atrophy and become nonfunctional. Other viruses may cause the same complication. *Radiation* (by X-ray or radioisotopes) is a notorious cause of testicular damage and many *drugs* interfere with testosterone production. These include alcohol, marihuana, spironolactone (a diuretic), cimetidine (an antiulcer drug) and certain chemotherapeutic agents. *Trauma* and *torsion* (twisting of the testicular cord with impairment of blood supply) are other causes. Finally bacterial *infections* and loss of testicular function due to *autoantibody formation* can both result in loss of secondary sexual characteristics and cause infertility.

Treatment of hypogonadism depends on the cause. If LH and FSH are low, they are replaced by injection of exogenous gonadotropins which stimulate testicular production of testosterone. If LH and FSH are normal, or high, indicating primary testicular disease, testosterone is given by injection in a depot form that exerts its effects over days to weeks. Either treatment will cause appearance of masculine features and often restore libido but will not cause sperm to be produced: fertility is not repaired.

PRECOCIOUS PUBERTY

Precocious puberty in the male is defined as development of sexual characteristics before the age of 10. As in the female the disorder may occur in the absence of recognizable cause. Other etiologies include brain tumors located in or near the hypothalamus, the adrenogenital syndrome and tumors of the adrenal glands or testes.

GYNECOMASTIA

Gynecomastia refers to enlargement of the male breasts because of glandular hypertrophy which is palpable on physical examination. It occurs normally during puberty in every male. Adolescent gynecomastia may be unilateral or bilateral; normally it regresses by age 20. The condition may also be normal in the aging male. In reproductive adult life gynecomastia usually indicates an abnormal state. It is the consequence of any condition in which estrogen production increases relative to that of testosterone. An increase in the estrogen: androgen ratio may be due to an absolute increase in estrogen synthesis, the ingestion of exogenous estrogens[21] or to impaired testosterone synthesis in the face of normal rates of estrogen formation. The latter is probably the major mechanism. Causes of gynecomastia include *Klinefelter's syndrome, the pseudohermaphroditic states, estrogen-producing testicular and adrenal tumors, testicular failure* of any cause, *liver disease, hyperthyroidism, drugs* (e.g., alcohol, marihuana, digitalis, spironolactone, cimetidine and certain antidepressants) and some types of *cancer of the lung.*

Treatment involves removal of the underlying cause. Occasionally the breasts become so large as to require surgical removal to avoid embarrassment to the patient. If the

[21] Some homosexual men take estrogens deliberately to increase breast growth. All transsexual men undergoing sex reversal operations are also given female hormones. Sometimes the source of estrogens is not obvious. I once saw an airline pilot with gigantic enlargement of the breasts and high estrogen levels in the blood. Initially an estrogen-secreting tumor was suspected, but it turned out that his wife, learning of an extramarital affair, had been secretly putting estrogen in his morning coffee.

enlargement is unilateral, biopsy may be required to rule out cancer.

INFERTILITY

Male infertility due to *failure of sperm production* may be caused by any condition leading to hypogonadism. A rare form of hypogonadism not mentioned earlier is the *Sertoli-cell-only* syndrome in which men have no sperm production, testes that are near normal size and elevated FSH levels in plasma. Germ cells (from which sperm are normally formed) are absent and only Sertoli cells (which are support cells) are seen on testicular biopsy. The most common treatable cause of infertility in men is a condition called *varicocele* in which the veins surrounding the testis become dilated and enlarged (varicose veins of the testes). The mechanism by which sperm formation is impaired is not known. One theory (not universally held) is that increased blood flow through the dilated veins raises scrotal temperature and stops sperm formation. (Sperm production is known to be exquisitely sensitive to heat; the probable reason testes are suspended in the scrotum is that its temperature is 2 degrees lower than the rest of the body.) Whatever the reason, correction of the varicocele restores fertility in a significant portion of patients. Infertility due to decreased gonadotropin production may be restored by gonadotropin administration or clomiphene treatment. The only hope for pregnancy with testicular failure is artificial insemination of the wife.

TUMORS OF THE TESTES

Testicular tumors are relatively rare (about 2 to 2.5 per 100,000 men per year) and account for less than 1 percent of male cancer deaths. The presence of an undescended testis (one that does not migrate normally from abdomen into the scrotum) predisposes to tumor formation, but normal glands also develop malignancies. Most tumors are of germ cell origin but neoplasms can develop from any cell type. They may manifest themselves as a discrete mass or general enlargement of the involved testis. A number of the tumors produce hormones and if estrogen production is increased, feminization with gynecomastia, decreased beard growth and a feminine distribution of body fat may result.[22] One hormone, the *beta subunit of*

[22] The other major cause of feminization in a previously normal male is an estrogen-secreting carcinoma of the adrenal gland.

human chorionic gonadotropin, is a reliable marker of tumor when present but is only synthesized by about a fourth of testicular neoplasms. Tumors of the testis metastasize early, particularly to lung.

Treatment consists of surgical removal of the involved gland followed by X-ray. If the tumor is localized to the testis, 5-year survival rates are excellent, although this is dependent on the cell type. The best prognosis is with *seminoma,* the most common testicular neoplasm in adults. Metastatic disease is treated by chemotherapy. An excellent new agent is a derivative of platinum (*cis-diamminedichloroplatinum*).

INFECTIONS OF THE REPRODUCTIVE SYSTEM

The primary infections of the reproductive organs are the venereal diseases. They are discussed in chapter 16.

FUNCTIONAL DISORDERS OF SEX

Sexual dysfunction in women has traditionally been called *frigidity.* This term is now used infrequently and dysfunctional states are divided into three classes. *Excitement phase dysfunction* refers to an inability to experience or sustain sexual arousal. As a result vaginal lubrication and pelvic congestion, the physiologic accompaniments of sexual excitement, do not occur. *Orgasmic phase dysfunction* means that arousal occurs normally (and can be sustained) but that culmination of intercourse in orgasm does not occur. (Such patients may have orgasms in response to masturbation or other sexual activity, or never have orgasm under any circumstance.) *Dyspareunia* indicates pain on intercourse. The pain is usually due to lack of vaginal lubrication, but a rare variant is *vaginismus,* painful muscular contractions of the vagina induced by penetration of the penis. Dissection of the causes of these disorders is complicated, but a high percentage are due to subconscious psychological or psychosocial conflicts. In other cases the problem is clearly external. For example, arousal defects may be the response to a boorish, sexually ignorant or unfeeling (unloving) marital partner. Similarly, depression or anxiety in response to illness or economic problems normally makes sex a low priority item and interferes with both arousal and orgasmic phases. Organic (physical) causes of sexual dysfunction are rare in women. Many sexual problems can be dealt with by the sympathetic physician, but some require more intensive treatment by a psychiatrist or trained sex counselor.[23]

The blanket term for sexual dysfunction in the male is *impotence*. It is generally divided into two categories; *erectile impotence* and *ejaculatory impotence*. *Erectile impotence*, by far the most common problem, means that the patient cannot achieve or maintain an erect penis in sexually stimulating circumstances. The term is reserved for persistent failure of erection since essentially all men have transient episodes of inadequacy induced by fatigue, preoccupation with work or stress. *Organic erectile impotence* refers to erectile failure due to a physical cause. The erection process is due to engorgement of the penis with blood and is dependent on normal nerve and blood supply to the genitalia. Common interfering mechanisms include abnormal nerve function (e.g., spinal cord injury, multiple sclerosis, involvement of the nerves by diabetes), blockade of blood flow to the penis (e.g., arteriosclerosis, clot formation in the aorta or arteries of the penis), and toxic effects of drugs (alcohol, tranquilizers, antihypertensive agents). *Functional erectile impotence* means that the biological apparatus controlling erection is intact but not operational. It is, for practical purposes, always due to subconscious intrapsychic conflict. If the patient is able to obtain erections at some times, but not others, organic impotence is unlikely. Distinction between organic and functional causes can be made by measuring *nocturnal penile tumescence*. Normal men have 3–5 erections per night, each lasting 15 to 20 minutes. These can be measured and recorded by a special instrument that does not interfere with sleep. Absence of nocturnal erections implies organic erectile impotence while normal erections indicate a functional (emotional) disorder.

Potency can often be restored by counseling, psychotherapy

[23] If sexual dysfunction is a source of unhappiness in the patient's life, therapy is probably indicated. A warning is in order, however. Popularization of "sex therapy" has resulted in the proliferation of many clinics (some run by doctors) in which the training and experience of the therapists is minimal or nil. The best procedure is to ask one's personal physician for advice and referral.

or conditioning (sex therapy) techniques. Failing this it is now possible to surgically implant a prosthesis to allow intercourse. Two types are available. The first is a semirigid rod which keeps the penis permanently distended (a definite disadvantage). The second is an inflatable prosthesis which can increase penile size on demand through a valve system placed in the scrotum. It is physiologically superior but is subject to mechanical failure; moreover, since the surgery is more difficult and the device more expensive, the cost is considerably greater than the semirigid implant.

Ejaculatory impotence is of two types. By far the most common variety is premature orgasm and ejaculation: climax is reached shortly after entry into the vagina, before the partner has had time for response. Less common is failure to achieve orgasm despite sexual arousal and erection. The disorders can often be overcome by counseling and conditioning techniques.

A COMMENT ON "THE SEXUAL SOCIETY"

Contemporary American society seems to be obsessed with sex. It is widely suggested that sexual activity is the key to happiness and that every sexual encounter should end in an orgasm of exquisite intensity. Patients whose experience does not conform to this picture frequently conclude that something is missing from their life or that something is wrong with them. To such persons I would like to say that most of what is written and portrayed on stage, film and television regarding sex is a myth. There are some positive benefits from the sexual revolution. It is very healthy to have sex openly recognized as an important part of life; it is an advance for men and women to know that sensual sexual fantasies and dreams are part of the secret life of most individuals and that they should not be a source of guilt.[24] But it is a misrepresentation of the worst type to suggest that happiness flows exclusively (or even significantly) from unlimited sexual activity or that every orgasm should be accompanied by bursting sky rockets and heavenly visions. Ecstasy may occasionally occur during sex but more

[24] I find this to be a particular problem in highly moral and religious people who are often consumed with guilt over something arising in the imagination even though the fantasy is never acted out.

often the experience is a pleasant episode and nothing more.[25] Sex is not nothing—one would hate to conceive of a world without it—but it also is not everything. Those whose lives reflect this view are not deprived (as the purveyors of sexual hype imply) but simply sane.

[25] Such pleasant episodes are transformed into something more lasting if the shared moment of pleasure is an expression of respect and love in which the gift of receiving is indistinguishably intertwined with the gift of giving.

13

Diseases of the
Musculoskeletal System

In one sense disease of muscle, bone and joints is less severe than disease in other organ systems simply because dysfunction of the structural support system does not acutely threaten life. On the other hand musculoskeletal disorders cause enormous disability and much pain; since in aggregate the number of patients affected is very large, it follows that they account for a very significant fraction of illnesses requiring the attention of the physician. In some cases, especially the muscle-wasting diseases and collagen-vascular syndromes, the illness not only causes disability but directly leads to death.

DIAGNOSTIC PROCEDURES

MUSCLE DISEASES

Three general types of diagnostic tests are used in muscle disease. The first is the *measure of muscle constituents in blood*. Many diseases that cause damage to or death of muscle cells manifest themselves by leakage of these components into the circulation. Most important are the enzymes *creatine phosphokinase* (CPK), *lactic dehydrogenase* (LDH), *aldolase* and *transaminase*. Increased enzyme levels can also occur with disease of the heart and liver so that evidence must be adduced that these organs are normal before it can be assumed that the enzymes are coming from muscle. More specific is the muscle pigment called *myoglobin*. This material is a sensitive sign of muscle cell lysis (destruction) and in high concentrations causes renal failure. The second type of diagnostic test is the *electromyogram* (EMG). In this test the electrical response of muscle is recorded after insertion of a needle electrode into the tissue. The pattern of activity can be used to differentiate primary muscle disease from neurological abnormalities that affect the muscle. Finally, *biopsy* of muscle allows differentiation of the cause of muscle weakness in many instances.

BONE DISEASE

The initial diagnostic test for bone disease usually involves *X-ray examination*. Loss of bone structure, tumors, fractures and cysts can often be identified. *Bone scans*, in which radioactive isotope uptake in bone is assessed, are helpful in identifying and localizing tumors of bone (primary or metastatic). Bone density is measured by a technique called *photon absorptiometry* in which photon passage through the bone is inversely related to the bone mass. *Direct biopsy* is sometimes required to definitively identify an abnormal bone process. *Chemical tests* in the blood are also important. These include the measurement of calcium and phosporus (the major minerals from which bone is constructed), alkaline phosphatase (an enzyme whose activity goes up when bone formation is active), vitamin D and its active metabolites (25-hydroxy- and 1,25-dihydroxycholecalciferol) and parathyroid hormone (which regulates the metabolism of calcium, phosphorus and vitamin D). Finally, *urine tests* may be required. These include assessment of calcium, phosphorus, cyclic AMP (an indirect marker of parathyroid hormone action on the kidney) and hydroxyproline (an amino acid whose excretion is an indication of increased bone destruction).

JOINT DISEASE

As in bone disease, *X-rays* usually represent the first diagnostic test done when arthritis or other disease of the joints is present. *Aspiration and examination of joint fluid (synovial fluid)* is useful in the diagnosis of gout, bleeding into the joints,

infections and rheumatoid arthritis. Microscopic examination
(for cells, crystals, bacteria), measurement of glucose content,
assessment of capacity to clot and culture for infective organisms are routinely carried out. A variety of *immunological tests*
are important in the diagnosis of rheumatoid arthritis and the
collagen-vascular diseases, appearing in varying combinations
in each syndrome. These include the *rheumatoid factor,* the
lupus erythematosus cell test (a marker of the disease of that
name but also present in other conditions), *antinuclear antibodies* and *cryoglobulins* (antibodies which clump and settle
out of solution in the cold). Cryoglobulins occur most commonly in the disease called *multiple myeloma* (see chapter 14)
but may also be present in lupus and related conditions. The
erythrocyte sedimentation rate, a measure of the rapidity with
which red blood cells settle to the bottom of a tube after blood
is thoroughly mixed, is a nonspecific test which becomes abnormal in most inflammatory diseases. It tends to be very high in
rheumatoid arthritis and the collagen-vascular syndromes.

MUSCLE DISEASES

THE MUSCULAR DYSTROPHIES

The muscular dystrophies are a group of diseases characterized by progressive weakness and atrophy of skeletal and other
muscles. Clinical syndromes range from mild affectation to permanent disability and death. Each variant is known to be genetically determined, but in no case has the cause of the muscle
disintegration been discovered.

Duchenne Type. This variant begins in infancy or childhood
and is the most feared form of the disease. The genetics are
complicated and two patterns of inheritance have been identified. The first is *sex-linked recessive* wherein females transmit
the disease but are not themselves clinically affected. Some
patients with this pattern have early onset of symptoms with
severe and rapidly progressive disease while others have a later
onset and milder course. The pattern tends to be consistent in
a given family. The serious form is eight or nine times more
common. The second mode of inheritance is *autosomal recessive* and the disease produced is similar to the mild type of
sex-linked illness. The severe form of sex-linked disease may

be demonstrable at birth or appear in the early childhood years. Weakness begins in the large muscles of the thighs and pelvis such that walking, climbing stairs and rising from the floor is difficult. Characteristically the children raise the upper body by "climbing up the legs"; i.e., they brace the hands over the lower legs and then push up, moving the hands as though climbing a ladder. Early on the muscles of the lower leg are not involved and appear hypertrophied. The gait is waddling, the abdomen is protuberant and curvature of the spine is common (due to involvement of back and shoulder muscles). Facial muscles are always spared. Most patients are bedridden by the early teens. Death results from pneumonia, respiratory insufficiency (because weakness of the chest muscles interferes with chest wall expansion and movement of the diaphragm) or heart failure (the heart muscle itself is affected by the disease).

Fascioscapulohumeral Type. The fascioscapulohumeral variant is inherited as an autosomal dominant trait. Males and females are equally affected. It usually begins later than the Duchenne type (on average in the early teens); symptoms may be mild or severe but most patients live a normal life span, becoming incapacitated late (if at all). The muscles involved are quite different than in Duchenne disease: the shoulders, upper arms and face are primarily affected. Patients are usually first identified by an inability to raise their arms above their heads. The facial weakness results in an expressionless appearance and a specific inability to pucker the mouth or whistle.

Limb-Girdle Type. This autosomal recessive disease usually appears during the second or third decade of life. Progression is slow. Muscles in the pelvic area or shoulder are generally affected and facial muscles are spared. Some authorities believe this disease is really identical to the mild, autosomally inherited type of Duchenne's dystrophy, differing only in age of onset.

Distal Dystrophy. This rare form of the disease, probably transmitted as a dominant disorder, involves progressive atrophy of the muscles of the hands and feet. It begins in middle age and usually causes only mild to moderate dysfunction.

Myotonic Dystrophy. Myotonic dystrophy differs dramatically from the previous disorders in that patients characteristically demonstrate *myotonia* (the failure of a muscle to relax after contraction) in addition to weakness and muscle wasting.[1] Myotonia is best demonstrated by the patient's inability to let go after shaking hands. Afflicted subjects have a uniform appearance which is readily recognized. There is frontal balding (in both men and women) and drooping of the eyelids (*ptosis*) which requires the patient to tilt the head backward in order to see. The face is flat and expressionless, and atrophy of muscles at the temples and in the anterior neck give the head a skull-like appearance. Cataracts are common and in males the testes atrophy. Eventually most of the muscles of the body, including the heart, are affected. Diagnosis is usually easy because of the striking clinical picture but can be confirmed by electromyography which shows a waxing and waning pattern of continuous electrical discharges when the muscle is stimulated.[2]

There is no treatment for the muscular dystrophies. Asymptomatic carriers can often be identified by finding elevated levels of muscle enzymes in the blood, making genetic counseling possible (to avoid birth of affected children). Myotonic symptoms are partially relieved by quinine (the antimalarial drug), but appearance of muscle atrophy is not delayed.

MYASTHENIA GRAVIS

Myasthenia gravis is an extraordinary disease, the central feature of which is *decremental muscle weakness* with exertion: the first contraction of a muscle group is stronger than the second which is stronger than the third and so on. Muscle strength returns to the basal state with rest. As the disease progresses, weakness (with profound feelings of fatigue) is present even at rest, although exacerbation by exercise remains demonstrable. Early signs include drooping of the eyelids, double vision (because weakness of eye muscles prevents coordinated movement) and difficulty in swallowing food. The voice tends to be feeble and the mouth frequently hangs open (the "hanging jaw"

---

[1] Two related diseases may be confused with myotonic dystrophy. The first is *myotonia congenita,* a condition of lifelong myotonia in which attacks of stiffness (failure of muscle to relax) are most prominent after prolonged rest. With exercise ("warming up") the myotonia improves. The second condition—quite rare—is *paramyotonia congenita* in which the myotonic syndrome is induced by cold temperatures.

[2] Ordinarily the electromyograph is connected to an audio as well as a visual recorder. Electrical discharges (action potentials) result in a popping noise somewhat like static on a radio. In myotonia the runs of repetitive discharge sound like the engine of a diving airplane (the "dive bomber" sign).

sign). Muscle atrophy, if it occurs, is a late phenomenon. Myasthenia may be mild or run a fulminant course with early death. Demise is usually caused by respiratory failure due to paralysis of the muscles of respiration or aspiration of fluids into the lungs (with subsequent pneumonia) because of weakness of throat muscles.

Recent investigations have clarified the nature of the defect in myasthenia. Muscle contraction is initiated by a nerve impulse which releases a chemical called *acetylcholine* from the nerve ending. Acetylcholine then binds to a receptor located in specialized areas of the muscle called *motor end plates,* thereby changing their electrical potential and inducing a contractile response. Patients with myasthenia have antibodies in the plasma that attach to the acetylcholine receptor and block access of the neurotransmitter to its binding site, thereby preventing transmission of nerve impulses to the muscle.[3] Most patients also have a defect in the release of acetylcholine from the nerve, compounding the difficulty.

Diagnosis is made from the clinical picture and from electromyography showing decreasing size of the electrical response during repetitive stimulation. Confirmation is provided by administering a drug called *edrophonium chloride* intravenously and demonstrating marked improvement in electromyographic response and muscle strength. This short-acting drug inhibits the breakdown of acetylcholine, thereby increasing its concentration at the motor end plate; presumably the higher concentration allows the antibody-induced block to be overcome. Longer-acting agents of the same type (*neostigmine, pyridostigmine*) are used for chronic treatment.[4] Acute exacerbations of the disease (*myasthenic crisis*) are treated with large doses of *ACTH* (adrenal-stimulating hormone) or *prednisone.* Many patients improve with surgical removal of the thymus gland, especially if a tumor of the thymus is present. Recent reports indicate striking response to *plasmapheresis,* a technique in which blood is withdrawn, the plasma removed (presumably

[3] These abnormal antibodies to the patients' own tissues (autoantibodies) also cause *neonatal myasthenia* in some infants born to myasthenic mothers. The antibodies pass to the fetus through the placenta. Symptoms last for several weeks (until the antibodies are destroyed) after which time the children are normal.

[4] Overdosage with these drugs also causes profound weakness. Management of myasthenic patients is therefore very tricky; they are weak if they don't receive enough medication and also weak if they get too much.

eliminating circulating antibodies) and the red cells transfused back into the patient. *Azathioprine*, a chemotherapeutic agent that suppresses antibody formation, is given simultaneously.

POLYMYOSITIS

Polymyositis, a disease of unknown etiology, causes weakness that usually begins in hip, thigh and pelvic muscles; initial symptoms include difficulty in walking, climbing stairs or rising from the squatting position. Weakness may spread to any muscle group, although the face is usually spared. Symptoms appear fairly rapidly over a period of weeks to months; involved muscles are painful in only a fraction of cases. A subset of patients have concomitant skin lesions, in which case the disease is called *dermatomyositis.* A lilac-colored rash over the cheeks and nose (*heliotrope rash*) is highly suggestive of the diagnosis. Dermatomyositis (more often than polymyositis) may be accompanied by signs of arthritis, swelling of the salivary glands, difficulty in swallowing and painful discoloration of the fingers on exposure to cold, symptoms suggestive of collagen-vascular disease (see page 276). About 10 percent of patients have an underlying cancer.

Diagnosis is made by demonstrating elevated concentrations of muscle enzymes in the blood and a characteristic picture of inflammation on microscopic examination of the muscle biopsy. The microscopic changes are quite distinct from those of muscular dystrophy, which might be confused with polymyositis that begins early in life. Polymyositis also has to be differentiated from muscle weakness (*myopathy*) due to alcohol, drugs, metabolic diseases and trichinosis. (The latter is contracted by the ingestion of inadequately cooked pork; localization of the *Trichinella* parasite in muscle causes marked pain, tenderness and weakness.)

The only effective treatment for polymyositis and dermatomyositis is *prednisone.*

RHABDOMYOLYSIS

Rhabdomyolysis refers to acute destruction of muscle fibers with release of cellular contents (enzymes, myoglobin) into the blood. Weakness and muscle pain are characteristic, but the most important consequence is acute renal failure due to toxic effects of myoglobin. With large-scale muscle necrosis, sufficient myoglobin is released to turn the urine brown (*myoglobin-*

uria), but damage to the kidneys can occur with levels of the pigment too low to discolor either plasma or urine. The causes of rhabdomyolysis are many. Statistically alcoholism is most important, but other drugs (including barbiturates and heroin) can produce the syndrome. Crush injuries, electrical shock, occlusion of the blood supply to muscles, severe exercise in poorly conditioned individuals, polymyositis and genetically determined deficiencies of muscle enzymes (that interfere with muscle energy metabolism) can all induce muscle necrosis. The diagnosis is made definitively by demonstration of elevated concentrations of myoglobin in plasma or urine although it can be suspected by finding increased muscle enzymes on routine blood examination in patients with a predisposing condition. Treatment is directed toward prevention of renal failure and involves administration of intravenous fluids containing sodium bicarbonate in an attempt to prevent myoglobin precipitation and cast formation in the kidney.

PERIODIC PARALYSIS

Periodic paralysis is a dramatic disease characterized by the episodic appearance of muscle weakness that may be so extensive as to completely immobilize the victim. Attacks last from a few minutes up to several days and tend to be precipitated by excessive exertion or ingestion of a high-carbohydrate meal. Between episodes the patients are perfectly normal. The mechanism of paralysis is not known although a sharp fall in plasma potassium concentration (due to a shift of potassium into cells) almost always precedes the attack. The syndrome occurs as a dominantly inherited disease but can also develop as a complication of hyperthyroidism (overactivity of the thyroid gland). An identical clinical picture is produced in *hyperkalemic periodic paralysis*, a condition in which the plasma potassium paradoxically rises with onset of symptoms. Treatment of the common low-potassium form involves the administration of potassium salts while the hyperkalemic form is managed by diuretic drugs that keep the plasma potassium on the low side. Periodic paralysis in hyperthyroidism disappears with treatment of the underlying disease.

SECONDARY MYOPATHIES

Muscle weakness may be the consequence of disease elsewhere in the body. While any debilitating disease with weight loss decreases body strength, some diseases cause specific syndromes of weakness out of proportion to any loss of muscle mass. The two most common are *hyperthyroidism* and *Cushing's syndrome* (overactivity of the adrenal gland). *Cancer of the lung* produces both primary muscle disease (*Eaton-Lambert syndrome*)[5] and weakness due to involvement of peripheral nerves. *Drugs* may also cause myopathy. Notorious in this regard are steroid hormones given in large doses and clofibrate, an agent used for treatment of elevated blood triglycerides. *Hypokalemia* (low plasma potassium) results in profound muscle weakness regardless of how produced. Diuretic drugs (which cause loss of potassium in the urine) are most commonly responsible, but diarrhea and vomiting (which cause loss of potassium-containing intestinal fluids) are close behind. Hypokalemia due to urinary loss of potassium is also seen in renal tubular acidosis, Cushing's syndrome and hyperaldosteronism (excessive release of the hormone aldosterone secondary to adrenal tumor or glandular overactivity).

DISEASE OF BONE

Bone, like all other tissues in the body, undergoes constant turnover; despite the fact that it is the hardest and strongest of tissues, appearing fixed and unchanging, in fact it is constantly being broken down and built up again. This remodeling process is carried out by specialized cells called *osteoclasts* (which tear down) and *osteoblasts* (which build up). Bone synthesis begins with production of a ground substance or *matrix* (composed primarily of *collagen*, the major protein building block of connective tissue) which then is hardened into bone by the deposition of calcium phosphate salts. If bone mass decreases but the ratio of mineral (calcium phosphate and its derivatives) to matrix is normal, *osteoporosis* (bone thinning) is said to be present. If matrix is present in relatively normal amounts but mineralization is impaired (the ratio of calcium salts to matrix is low), the condition is called *osteomalacia*. Lack of mineraliza-

---

[5] The *Eaton-Lambert syndrome* has been called "reverse myasthenia" because weakness tends to improve with repetitive muscle contraction. Electromyography shows a stepwise increase in the voltage of the action potential with recurrent stimulation, a pattern opposite to that seen in myasthenia.

tion is usually due to low levels of calcium and/or phosphorus in the plasma, the chemical hallmarks of osteomalacia. Other diseases of bone are due to remodeling abnormalities (*Paget's disease*), increased resorption of calcium salts (*hyperparathyroidism*), infection and tumor formation.

OSTEOPOROSIS

Osteoporosis, by far the most common of bone diseases, occurs primarily in aging women. The disorder appears to be produced by or associated with the loss of female hormones that occurs at menopause. How the hormone deficiency exerts its effect is not known, but regardless of mechanism bone resorption exceeds synthesis such that its density decreases.[6] A number of systemic diseases cause osteoporosis as part of their clinical picture; these include *genetic disorders*,[7] *endocrine and metabolic diseases* (hyperthyroidism, Cushing's syndrome, diabetes mellitus, acromegaly), *renal failure* and a variety of *drugs* (phenytoin, steroid hormones, immunosuppressive agents). Interestingly *chronic alcoholism* also appears to predispose to loss of bone mass. Osteoporosis is not a prominent feature of aging in men and when it occurs is almost always secondary to one of the aforementioned conditions.

The symptoms produced by osteoporosis are *chronic back pain, fractures of the hip and vertebrae* (occurring spontaneously or with minimal trauma) and *loss of height*. The spine often becomes convexly curved (*kyphosis*) due to narrowing and collapse of vertebrae. Sudden worsening of chronic back pain in a patient with osteoporosis strongly suggests vertebral fracture. Diagnosis is made by X-ray and measurement of bone density by absorptiometry. Plasma calcium and phosphorus are normal, but alkaline phosphatase may be elevated.

---

[6] Three theories have been proposed to account for osteoporosis: (1) diminished formation of 1,25-dihydroxycholecalciferol, the active form of vitamin D; (2) subtle hyperparathyroidism leading to increased resorption of bone; and (3) a "leak" of calcium in the urine. Whatever the cause the important point is that mineralization and matrix formation are decreased proportionately such that remaining bone is normally calcified—there is simply less of it.

[7] The most interesting of the genetic diseases is *osteogenesis imperfecta*, an autosomal dominant condition in which children have osteoporosis coupled with deafness and blue scleras (the sclera is that part of the eye which is normally white). Other genetic causes of osteoporosis include the *Turner syndrome, homocystinuria* (a disorder of amino acid metabolism leading to mental retardation, displaced lens of the eye and early atherosclerosis) and *Ehlers-Danlos syndrome* (described on page 280).

Neither prophylaxis nor treatment is satisfactory. Estrogen therapy probably slows (or prevents) progress of the disease in postmenopausal women but is associated with the risk of uterine cancer. For this reason hormone replacement is indicated only when osteoporosis appears to be rapidly progressive. Some investigators recommend the use of small doses of vitamin D in conjunction with administration of calcium supplements, but this therapy is unproven. Fluoride has been tried but the benefit is questionable.

OSTEOMALACIA

Traditionally failure of mineralization in bone has been called *rickets* when it occurs in childhood and *osteomalacia* when adults are affected. Such a definition is somewhat misleading since the basic mechanism—failure of deposition of calcium phosphate crystals in the newly formed matrix—is similar regardless of age of onset. Clinically the distinction may be justified since demineralization during the growth phases of childhood results in skeletal deformity while onset of disease after growth has ceased does not. Historically the preeminent cause of rickets was vitamin D deficiency. Dietary rickets is now quite rare in Western society since almost all children are given vitamin supplements in infancy and receive extra vitamin D in milk and other foods through the childhood years. As a consequence rickets and osteomalacia due to vitamin D deficiency now occur almost exclusively in *malabsorption syndromes* (cystic fibrosis in children, chronic pancreatitis and sprue in adults). When osteomalacia occurs in the face of normal vitamin D intake and absorption, the cause is almost always *disease in the kidney*. Since bone mineralization does not proceed normally despite adequate amounts of the vitamin, such patients are considered to be *vitamin D resistant*.[8] Finally, osteomalacia may be caused by *hypophosphatasia,* a rare disease in which the enzyme alkaline phosphatase is deficient.

[8] The terminology of the vitamin D-resistance syndromes is complicated. Three distinct illnesses are recognized. *Vitamin D-dependent rickets* is an autosomal recessive disease characterized by low plasma calcium, low or normal plasma phosphorus and severe rickets. *Hypophosphatemic rickets* (vitamin D-resistant rickets) is an X-linked disorder accompanied by normal plasma calcium levels, very low plasma phosphorus, dwarfism and moderate to severe rickets. Patients with this defect are unable to reabsorb phosphorus in the renal tubule and have a continuous "phosphate leak." *Hypophosphatemic bone disease* is an autosomal dominant illness with normal calcium but low phosphorus levels in plasma. Bone disease is present, but the deforming changes of rickets are absent.

The characteristic skeletal deformities of rickets are: short stature, bowed legs and arms and knobby excrescences on the anterior chest. Similar features may be seen in renal rickets due to disease of the kidney tubules. In adults the usual manifestations of osteomalacia are bone pain, muscle weakness and fractures.

Differentiating the diseases that cause osteomalacia is sometimes difficult and usually requires measurement of calcium, phosphorus, alkaline phosphatase and vitamin D and its metabolites in plasma. Sophisticated tests of kidney function and assessment of stool fat are also necessary.

Treatment varies depending on which disease is present. In dietary rickets simple vitamin D replacement is sufficient; malabsorption syndromes require pancreatic enzymes as well as vitamin D. Vitamin D-dependent renal rickets generally responds to large doses of vitamin D or small quantities of its active metabolite, 1,25-dihydroxycholecalciferol. Hypophosphatemic rickets is resistant to all forms of D therapy. Currently recommended treatment is oral phosphate salts (with or without 1,25-dihydroxycholecalciferol supplements).

PAGET'S DISEASE OF BONE

Paget's disease (*osteitis deformans*) occurs in around 3 percent of persons over the age of 40. Affected bone shows an alternating pattern of increased resorption and accelerated formation; the latter, ultimately, causes significant bony overgrowth. The cause of the disease is unknown. It may involve only one bone (*monostotic*) or be generalized (*polystotic*). The latter form produces a striking and unmistakable clinical picture. The head enlarges, the tibias (shin bones) bow anteriorly, the femurs (thigh bones) bow laterally, the spine shows posterior curvature and the height shrinks. Bony overgrowth in the skull often causes deafness by trapping the auditory nerve or directly involving the tiny conducting bones of the inner ear. Increased blood flow occurs in involved areas and overlying skin may be warm to touch. Bone pain can be severe. Three complications are noteworthy. First, fractures are common. Second, the disease appears to predispose to development of bone cancer (*osteogenic sarcoma*). Third, because of the increased blood flow, patients with generalized disease may develop a form of heart failure (*high output failure*) in which the heart is not diseased but simply cannot meet the increased circulatory demands placed upon it by the wide open vessels of diseased areas.

Diagnosis of Paget's disease is made from the characteristic X-ray picture. Plasma calcium and phosphorus are normal, but the alkaline phosphatase is elevated in active phases, reflecting the extensive bone remodeling and increased osteoblastic activity that are its primary features.[9]

Several forms of treatment are now available for use in symptomatic patients with generalized Paget's disease. *Calcitonin,* a hormone normally produced in specialized cells of the thyroid gland, is very effective. The commercial preparation is obtained from salmon. Another drug that appears to be helpful is *disodium etidronate.*

HYPERPARATHYROIDISM

Hyperparathyroidism is considered in the chapter on endocrine and metabolic diseases (chapter 15). It produces a type of bone disease called *osteitis fibrosa cystica.* Mild forms cause resorption of the bone at the tips of the fingers and at the base of the teeth. With more severe disease generalized demineralization of the skeleton is produced. In this state X-rays of the skull show extensive punched-out lesions that give a "salt and pepper" appearance. Spontaneous fractures may occur. Diagnosis is made by finding elevated plasma parathyroid hormone levels and increased urinary cyclic AMP values in patients with hypercalcemia.

OSTEOMYELITIS

Osteomyelitis refers to bacterial infection of bone and is usually due to the *staphylococcus.* The infection may begin as a consequence of trauma (a fracture or surgery on the bone) or the result of bloodstream dissemination from a local infection such as a boil. The symptoms are *bone pain, fever* (often with chills), *redness of the overlying skin* and an *elevated white blood cell count.* Occasionally bacteria other than staph are involved; for example patients with sickle cell anemia may de-

[9] If the patient with Paget's disease is put to bed, the plasma calcium may rise precipitously and lead to coma and death. For reasons that are not clear, absence of weight bearing causes resorption of calcium from bone. (By way of example, astronauts in space, freed from the effects of gravity and thus effectively much lighter in weight, all show excess mobilization of bone calcium.) The effect is multiplied if there is a disease present which itself leads to bone resorption.

velop osteomyelitis due to salmonella strains (which ordinarily cause typhoid fever and bacillary dysentery). Cure requires intensive antibiotic therapy. Occasionally surgical removal of infected bone is necessary. Chronic osteomyelitis is a difficult problem and may be accompanied by draining fistula formation from bone to skin.

TUMORS
The bone is subject to primary tumor development and is also an extremely common site of metastasis from tumors elsewhere (breast, lung, prostate, thyroid, etc.). *Osteogenic sarcoma* is the most common primary malignant tumor. It usually arises in the legs of individuals in the second and third decade of life, manifesting itself by pain and swelling. The tumor metastasizes rapidly, usually to lung. Even with radical amputation of the involved leg, cure is rare and death is expected within 6 months to a year. Aggressive chemotherapy has produced a more prolonged course in some patients, but basically osteogenic sarcoma must be considered a fatal disease. X-rays, bone scans and biopsy are utilized in diagnosis.

DISEASE OF THE JOINTS

Disease of the joints produces pain, stiffness, swelling and limitation of motion. If the process is inflammatory in nature, heat, redness and fluid accumulation may also be present. Arthritis may occur in isolation or be only one manifestation of a systemic disease. Both types of disorders will be discussed.

DEGENERATIVE JOINT DISEASE (OSTEOARTHRITIS)
This disorder, a type of wear-and-tear arthritis, is the most common form of joint disease; it affects some 40 to 50 million people in the United States (85 percent of persons over the age of 70) and can be considered an inevitable accompaniment of aging. The disease can best be understood if normal joint structure is briefly described.

When two bones articulate with each other, their ends are separated by a layer of cartilage that functions as a sort of cushion or shock absorber to keep them from scraping when bearing weight. The joint is lined by the *synovial membrane* which produces small amounts of lubricating fluid to facilitate friction-free movement. In degenerative joint disease, the cushioning cartilage degenerates, the joint space narrows and bony overgrowth is stimulated. Irritation of the synovial membrane may result in fluid accumulation ("water on the joint"). A characteristic finding is knoblike deformity of the distal fingers (*Heberden's nodes*). The large weight-bearing joints of the spine and legs are usually first involved, but osteoarthritis can be produced in any location by activity that increases trauma to the joints; for example, jackhammer operators develop symptoms first in the elbows and shoulders while runners damage ankles and knees. Obesity is a major contributing factor. The primary symptom is aching pain that is made worse by activity and relieved by rest. In advanced disease the joint may be so severely damaged that all capacity for motion is lost.

Diagnosis is made by the typical X-ray picture and the absence of signs of inflammatory arthritis. The best treatment is large amounts of aspirin, although indomethacin and other nonsteroidal anti-inflammatory agents (ibuprofen) are used in resistant cases. Great progress has been made in the surgical treatment of degenerative arthritis, and successful replacement of destroyed hip and knee joints is now possible. The replacement joint is most often a prosthesis, but human joints can also be used when available (from accident victims).

RHEUMATOID ARTHRITIS

Rheumatoid arthritis is a destructive, deforming arthritis of unknown etiology that can affect any joint in the body but most often begins in the hands and feet. Most cases occur in adults but the disease can also strike young children (*juvenile rheumatoid arthritis*). Affected joints are tender, hot, red, swollen and often contain fluid. As the disease progresses the involved areas become deformed and dysfunctional. Classically the hands become fixed in a partially closed position with the fingers extended and deviated away from the thumb side (*ulnar deviation*). There is marked atrophy of the muscles around the joints, and sunken spaces are seen between the bones of the hands (*interosseous atrophy*). While the disease begins as an arthritis, it really is a generalized illness. Other features include nodules over bones, tendons and pressure points of the skin (*subcutaneous nodules*); dryness of the mucous membranes of mouth and eyes (*Sjögren's syndrome*) which interferes with swallowing and produces ocular burning and itching; *lung disease* characterized by nodule formation, scarring and (occasionally) pleural effusions; and *heart disease* which may vary from pericarditis to incompetence of the aortic valve. In the acute phases systemic symptoms such as *fever* and *muscle weakness* are frequent.

Laboratory examination shows a markedly elevated erythrocyte sedimentation rate, anemia, leukocytosis and (often but not invariably) a positive test for the rheumatoid factor. Other immunologic tests such as antinuclear antibodies and the lupus erythematosus cell test (LE test) are positive a significant percentage of the time, indicating a close relationship between rheumatoid arthritis and the collagen-vascular diseases.

Treatment is complicated. Mild disease usually responds to *aspirin* in high doses. Other useful agents include *phenylbutazone, ibuprofen* and *chloroquine.* An effective form of therapy in many patients is the injection of *gold salts,* usually gold sodium thiomalate. While gold may cause a serious skin rash and damage the kidneys, its benefits are clearly worth the risk. Steroids such as *prednisone* have dramatic effects in reducing the pain and inflammation of rheumatoid arthritis but are usually prescribed only in cases that cannot be managed by other measures because prolonged use produces undesirable side effects. When needed they should not be withheld, however. Immunosuppressive drugs such as *azathioprine* have also been used with some benefit.[10] Recently D-penicillamine was approved for treatment of rheumatoid arthritis in the United States. It appears to be a very effective agent. Three to six months of treatment are required before signs of improvement appear, and side effects (abnormal taste, nausea, vomiting, skin rashes, protein in the urine) are not infrequent. Nevertheless, because of its effectiveness, it seems likely that penicillamine may soon be the drug of choice in most severe cases of rheumatoid arthritis. Physical therapy is helpful and reconstructive surgery plays an important role in restoring function to severely deformed joints.

[10] The current feeling is that rheumatoid arthritis and the collagen-vascular diseases are autoimmune in origin. Presumably destructive autoantibodies are diminished by these drugs.

ANKYLOSING SPONDYLITIS

Ankylosing spondylitis is a progressive arthritis involving the joints of the spine. Symptoms begin with pain and end with a completely rigid vertebral column which will not bend. A diagnostic picture is seen on X-ray where bony bridges between vertebrae give the appearance of a *bamboo spine*. The disease most often affects young men in the twenties. Peripheral arthritis can occur but is not common. Pain radiating into chest, leg and other areas is due to nerve entrapment by the involved vertebrae. For reasons that are not clear, *uveitis,* an inflammation of the anterior chambers of the eyes (which may lead to blindness), occurs in 20–30 percent of patients. Heart disease involving the aortic valve is more common than in rheumatoid arthritis, occurring in 3 percent of cases. The cause of the disease, which may be mild or severe, is not known but the presence of the histocompatibility antigen HLA–B27 appears to predispose to its development.[11] Treatment is similar to that of rheumatoid arthritis.

THE COLLAGEN-VASCULAR DISEASES

The collagen-vascular diseases are progressive systemic diseases that are usually fatal. While clinically distinct, they have certain features in common, especially arthritis or arthralgias (pain in the joints without deformity). The four major entities are *lupus erythematosus, scleroderma, polyarteritis nodosa* and *mixed connective tissue disease.*

Lupus Erythematosus. This disease occurs primarily in women (female:male ratio, 9:1). The primary manifestations are *arthritis* (or arthralgias), a typical *butterfly-shaped skin rash* over the nose and cheeks,[12] *pleurisy* (pain and fluid accumulation in the chest cavities), *neurologic dysfunction* (emotional

[11] The histocompatibility (HLA) antigens are a set of determinants on the 6th chromosome which have to do with rejection or acceptance of grafts and transplanted organs. Transplants are more easily accepted if the HLA makeup between donor and recipient is similar than if it is disparate. New knowledge indicates an association between various HLA phenotypes and specific diseases. One of the first associations discovered was ankylosing spondylitis and the HLA-B27 antigen.

[12] This skin rash can occur in isolation, in which case the disease is called *discoid lupus.* The lesion is accompanied by scaling of the skin, scarring and depigmentation (*vitiligo*). Involvement may spread to neck, arms and scalp. In the latter area it causes baldness. How often discoid lupus converts to systemic lupus (if ever) is an unsettled question.

lability, loss of reasoning capacity, psychosis, convulsions), *heart disease* (pericarditis, valve disorders, myocarditis) and *renal failure* (the most common cause of death). Systemic symptoms include *fever, loss of appetite* and *weight loss. Raynaud's phenomenon* is often present; in this condition exposure to cold results in painful blanching of the fingers followed by a bluish then a red discoloration (the triphasic color response). Diagnosis is made by laboratory exam which shows anemia, elevated sedimentation rate, positive LE cell test and high levels of antinuclear antibodies. Cryoglobulins may also be noted. Interestingly the lupus syndrome, which most often occurs spontaneously, can be produced by certain drugs. *Hydralazine* (used to treat high blood pressure) and *procainamide* (an agent used to control irregularities of cardiac rhythm) are the outstanding examples.

Polyarteritis Nodosa. Polyarteritis (also called *periarteritis nodosa*) is an inflammatory disease of arteries throughout the body; [13] associated nerves and veins are also involved. Men are more commonly affected than women. Symptoms vary depending on the primary organ system affected but most patients have *fever, arthralgias, muscle aches, weight loss* and *pain in the abdomen or chest. Kidney disease* is common and *involvement of the coronary arteries* may lead to heart attacks. *Pleurisy* and *pericarditis* are not unusual. *Bleeding* into the skin and gastrointestinal tract is frequent. *Neurologic symptoms* such as numbness, tingling of the extremities or even paralysis may accompany the picture. Diagnosis can only be made by demonstrating the characteristic vascular lesions in biopsy material.

Scleroderma. Scleroderma usually begins with *arthralgias* and *Raynaud's phenomenon*, following which the *skin becomes thickened and tightly attached to underlying structures*, giving a hidebound appearance particularly over the hands. Ulcers develop on the tips of fingers and the skin is darkly pigmented. Calcium salts may be deposited, increasing the hardness. Di-

---

[13] A number of similar vascular syndromes are known, differing slightly in clinical picture and the type of vessels involved on microscopic examination. *Hypersensitivity angiitis* affects small vessels and often follows allergic response to drugs (e.g., penicillin) or infectious organisms. *Wegner's granulomatosis* is a rapidly fatal arteritis involving the lungs (which usually are spared in polyarteritis), sinuses and upper airways and kidneys. *Temporal arteritis* occurs in elderly patients who develop severe headache and palpable tender arteries in the temples of the head. Blindness may result. Despite the name arterial involvement may be generalized.

lated blood vessels (*telangiectasis*) are common. A characteristic feature is *esophageal disease* which causes difficulty in swallowing. *Lungs, heart* and *kidneys* are usually affected and death results from involvement of these vital organs. Diagnosis is usually clear from the clinical picture, but biopsy of the skin may be confirmatory.

Mixed Connective Tissue Disease. Patients with this illness have overlapping features of lupus, scleroderma and polymyositis. Diagnosis is made by the finding of high concentrations of *antinuclear antibodies* coupled with the presence of a material called *extractable nuclear antigen* in the blood.

INFECTIOUS ARTHRITIS

Arthritis due to bacteria is usually abrupt in onset and characterized by *fever, chills* and *red, swollen, painful joints.* Many organisms can be involved, but the most common is the *gonococcus* (the causative agent of gonorrhea).[14] Indeed, gonococcal arthritis is the leading cause of arthritis in young adults. The diagnosis of infectious arthritis is made by aspiration of joint fluid with demonstration of leukocytes and bacteria. Culture confirms the presence of infection and identifies the type of bacteria present. (The gonococcus is particularly difficult to grow and may elude culture in over half the cases.) In men a condition called *Reiter's syndrome* may be confused with gonococcal arthritis. Affected patients have a triad of symptoms consisting of *urethral discharge* (suggesting gonorrhea), *arthritis* and *conjunctivitis* (an inflammation of the eyes). Like ankylosing spondylitis, Reiter's syndrome occurs almost exclusively in patients bearing the HLA–B27 histocompatibility antigen. Gonococcal arthritis responds rapidly to penicillin therapy while Reiter's does not. Other illnesses that may mimic bacterial arthritis are acute rheumatic fever, rheumatoid arthritis and gout.

GOUT

Gout, often called the "disease of kings," actually cuts across all socio-economic strata. It is caused by elevated concentra-

---

[14] Gonococcal arthritis occurs more frequently in women and in male homosexuals than it does in heterosexual males who recognize they have the disease from the urethral discharge (*clap*) that usually develops shortly after exposure and thus receive treatment early. Women and male homosexuals (who practice anal intercourse) often do not realize they are infected and thus get systemic gonococcal symptoms.

tions of uric acid in the blood. Uric acid is a normal constituent of blood and other body fluids but causes difficulty only when concentrations exceed solubility limits in the plasma. Under these circumstances crystals of uric acid precipitate, initiating the symptoms that characterize the illness. Acute attacks involve the sudden onset of *excruciating joint pain,* often in the big toe (*podagra*) accompanied by *fever* and *chills.* Affected joints are so sensitive that the patient cannot tolerate the weight of a bedsheet or even the vibration produced by someone's walking in the room. Untreated, attacks last from a few days to a few weeks and then disappear only to return at a later time. As the disease progresses, joints become chronically involved and progressively destroyed. Tumorlike depositions of uric acid (*tophi*) are often found in the ears and over pressure points. *Kidney stones* (of uric acid) are common, and in the absence of treatment, *kidney failure* results from renal deposition of the chemical.

There are many causes of the gout syndrome. *Primary gout* can be due either to an overproduction of uric acid or its under-excretion by the kidney. The cause is unknown in most instances, but some cases are due to enzyme defects. The most striking example of the latter is the *Lesch-Nyhan syndrome* in which mentally deficient children with cerebral palsy mutilate themselves by biting off their tongues and fingers. Uric acid levels are high and both gout and renal stones may develop. In severe forms death occurs from renal failure, usually by age 10. Why deficiency of a single enzyme involved in uric acid metabolism (*hypoxanthine-guanine phosphoribosyltransferase*) causes this picture is an unsolved mystery. *Secondary gout* refers to elevations of uric acid caused by drugs (most often diuretics of the thiazide class) or another disease. Kidney failure and disorders of blood such as polycythemia, leukemia and hemolytic anemia (see chapter 14) are examples of predisposing conditions. The mechanism is an increased turnover (breakdown and synthesis) of red and white blood cells. Uric acid is a degradative product of cellular nucleic acids in such cases.

Diagnosis of gout is suggested by the clinical picture and confirmed by the presence of elevated uric acid concentrations in the blood or the demonstration of uric acid crystals in joint fluid. A disease called *pseudogout* closely mimics gout and can only be differentiated by showing that joint fluid contains calcium pyrophosphate rather than uric acid crystals.

Treatment depends on the phase of the disease. Acute gout responds dramatically to a drug called *colchicine* and may also be alleviated by *phenylbutazone* and *indomethacin*. For prevention of the acute attack, *allopurinol*, which blocks synthesis of uric acid, is the drug of choice. *Probenecid* or *sulfinpyrazone* act by causing increased urinary excretion of uric acid and are prescribed when tophi are present (indicating increased tissue stores of uric acid).

OTHER FORMS OF ARTHRITIS

Arthritis and arthralgias may be seen as a component of a variety of other diseases. *Psoriasis,* a generalized skin disease, frequently has arthritis as a complication. Many *viral illnesses* (e.g., hepatitis) cause joint pains as do certain *systemic infections* (such as brucellosis). A destructive form of arthritis results from bleeding in the joint space as is common in *hemophilia.* Joints can also be destroyed as a consequence of loss of nerve supply in which case the term used is *Charcot joint.* The most common causes are *syphilis, diabetes mellitus* and *leprosy.* Because the patient has lost the sensation of pain and position sense, the joint is continually traumatized and eventually loses all structure. It is important to recognize that all pain near joints is not arthritis. *Bursitis,* an inflammation of the cushioning pads (*bursae*) located beneath tendons and muscles, is common, as is *tendinitis,* inflammation of the muscular tendons. These conditions can usually be differentiated by careful physical examination.

DISORDERS OF CONNECTIVE TISSUE

Connective tissue diseases are genetically determined and quite rare. The most common is probably the *Marfan syndrome* which has been discussed as a cause of dissecting aneurysm of the aorta (see chapter 6). The only other disorder that should be mentioned (simply for interest) is the *Ehlers-Danlos syndrome.* Patients afflicted with this disease are the so-called *India rubber men* whose skin is so elastic that it can be pulled away from the body like a sheet of rubber, returning to its original position as soon as released. The connective tissue of the skin is biochemically abnormal, accounting for the hyperelasticity. The joints are also hyperdistensible. It is not unusual for the subject to be able to fold the fingers and thumbs backward to touch the wrist or to bend backward at the waist and touch the floor. At least seven variants are known, varying slightly in the clinical picture. There is no known treatment.

14

Diseases of Blood

Blood contains three types of cellular elements (red blood cells, white blood cells and platelets) suspended in the plasma. *Red blood cells* (erythrocytes) function primarily in the transport of oxygen and carbon dioxide between tissues and lungs; *white blood cells* protect against infection by engulfing invading bacteria and producing protective antibodies; *platelets* represent the first line of defense against hemorrhage. All noncellular, blood-borne substances (fuels, hormones, antibodies, etc.) are dissolved in and transported by the plasma. The only plasma components to be considered in this chapter will be the *coagulation factors* which allow blood to clot (and keep it from clotting abnormally). The lymph nodes and spleen function in close relation to the *hematopoietic system* (blood-forming system), and their diseases are therefore ordinarily classified with the primary disorders of blood.

The cellular elements of blood are normally synthesized in the bone marrow which is located in the inner core of most bones. Production goes on continually to replace senescent cells that are removed from the circulation. Cellular synthesis is thought to proceed from primitive (nondifferentiated) *stem cells* that develop into the various cell lines under the influence of hormonal and other signals. Following maturation in the marrow, finished cells are released into the circulation. Red cells and platelets remain confined to the blood vessels while white cells have the capacity to pass from the blood into the tissues, a process that is accelerated by the presence of invading infective organisms or tissue damage of any cause.

Clotting factors, in contrast to blood cells, are synthesized in the liver. Prevention of blood loss when capillary or larger vessels are cut or disrupted by disease (*hemostasis*) thus requires the combined action of a bone marrow factor (platelets) and protein products of the liver. Disease in either organ may lead to a bleeding tendency.

Anemia is the most common manifestation of disease in the hemopoietic system, but overproduction of red blood cells (*polycythemia*) can also occur. Serious *leukocyte* (white blood cell) abnormalities are of two types: deficiency (*leukopenia*), which predisposes to infection, and malignant overproduction (*the leukemias*). *Depression of platelet number or function* manifests itself by abnormal bleeding while an *excess of platelets* can cause clot formation and strokes. The most frequent disease of the lymph system is tumor formation (*the lymphomas*).

DIAGNOSTIC PROCEDURES

EXAMINATION OF BLOOD

A high percentage of the diseases to be discussed in this chapter are first suspected (or diagnosed) by routine examination of the peripheral blood. In the *CBC (complete blood count)* red and white blood cells are counted, the concentration of hemoglobin in the blood is determined and the hematocrit is measured. The latter is done by spinning a sample of blood in a centrifuge and recording the volume of packed red cells as a percentage of the total blood volume. A low hematocrit is probably the best indicator of the presence of anemia, but the hemoglobin is also reliable. A smear of blood is then made; after staining, the percentage of various white blood cells is determined: polymorphonuclear (neutrophilic) leukocytes, lymphocytes, monocytes, eosinophils and basophils (*differential count*). In addition red cell size and shape is examined and a search is made for abnormal cells (e.g., leukemic forms). With the automated equipment now used in most hospitals, the CBC usually also includes *the red blood cell indices:* mean corpuscular volume (*MCV*), mean corpuscular hemoglobin (*MCH*) and mean corpuscular hemoglobin concentration (*MCHC*). The

MCV gives an estimate of red cell size while the MCH and MCHC indicate the hemoglobin content of the cells. Various anemias produce typical changes in the indices that are helpful in diagnosis. *Platelets* are counted separately from other elements, although an estimate of their prevalence can be obtained by looking at the blood smear. The *reticulocyte count* refers to staining for very young red blood cells. If the reticulocyte count is high, it means that the bone marrow is overproducing red cells in an attempt to compensate for anemia.

Other tests commonly done in blood include measurement of plasma *iron, vitamin B_{12}* and *folic acid,* all important for normal blood formation. On occasion the red blood cells are tested for antibodies that bind to their surface and decrease their life span (*Coombs' test*). When polycythemia is suspected, the *total red cell mass* can be directly determined by labeling a sample of the patient's red cells with radioactive chromium and reinfusing them. Assessment of the dilution of radioactive by nonradioactive cells allows calculation of the total number of red cells in the body. *Red cell life span* can be determined from the rate of disappearance of radioactive cells.

EXAMINATION OF THE BONE MARROW

In almost every form of blood disease, examination of the bone marrow is required. The sample is usually obtained by placing a special needle into the sternum (breastbone) or iliac crest (the upper part of the pelvic bone that surrounds the lower abdomen). The specimen is removed by suction and smeared for microscopic examination (after staining). The procedure is quite simple and takes only a few minutes. The type of cells present (normal, abnormal, malignant) and their percentage distribution is determined, and the amount of iron available for hemoglobin formation is assessed. If marrow cannot be obtained by aspiration, biopsy (removal of bone with contained marrow) is required. Culture of the bone marrow is often done in obscure cases of infection since bacteria, fungi and the organisms causing tuberculosis tend to be trapped in the bone marrow core.

BIOPSY

The primary biopsy applicable to hematologic diseases is lymph node removal. Lymphomas and other tumors of the lymph system ordinarily begin with lymph node enlargement, and microscopic examination of the nodes reveals the diagnosis. Tissue from liver and spleen is also occasionally helpful.

RADIOLOGIC PROCEDURES

Routine chest X-ray is often helpful in showing enlarged lymph nodes in the central chest (mediastinum) or near the hilum (root) of the lung in patients with lymphomas. *Lymphangiograms* and radioactive *gallium scans* are useful in clarifying the presence and extent of disease in lymph tumors. In the former radiopaque material is injected in the lower extremity, outlining the ascending lymph chains and any enlarged nodes; in the latter isotopic gallium, which concentrates in tumor tissue, is utilized to identify intra-abdominal and intrathoracic tumor masses.

TESTS OF BLEEDING FUNCTION

Identification of the cause of abnormal bleeding is quite complicated. A simplified description of hemostasis is as follows. When a vessel is cut *platelets* are attracted to the site of disruption and form a plug that slows or stops the bleeding. The platelet plug is stabilized by production of a substance called *thrombin* which both fuses the aggregated platelets and stimulates the laying down of a threadlike network of *fibrin*. The fibrin threads merge together (*polymerize*) to form the bulk of the clot. Without clot formation the platelet plug becomes inadequate to maintain hemostasis and hemorrhage supervenes. In short, the platelet plug temporarily stops bleeding but is not sufficient to permanently stanch blood flow. The clotting mechanism, sometimes called the *coagulation cascade*, involves a number of protein clotting factors (enzymes) which circulate in inactive (precursor) form. These factors are sequentially converted to functional molecules as clotting is initiated: each activated enzyme acts on the next precursor in the chain to make it active. Most of the factors bear Roman numerals; normally clotting factor XII is activated at the time of tissue injury to initiate the sequence XII→XI→IX→VIII→X. Activated factor X then converts *prothrombin* to *thrombin* in the presence of factor V, and thrombin completes the sequence by converting *fibrinogen* to *fibrin*. This pathway is called the *intrinsic pathway*. A short loop system, more rapidly operable, activates factor X via factor VII and bypasses factors XII, XI, IX and VIII. It is called the *extrinsic pathway*. Calcium and platelets are required for proper functioning of both pathways. A deficiency of any of the coagulation factors can lead to clotting difficulty. For example, hemophilia is due to a deficiency of factor VIII. There is also an opposing system designed to keep blood fluid and prevent abnormal clotting. Called the *fibrinolytic system*, it rapidly dissolves unnecessary clots. Against this background the major bleeding tests can be described.

Bleeding Time. In this procedure a standardized nick is made in the skin, and the time to cessation of bleeding is measured. The test is abnormal when platelets are deficient in number or function inadequately. The bleeding time is normal in disorders of the coagulation cascade.

Clotting Time. This is the time required for 1 milliliter of whole blood to clot at 37°C when exposed to a glass tube. It becomes abnormal when coagulation factors are deficient. Clotting time is also used to assess the effectiveness of the anticlotting agent *heparin*.

Partial Thromboplastin Time. This test measures the effectiveness of the intrinsic clotting pathway (the entire sequence of reactions from factor XII to fibrin). If the partial thromboplastin time (PTT) is abnormal but the prothrombin time is normal, it follows that the defect is due to deficiency or abnormality in factors XII, XI, IX or VIII.[1]

Prothrombin Time. The prothrombin time is a measure of the extrinsic clotting pathway. It identifies deficient function of factors VII, X, V, prothrombin, thrombin, fibrinogen and fibrin. Therapeutically the test is used to monitor anticoagulation with the oral anticlotting agents *bis-hydroxycoumarin* and *warfarin*.

Thrombin Clotting Time. This test reveals the presence of abnormalities in terminal clot formation, the conversion of fibrinogen to fibrin.

Platelet Function. A variety of tests are used to evaluate platelet function. The most common is *clot retraction* (the process by which the newly formed clot extrudes fluid and tightens

---

[1] A clue as to which factor is missing can be obtained by adding other plasma samples known to be deficient in a given coagulation protein. For example, if a prolonged PTT is restored to normal by the addition of plasma from a hemophiliac, which is deficient in factor VIII, it follows that the cause of the abnormality in the patient's plasma was not factor VIII deficiency.

down), but *platelet aggregation* (the clumping response of platelets to various stimulating agents) and the *platelet release reaction* (the discharge of platelet chemicals into the blood to accelerate aggregation of additional circulating platelets) can also be assessed.

ANEMIA

There are three general causes of anemia: *underproduction of red cells, increased destruction of red cells (hemolysis)* and *blood loss. Underproduction* may be due to a deficiency of iron or vitamin cofactors, diminished availability of erythropoietin (the red blood cell stimulating hormone) or primary disease of the marrow itself. *Increased destruction*, which is far less common than underproduction, may be due to inherited abnormalities of the red cell membrane or hemoglobin molecules, anti-red cell antibodies or acquired disease in the blood vessels or spleen. Anemia due to *blood loss* may occur following trauma but most often is due to hemorrhage in the gastrointestinal tract. A simple reticulocyte count is usually the first step in deciding between mechanisms, since a low count indicates underproduction while hemolysis and blood loss are accompanied by high values.

Regardless of etiology anemia causes *weakness, fatigue* and *pallor* as primary symptoms. In severe disease *rapid heart rate, shortness of breath on exertion, headache, dizziness, fainting* and *roaring noises in the ear* may be present. Occasionally *heart failure* may appear with pulmonary congestion and edema.[2]

ANEMIA DUE TO UNDERPRODUCTION OF RED BLOOD CELLS

Iron Deficiency Anemia. Iron deficiency is by far the most common cause of anemia in the world. Iron is necessary for the formation of hemoglobin and in its absence anemia supervenes. Women are more vulnerable to iron deficiency than men. Normally 10 to 20 milligrams of iron are ingested daily but only 1

[2] Symptoms depend to a large extent on the speed with which anemia develops: a rapid fall in hematocrit produces severe distress while an equivalent anemia developing gradually may cause no symptoms at all.

to 2 milligrams are absorbed. Men and nonmenstruating women lose about 0.5 to 1 milligram of the metal a day in cells cast off from the intestine and skin. Menstruating women, on the other hand, lose, on average, 1.5 milligrams per day because of the blood discharged during each menstrual period. (Red blood cells have a high iron content and so the menses represent a constant iron drain from the body.) Since total monthly iron loss is close to iron absorbed, iron balance is precarious throughout menstrual life. There is normally a reserve store of iron in the body which can be mobilized during periods of negative balance (when outgo is greater than intake). However, this pool is smaller in women than men. Moreover, it is easily depleted by pregnancy (which requires an extra 700 milligrams of iron for development of the fetus) or by excessive menstrual flow which may not be enough above normal to alert the patient to the fact that she is in a negative iron drain.

Iron deficiency can also be produced in both men and women by hidden (*occult*) blood loss, usually in the gastrointestinal tract.[3] A search for occult bleeding is absolutely required whenever iron deficiency is found. Such blood loss occurring in an asymptomatic patient has a high chance of being cancer of the colon, although other forms of cancer, silent duodenal ulcers, parasites (such as hookworm) or hemorrhoids may be the cause. Aspirin overuse can also result in occult bleeding.

In addition to the symptoms produced by any anemia, iron deficiency causes a *sore, smooth tongue* (the normal bumps or *papillae* are missing), *flattening* (spooning) and *ridging of the fingernails, dryness* and *wrinkling of the skin* and (sometimes) *difficulty in swallowing.*

The blood picture is characteristic. Small, hemoglobin-deficient (*microcytic, hypochromic*) red cells are seen on smear and all three red cell indices (MCV, MCH and MCHC) are low. Serum iron concentrations are depressed while the iron-binding protein of plasma is increased. Iron is absent from the bone marrow. Treatment requires the administration of iron salts (fer-

---

[3] Anemia can be produced by bleeding in two ways. Hemorrhage causes anemia because large volumes of blood are lost so rapidly the bone marrow cannot compensate. This type of bleeding is easily recognized because it is visible. In slow bleeding, as in oozing from a gastrointestinal cancer, the bone marrow is able to compensate, and anemia does not develop until iron stores are depleted. Slow bleeding is usually not grossly visible (hence, *occult*) and has to be demonstrated by doing a chemical test for blood on the stool or gastric contents.

rous gluconate or ferrous sulfate) by mouth until the bone marrow deficit is repaired and tissue stores are repleted.

Anemia of Chronic Inflammation. Long-standing infections and chronic systemic diseases (such as the collagen-vascular diseases) are accompanied by mild to moderate anemia which on the surface may mimic iron deficiency since plasma iron tends to be low. However iron stores in the *reticuloendothelial system* (RE system), which is responsible for red blood cell breakdown, are actually increased. This iron is normally reutilized for new blood synthesis in the bone marrow, but inflammation apparently causes a block in transport of iron between the RE system and marrow. The condition has thus been termed an "iron reutilization defect." Red cell survival is also slightly decreased in inflammatory diseases and erythropoietin levels are depressed.

Pernicious Anemia and the Megaloblastic States. The term *megaloblastic anemia* refers to a condition in which maturation of red blood cells in the bone marrow is impaired. Large red blood cells with increased volume (increased MCV) are characteristic. The most common cause of the condition is *folic acid* deficiency and the most frequent cause of folic acid deficiency is chronic alcoholism.[4] *Pernicious anemia*, due to a deficiency of *vitamin B_{12}*, is the second major cause. B_{12} deficiency does not result from inadequate dietary intake of the vitamin but from an inability of the patient to absorb it. Absorption of vitamin B_{12} requires binding to a carrier protein, made in the stomach, called *intrinsic factor.* Intrinsic factor carrying the vitamin passes to the small intestine where it binds to a specific receptor that allows B_{12} transfer across the intestinal wall. Pernicious anemia is due to spontaneously arising autoantibodies of two types: the first attacks the stomach lining, preventing production of intrinsic factor, while the second binds to intrinsic factor itself, interfering with its function. In addition to anemia, patients with pernicious anemia have *severe neurological symptoms* which may vary from numbness and tingling of the extremities to loss of position sense and difficulty in walking. *Sore tongue* and a *yellowish cast to the skin* are characteristic. Vitamin B_{12} deficiency can also be produced by surgical re-

---

[4] Folic acid deficiency can also occur in pregnancy, malabsorptive states, with drugs (particularly anticonvulsants and chemotherapeutic agents) and as a consequence of food faddism.

moval of the stomach and small intestine or by intestinal disease, all of which result in decreased absorption.

The diagnosis of megaloblastic anemia is made from examination of peripheral blood and bone marrow smears which show giant red cells, enlarged (and hypersegmented) polymorphonuclear leukocytes and bizarrely shaped platelets. Measurement of folic acid and B_{12} levels in the plasma indicates which vitamin deficiency is involved. Repair of folic acid deficiency is easily accomplished by oral administration of the vitamin, but B_{12} has to be given by monthly injection for life.[5]

Aplastic Anemia. Aplastic anemia refers to a condition in which the production of red blood cells, white blood cells and platelets ceases (or becomes markedly impaired) because the producing cells of the bone marrow are damaged or destroyed. Failure of all elements is called *pancytopenia*. While the condition can occur without apparent cause, it most often develops secondary to the toxic effects of drugs and other chemicals. If the chemical produces bone marrow damage in all recipients given a large enough amount, the reaction is called *dose dependent*. The prototypic dose-dependent chemical is *benzene,* a solvent used in paint removers and degreasing compounds, but arsenic derivatives and cancer chemotherapeutic agents can cause the disease. Other drugs cause aplastic anemia *idiosyncratically,* meaning that only a few persons exposed will be affected; these reactions are independent of dose. The best known cause is the antibiotic *chloramphenicol,*[6] but gold salts, phenylbutazone (an antiarthritis drug), propylthiouracil (used in the treatment of hyperthyroidism) and a variety of insecticides can also produce the syndrome.

Patients with this disorder have symptoms of *anemia, abnormal bleeding* (because of the platelet deficiency) and *recurrent infection* (due to insufficient numbers of white cells). In severe disease the latter is usually the cause of death. Diagnosis is suspected when pancytopenia is accompanied by a "dry tap" on

---

[5] It is an interesting fact that folic acid in large doses will reverse the anemia of pernicious anemia while neurologic disease progresses; permanent paralysis has been produced under such circumstances. Obviously care must be taken not to confuse the two states.

[6] Chloramphenicol is a superb antibiotic, but because of this problem, it is now used only in conditions where a life-threatening infection is present (e.g., brain abscess, bloodstream infection with resistant organisms). It is interesting that chloramphenicol causes bone marrow depression by both dose-dependent and idiosyncratic mechanisms. The former is reversible on stopping the drug; the latter is unrelenting.

bone marrow aspiration. Bone marrow biopsy then shows only a few cells with the remainder of the tissue replaced by fat.[7]

Treatment is complicated. The first step is withdrawal of the inducing agent. Mild disease may respond to male sex hormones (androgens) which have the capacity to stimulate remaining cellular elements. In severe cases the only hope is *bone marrow transplantation* from an appropriate donor. This procedure can be done only in a few centers in the United States. Unless the donor is an identical twin, the recipient must have his immune system completely suppressed (or destroyed) by total body X-ray and/or immunosuppressive agents. The donor marrow is then infused intravenously to recolonize the empty bone marrow sites. The patient must be isolated in a completely sterile (germ free) environment until the marrow takes.[8]

Other Anemias Due to Underproduction of Red Cells. Sideroblastic anemias are a group of disorders characterized by red blood cells that appear hypochromic (resembling those of iron deficiency) and a type of precursor red cell in the bone marrow that has a ring of iron containing granules around the nucleus (*ringed sideroblasts*). Total iron in the body is increased, but its utilization is impaired. The most common cause is deficiency of *pyridoxine* (vitamin B_6), but the same picture can be produced in lead poisoning, certain forms of cancer and with a variety of drugs. Anemia due to failure of production is also a feature of a number of systemic diseases. Outstanding examples are *kidney failure, liver disease* and *endocrine disorders* (hypothyroidism, adrenal insufficiency, hypopituitarism, hypogonadism).

ANEMIA DUE TO INCREASED RED BLOOD CELL DESTRUCTION

There are three general causes for decreased red cell survival. *First,* abnormalities in the environment may mechani-

[7] Two other conditions may give the picture of pancytopenia with an abnormal bone marrow. In the first the marrow is replaced by metastatic cancer cells or advanced infection such as tuberculosis. This phenomenon is called *myelophthisic anemia*. The second cause is *myelofibrosis,* in which the bone marrow is replaced by fibrous tissue (see myeloproliferative disorders).

[8] In the usual type of transplantation (kidney, liver, heart), the major problem is rejection of the transplanted organ. With bone marrow transplantation the difficulty is *graft vs host disease.* Since the bone marrow transplant contains cells capable of making antibodies while the host's immune response has been paralyzed, the transplant rejects (attacks) the host tissues rather than *vice versa.*

cally injure normal cells. Examples include the implantation of artificial heart valves (the hard surface of the prosthesis does the damage), enlargement of the spleen (which distorts red cells and retards their passage in the filtering spaces through which they normally pass) and narrowing of small arteries by fibrin deposition and clot formation as occurs in diffuse intravascular coagulation (described later in this chapter). *Second,* hemolysis may result from structural or functional abnormalities of the red cell membrane itself. Such defects may be congenital or acquired. The latter are most frequently due to antibodies that attack the cell membrane (*immune hemolytic anemias*), but acquired mutations that result in weaknesses in membrane structure are also known.[9] A rare cause is the bite of poisonous snakes; their venom essentially dissolves the red cell membrane. *Third,* diminished life span may be produced by internal (nonmembrane) defects in the erythrocyte. These include abnormal hemoglobins (*hemoglobinopathies*) and enzyme deficiencies.

In most cases the damaged red cells are removed in normal disposal sites such as the liver and spleen (the reticuloendothelial system), but occasionally red cell breakdown occurs in the blood vessels themselves. The former is called *extravascular hemolysis* while the latter is designated *intravascular hemolysis*.

The primary symptoms of hemolytic anemia are *anemia* and *jaundice;* the latter is due to the fact that the liver cannot adequately handle the increased loads of bilirubin presented to it by the accelerated erythrocyte breakdown. The blood smear shows *deformed red cells* and the *reticulocyte count is high.* With intravascular hemolysis *free* (not contained in red cells) *hemoglobin concentrations are elevated* in plasma and urine. *Haptoglobin,* the hemoglobin-binding protein of blood, is decreased since it is rapidly removed from plasma after attaching

[9] The classic example of an acquired mutation is *paroxysmal nocturnal hemoglobinuria,* a condition of red cell breakdown accompanied by leakage of hemoglobin into the urine that tends to undergo periodic exacerbation (hence, *paroxysmal*). The disorder appears to result from proliferation of an abnormal line (*clone*) of stem cells in the bone marrow which produce red cells with defective membranes. The altered red cell membrane abnormally binds a plasma component called *complement* which causes it to lyse. Affected cells are very labile in the presence of acid, which serves as the basis of diagnosis (*acid hemolysis test*). Patients with this disease may develop *acute myelogenous leukemia.* They are also prone to clot formation in blood vessels, and such thrombosis is the usual cause of death.

to free hemoglobin. Definitive diagnosis of hemolysis requires demonstration of decreased red blood cell survival by radioactive labeling of the cells. The common causes follow.

Hypersplenism. Hemolytic anemia (indeed, pancytopenia) can occur whenever the spleen is enlarged. Such increased extravascular destruction is called *hypersplenism.* The most common cause is probably congestion of the spleen secondary to cirrhosis of the liver, but lymphomas, leukemias and a variety of infections can produce the syndrome.

Hereditary Spherocytosis. This congenital disorder is transmitted as an autosomal dominant trait. The diagnosis is suggested whenever *anemia, jaundice* and *enlargement of the spleen* are found in a young person with a family history of anemia. On blood smear the red cells are seen to be rounded into spheres rather than maintaining the biconcave structure of the normal erythrocyte. Spherical red cells are not easily compressed as they pass through the spleen and as a consequence, their rate of destruction is increased. The spherical shape also makes them more susceptible to lysis when placed in hypotonic (low salt content) solutions; this increased *osmotic fragility* is helpful in confirming the diagnosis. Correct diagnosis is important since the disease can be completely cured by removing the spleen.

Immune Hemolytic Anemias. Destructive antibodies to red cells most often develop as a consequence of diseases involving the immune system. The leading offenders are *lupus erythematosus,* certain *lymphomas* and *chronic myelogenous leukemia.* The condition can also be produced by two common *drugs* which lead to antibody formation against red cells: methyldopa (used in the treatment of high blood pressure) and penicillin. Some hemolytic antibodies are only destructive to red cells at low temperatures. (*cold agglutinins*). Such antibodies are most often seen with *infectious mononucleosis,* pneumonia due to an organism called *mycoplasma, lymphomas* and as a rare complication of *syphilis. Hemolysis* can also occur after *incompatible blood transfusions;*[10] in this case, naturally occurring plasma antibodies in the recipient act to lyse mismatched red cells from the donor. Most reactions are due to antibodies

[10] The symptoms of a major transfusion reaction include restlessness, anxiety, rapid heartbeat, nausea, pain in the chest or flanks and finally shock. Renal failure is common and is due to both shock and direct damage by the hemoglobin molecule.

directed against antigens of the ABO and Rh systems, but they can occur against numerous other antigens carried in the red cell membrane. For reasons that are not clear, everyone possesses natural antibodies to all antigens not contained in his own erythrocytes but present in the red cells of others.

The laboratory test most indicative of immune hemolytic anemia is a positive *Coombs' test*. Therapy, as in most immune disorders, is prednisone.

Glucose-6-Phosphate Dehydrogenase Deficiency (G-6-PD deficiency). G-6-PD deficiency is an X-linked disorder in which hemolysis is caused by exposure to one of several *drugs* (sulfonamides, antimalarial agents, urinary antiseptics) or following *infection*. Some patients are sensitive to ingestion of the *fava bean*. The enzyme glucose-6-phosphate dehydrogenase is necessary for generation of a cellular chemical called *reduced glutathione* that protects the red cell membrane and hemoglobin from injury in the face of the aforementioned drugs, bacteria and viruses. In its absence, hemolysis occurs. The disease, expressed in males and carried by females, occurs mainly in blacks. Up to 20 percent of the black male population carry an abnormal G-6-PD gene, but not all variants cause hemolysis.

Hemoglobinopathies. Several hundred genetically abnormal hemoglobins have now been discovered, but only about a third are symptomatic. The most important is *sickle cell anemia* (SS disease), an illness of blacks characterized by *growth failure* in children, increased *tendency to infection* (particularly pneumonia due to the pneumococcus), *anemia* (with a red cell survival of about 2 weeks as opposed to the normal 100–120 days) and *recurrent episodes of excruciating pain* in the abdomen, chest and extremities (*sickle crises*). Other complications include jaundice, gallstones, heart failure, hematuria, osteomyelitis, chronic ulcers of the skin (especially over the ankles), strokes and convulsions. Many of the symptoms are thought to be due to occlusion of small blood vessels by the abnormally shaped cells (*sickle cells*). At present no specific treatment is available, and crises have to be managed by intravenous fluids and pain-relieving drugs. Transfusions are required when anemia is severe. Investigations continue into the possibility that the disease may be alleviated by chemical modification of the hemoglobin molecule.[11] *Sickle cell trait* (SA disease) is a largely asymptomatic condition in which the patient is heterozygous for sickle hemoglobin: he inherits a normal hemoglobin gene from one parent and the sickle gene from the other. *Sickle cell-C disease* (SC disease) is similar to sickle cell anemia but tends to be milder with fewer crises. While hemoglobin S (sickle hemoglobin) is a mutation due to substitution of the amino acid valine for the normal glutamic acid in position 6 of the beta chain of the hemoglobin molecule, hemoglobin C is the consequence of the substitution of lysine in the same position.[12] In SC disease the patient inherits an S beta chain from one parent and a C beta chain from the other. Patients with this disorder have *anemia, eye complications* (retinal detachment, hemorrhage, infarcts) and *hematuria* as primary symptoms. The *thalassemias* are congenital anemias found in persons of Mediterranean and Oriental descent. There are two major types, alpha and beta. The abnormal hemoglobin in these disorders is not due to single amino-acid substitutions but to abnormal synthesis of whole chains. In beta thalassemia the beta chain is deficient while in alpha thalassemia the alpha chain is missing or depressed. The most serious form is homozygous beta thalassemia (*Cooley's anemia*) in which the child receives a beta thalassemia gene from both parents. Affected children have *severe anemia, retarded growth, delayed puberty, dark skin* (due to jaundice and increased pigment deposition), *enlarged hearts, big livers* and *hypertrophied spleens*. The only treatment is transfusion when anemia becomes severe. Life expectancy is short.

ANEMIA DUE TO ACUTE BLOOD LOSS

It has already been noted that gradual loss of blood produces anemia by causing iron deficiency. When large amounts of blood are lost suddenly, the picture is quite different. The patient is *pale, restless, breathing rapidly, weak* and *sweating*.

[11] Treatment of sickle hemoglobin with sodium cyanate (*carbamylation*) alters the molecule such that it binds more oxygen and sickles less. Cyanate cannot be given directly to patients because it is toxic. However, blood can be removed from the patient for carbamylation outside the body followed by retransfusion of the treated cells. Preliminary studies show that this procedure decreases the incidence of painful crises by about 80 percent. Research in this area is continuing.

[12] Normal adult hemoglobin contains four chains of amino acids, two alpha and two beta.

The *pulse rate rises* and *blood pressure falls.*[13] All these are signs of acutely diminished blood volume. When blood is taken for determination of hemoglobin and hematocrit immediately after hemorrhage, *there may be no sign of anemia.* This is because both plasma and red cells are lost proportionately in contrast to the usual forms of anemia where plasma volume remains normal (or expands) as red cell mass decreases. The anemia becomes manifest as plasma volume is restored by intravenous fluids given while waiting for blood to be typed and cross-matched for transfusion.

When a patient has lost large amounts of blood, treatment of shock is the first consideration. As soon as conditions stabilize, the site of blood loss must be identified and attempts made to stop the hemorrhage. Apart from trauma (accidents, gunshot wounds, stabbings, etc.) the most common site of bleeding is the gastrointestinal tract; esophageal varices, ulcers, gastritis and cancer account for the bulk of cases. However, hemorrhage may be internal and nonvisible; e.g., rupture of a dissecting aneurysm into the chest or bleeding into the pancreatic bed secondary to acute pancreatitis.

POLYCYTHEMIA AND THE MYELOPROLIFERATIVE SYNDROMES

Polycythemia refers to the overproduction of red blood cells by the bone marrow; it is the mirror image of anemia and is characterized by an elevated hemoglobin concentration and hematocrit. The abnormality may be a *primary bone marrow dysfunction (polycythemia vera)* or *secondary* to other conditions, particularly diseases resulting in low oxygen tension in the blood (chronic pulmonary disease, congenital heart disease with intracardiac shunts). It may also be the consequence of cancer of the kidney. Symptoms are due to increased blood

---

[13] Initially the blood pressure may be normal if the patient is lying flat but will fall if the patient sits up or stands (*orthostatic hypotension*). A rough estimate of the degree of hemorrhage can be obtained from changes in the pulse and blood pressure. If the pulse rises more than 25 percent and the systolic blood pressure falls more than 20 millimeters of mercury, the chances are good that the blood loss is greater than 1000 milliliters. Under these circumstances shock, which usually occurs with acute blood loss of 1500 milliliters, is imminent.

volume with concomitant enhanced viscosity (stickiness or resistance to flow); they include *dizziness, headache, vertigo, blurred vision* and *stroke. Abnormal bleeding* is common. As the spleen becomes enlarged, *abdominal pain* and *fullness* may be noted. It is now thought that polycythemia vera represents one stage of a spectrum of hematologic disorders (the *myeloproliferative syndromes*) which also includes *myelofibrosis-myeloid metaplasia, chronic granulocytic leukemia* and *hemorrhagic thrombocythemia,* a condition in which bleeding occurs in the face of excess platelets. The precise relationship between these conditions is unknown, but it seems likely that *myelofibrosis* results as a late consequence of the marrow overgrowth that initially caused polycythemia. For unknown reason fibrous tissue (scar) is laid down, red cell overproduction diminishes, anemia develops and marrow cells proliferate in other sites (*myeloid metaplasia*) in an attempt to overcome the anemia. As a consequence liver and spleen enlarge and platelet and white cell production increase. In some patients white blood cell synthesis goes out of control and *leukemia* results. In others platelet overproduction results in *thrombocythemia.* The excess platelets predispose to spontaneous clot formation throughout the body and presumably cause bleeding by the mechanisms described under disseminated intravascular coagulation (see page 300).

Polycythemia vera is treated by *phlebotomy,* the regular removal of blood. In resistant patients chemotherapeutic suppression of the bone marrow or radioactive phosphorus therapy may be used. The latter is somewhat controversial because it increases the subsequent risk of leukemic transformation. Myelofibrosis-myeloid metaplasia is treated by androgen administration and occasionally splenectomy. Granulocytic leukemia and thrombocythemia require chemotherapy.

BLEEDING DISORDERS

PLATELET DISEASES

Diseases involving platelets, essentially all of which result in bleeding that is potentially dangerous, are of three types: *thrombocytopenia* indicates a decreased number of platelets; *thrombasthenia* refers to a state of abnormal platelet function despite normal numbers; and *thrombocythemia* indicates increased numbers of platelets.

Thrombocytopenia. Diminished platelet number is frequently due to bone marrow suppression by *drugs* such as chemotherapeutic (cytotoxic) agents used in the treatment of cancer. Thrombocytopenia is also part of the *aplastic anemia syndrome.* Defective maturation of platelets occurs in *vitamin B_{12}* or *folic acid deficiency* and in the congenital disease called the *Wiskott-Aldrich syndrome.* In the latter, precursor cells for the platelets (*megakaryocytes*) are normal but do not progress to platelet production. In addition, thrombocytopenia can result from *increased rates of platelet destruction.* A common cause is enlargement of the spleen (*hypersplenism*). In *idiopathic thrombocytopenic purpura* platelet destruction is due to auto-antibodies. The term *purpura* refers to bleeding in the skin, but hemorrhage can occur anywhere in the body. The disease is treated by administration of prednisone. Patients who do not respond to steroids undergo splenectomy (removal of the spleen) with an 85 percent cure rate. *Thrombotic thrombocytopenic purpura* is a fulminant, frequently lethal disorder in which thrombocytopenia and severe bleeding are accompanied by widespread clot formation, extensive neurologic (strokelike) lesions that may be transient or permanent, fever and kidney failure. Hemolytic anemia is severe, and bizarrely shaped or fragmented red cells are seen on blood smear. The cause of the disease is unknown. High dose prednisone therapy and emergency splenectomy are recommended, but the outlook is poor. Platelet number also falls in *disseminated intravascular coagulation.*

Acute bleeding episodes due to thrombocytopenia from any cause are treated by platelet transfusions.

Thrombasthenia. Thrombasthenia is a congenital disorder in which platelets do not aggregate at a bleeding site and do not undergo the release reaction to initiate clotting. Secondary impairment of platelet function can be produced by aspirin and other drugs.[14]

[14] Patients predisposed to developing clots, transient ischemic attacks in the brain (little strokes) and myocardial infarction have been treated with aspirin and sulfinpyrazone to induce a mild functional thrombasthenia. The hope is that thrombosis can be prevented. Preliminary results are encouraging, but firm conclusions regarding long-term benefits cannot yet be drawn. Interestingly beneficial effects have been seen only in men.

Thrombocythemia. This condition is usually a manifestation of myeloproliferative disease and has already been described. *Thrombocytosis* refers to the functionally insignificant rise in platelet number that often occurs following acute hemorrhage, general surgical procedures and splenectomy.

COAGULATION FACTOR DEFECTS

Coagulation factors may be congenitally absent or fall secondary to acquired disease. Factor VIII deficiency is by far the most common of the congenital disorders and is associated with two clinical syndromes: classical *hemophilia* and *von Willebrand's disease.* Defects in synthesis of factors IX, XI and fibrinogen are also known; they produce a hemophilialike state but are much rarer. Also infrequent are deficiencies of factors XII and XIII (a factor not previously mentioned which is necessary for stabilization of newly formed clots). The former is asymptomatic while the latter is associated with bleeding. Acquired insufficiency of coagulation factors may result from *vitamin K depletion, severe liver disease, disseminated intravascular coagulation and therapeutic administration of anticoagulant drugs.*[15] *Circulating anticoagulants* which block the action of coagulant factors are also known. Usually antibodies, they may arise spontaneously or be secondary to immune diseases such as lupus erythematosus.

Hemophilia and von Willebrand's Disease. Factor VIII is a large molecule which has two actions, one necessary for the clotting cascade and the other necessary for proper platelet function. In *hemophilia* the coagulant activity is deficient but the platelet-promoting function is intact. In *von Willebrand's disease* the platelet-promoting factor is primarily defective while coagulation activity is only moderately depressed. *Hemophilia* causes abnormal bleeding following mild trauma, especially into joints. Since platelet function is normal, bleeding from small cuts stops normally but failure to progress to clot

---

[15] The two most commonly used anticoagulants are *heparin* (which must be given by injection) and *coumarin derivatives* (which can be given orally). Heparin acts primarily by inactivating thrombin while the coumarins block the action of vitamin K. These drugs are very tricky to use, and bleeding complications often occur even when they are given under the strict supervision of a skilled physician. For this reason I recommend their use only in thrombophlebitis, pulmonary embolism and rarely in certain forms of heart disease known to predispose to clot formation with subsequent embolization (cardiomyopathies).

formation leads to delayed hemorrhage. While joints are most often involved, hemorrhage may occur from any site in the body. By contrast, patients with *von Willebrand's disease* bleed following minor cuts and bruise easily (because the initial platelet plug does not form) but ordinarily do not hemorrhage.

Treatment involves transfusion of whole blood for major blood loss and administration of fresh frozen plasma (which contains the clotting factors that are deficient in plasma stored in the normal way). Concentrated factor VIII preparations are also available but are very expensive. Hepatitis is common in patients with hemophilia because of the large number of transfusions required.

Liver Disease. Severe liver disease always results in abnormalities of the clotting system. Cirrhosis (alcoholic or postnecrotic) and severe hepatitis are the usual causes. Multiple coagulation factors are involved with fibrinogen deficiency being prominent. No effective therapy is available.

Disseminated Intravascular Coagulation (DIC). In certain clinical conditions widespread intravascular clot formation occurs followed by the appearance of extensive, uncontrollable bleeding. The outstanding causes are shock, invasion of the bloodstream by bacteria (septicemia), certain cancers, intrauterine fetal death and premature separation of the placenta in pregnancy, and severe liver disease. The apparent mechanism is precipitation of essentially all of the fibrinogen in the blood as a consequence of massive clotting. Breakdown of fibrin by the fibrinolytic system yields fibrin fragments that have anticoagulant activity. Platelets and other coagulant factors also fall. As a consequence blood begins to ooze from multiple blood vessels. Treatment is inadequate although heparin is given (to prevent further pathologic clotting) together with fibrinogen, platelet and whole blood transfusions. Despite such heroic measures the outlook is grim unless the predisposing process can be reversed.

THE LEUKEMIAS

The leukemias are malignant diseases of the bone marrow involving the stem cells from which mature blood cells are normally made. The four most common forms are *acute lympho-*

blastic, acute myelogenous, chronic lymphocytic and *chronic myelogenous leukemias.* Other leukemias, which occur much less frequently, show malignant proliferation of monocytes, eosinophils, basophils, erythrocytes or mast cells. Sometimes the leukemic cell is so primitive as to defy classification, in which case the term *stem cell leukemia* is used. Precise identification is important because chemotherapy varies drastically depending on the cell type.

The clinical picture in *acute leukemia* consists of the rapid onset of weakness, fever and abnormal bleeding. Patients are prone to infection, and neurologic findings are extremely common either because of leukemic infiltration of the brain, meninges or spinal cord or because of hemorrhage into these areas. Headache, vomiting, loss of consciousness and paralysis are the major manifestations of central nervous system involvement. Bleeding usually is due to deficient platelet number (their production is impaired in the leukemic bone marrow) while infection is the consequence of impaired white cell function. Symptoms in *chronic leukemias* develop much more slowly with anemia, weakness, weight loss, lymph node enlargement or pain in the abdomen due to an enlarged spleen being the primary complaints.

In the past acute leukemia was invariably and rapidly fatal. Remarkably, complete cures can now be achieved in 30 percent or more of children with acute lymphoblastic leukemia and prolonged survival has been achieved in those who are not cured.[16] Therapy is not as effective in acute myelogenous forms but even here is much better than in the past. Chronic lymphocytic leukemia is a slowly progressive disease which may need no therapy for prolonged periods. Chronic myelogenous leukemia always requires treatment but usually is responsive to chemotherapeutic drugs. However, the disease may suddenly shift into a phase resembling acute leukemia (a condition called *blast crisis*) in which case there is resistance to therapy. Remission of blast crisis can be achieved in only about 20 percent of cases.

---

[16] In addition to chemotherapeutic drugs, patients have to receive X-ray treatment to the brain and spinal cord. The cytotoxic agents do not penetrate the central nervous system, which has been called a "privileged sanctuary" for the leukemic cells. If they are not wiped out by X-ray, the disease recurs even if chemotherapy has effectively destroyed leukemic cells elsewhere. The chemotherapeutic regimens are quite complicated and involve multiple drugs; they will not be outlined here.

MULTIPLE MYELOMA

Multiple myeloma is a neoplastic disease (somewhat analogous to leukemia) in which the plasma cell becomes malignant.[17] Plasma cells are antibody-producing cells that are probably derived from lymphocytes. The disease manifests itself by attacking bone. X-ray shows multiple punched-out lesions and, in late stages, generalized thinning. The initial symptom is usually back pain. On examination the patient is found to be weak and anemic and to have high levels of calcium in the blood. Examination of plasma proteins shows a marked elevation of the IgG fraction (which normally contains circulating antibodies); this peak of IgG protein is called the M (myeloma) spike. Many patients have a protein in the urine called *Bence Jones protein*. Diagnosis is confirmed by bone marrow aspiration showing sheets of plasma cells replacing the normal marrow structure. Patients with myeloma are peculiarly susceptible to infection (especially pneumococcal pneumonia). Death is usually due to pneumonia or kidney failure. The latter results from deposition of myeloma proteins in the kidney tubules with obstruction to urine flow and subsequent tubular destruction. Myeloma may be complicated by the appearance of *amyloidosis*, in which another abnormal protein (*amyloid*) is deposited throughout the body damaging heart, nerves and kidney. Treatment consists of the administration of melphalan and cyclophosphamide, two chemotherapeutic agents that are usually quite effective.

LYMPHOMAS

The lymphomas are malignancies of the lymphatic system. The best known is *Hodgkin's disease*, but other tumors with different clinical presentations and distinct features on microscopic examination of biopsied tissue are also part of the lym-

---

[17] Other conditions associated with plasma cell abnormalities are known wherein different proteins accumulate in blood: *Waldenström's macroglobulinemia, gamma heavy-chain disease,* and *alpha-chain disease.* Clinically they tend to resemble lymphomas rather than myeloma.

phoma group. These are called *non-Hodgkin's lymphomas,* an imprecise term but one which is probably here to stay. The lymphomas are generally diagnosed when the patient notices painless enlargement of lymph nodes in the neck or elsewhere in the body; alternatively large lymph nodes may be identified in the chest by routine chest X-ray. Unexplained fever and generalized itching may signal the presence of the disease. Weakness and weight loss are usual in the late stages. Examination often shows enlargement of the liver and spleen. The bone is widely involved and often painful. Affected patients are peculiarly prone to infection, especially by funguses. Diagnosis is made by biopsy of involved lymph nodes or other tissues. Lymphangiography and gallium scans are occasionally helpful in obscure cases.

Treatment depends on the stage and spread of the disease. The critical issue is whether the tumor is localized or has spread into chest and abdomen. The first line of treatment is X-ray, since most lymphomas are radiosensitive. With disseminated disease, chemotherapy is required. Cure is now possible in many patients with Hodgkin's disease, and prolonged remission can be induced even in the more malignant non-Hodgkin's lymphomas.

15

Endocrine and
Metabolic Diseases

The endocrine glands are specialized tissues that have the capacity to synthesize and secrete *hormones* into the bloodstream.[1] These hormones, which chemically are usually either short chains of amino acids (*peptide hormones*) or cholesterol-like molecules (*steroid hormones*), do not act indiscriminately on all tissues; rather, they affect only certain *target organs*. Some hormones have only one target tissue while others act at multiple sites. As noted in chapter 2, hormones regulate the speed or rate at which chemical reactions in the body are carried out but do not themselves catalyze chemical transformations. How this regulatory activity is accomplished is just beginning to be understood. In general peptide hormones bind to receptors on the cell surface and thereby induce formation or release of a *second messenger* (often an important intracellular chemical called *cyclic AMP*) which then produces the expected biological effect. Steroid hormones, on the other hand, tend to bind to chromosomes in the nucleus of the cell, thereby inducing the synthesis of messenger RNA which codes for the syn-

[1] In the past it was thought that hormones acted only at a site distant to their point of origin. This is now known to be inaccurate. Many hormones also act in the tissues where they are made without ever passing into the bloodstream. Local hormone action is referred to as *paracrine function*, while the term *endocrine function* indicates an action away from the originating organ.

thesis of a specialized protein. This protein then becomes the final mediator of hormone action.

The endocrine glands include the *hypothalamus* and the *pituitary gland* (located in the brain), the *thyroid* and *parathyroid glands* (situated in the neck), the *pancreas* and *adrenal glands* (intra-abdominal organs) and the *testes* and *ovaries* (the sexual glands). Diseases of these glands are arbitrarily divided into two categories. Those disorders affecting the pancreas, parathyroid glands and the levels of cholesterol and triglyceride in the blood are designated *metabolic*[2] while diseases of the hypothalamus, pituitary, thyroid, gonads and adrenals are classified as *endocrine*. The number of endocrine and metabolic diseases is very large. In this chapter only the major dysfunctions will be considered. (Diseases of testes and ovaries are discussed in chapter 12.)

DIAGNOSTIC PROCEDURES

RADIOIMMUNOASSAY

Radioimmunoassay techniques have revolutionized endocrinology by making it possible to measure all hormones at the extremely low concentrations in which they are found in blood. In principle the procedure is quite simple and requires only a radioactive form of the hormone to be measured, an antibody which will bind the hormone (produced by immunizing animals with the desired hormone) and a method for separating free from antibody-bound material. Here is how it works. Radioactive hormone (H*) and antibody (Ab) are added to the sample to be tested and incubated. During this time a portion of the hormone binds to antibody according to the reaction.

$$(1) \; H^* + Ab \rightleftharpoons H^*Ab$$

(The double arrows signify that the reaction is reversible.) After the proper interval the antibody-bound hormone is isolated by one of a variety of techniques, and the radioactivity in free and

[2] Disorders of fat and cholesterol metabolism (the *hyperlipoproteinemias*) can result from disease of the endocrine glands but also may develop independently of hormonal dysfunction. Despite this fact they have traditionally been considered as metabolic diseases.

antibody-bound fractions is determined. If the plasma sample contains none of the hormone to be assayed, all hormone bound to antibody will be radioactive. On the other hand if natural hormone is present, the antibody will bind both radioactive (H*) and nonradioactive molecules (H):

$$(2)\ H^* + H + Ab \rightleftharpoons H^*Ab + HAb$$

The quantity of antibody added is deliberately kept insufficient to bind all the hormone present. Since the antibody cannot discriminate between radioactive and nonradioactive forms, there is competition between the two for binding. The higher the concentration of unlabeled hormone, the less radioactive hormone will be bound. As an illustration, in a control sample devoid of native hormone, the antibody is found to bind 10,000 counts per minute of radioactivity; after incubation with hormone-containing plasma, only 2000 counts per minute of antibody-bound radioactivity are recovered. From standard curves run with known amounts of pure hormone, the laboratory can determine how much hormone would have had to be present in the plasma sample to displace 8000 counts of radioactivity and thus calculate its concentration.

PROVOCATIVE TESTS

In addition to measuring hormone levels, it is often necessary to carry out provocative tests of endocrine regulation. Two general types are done: *stimulation* and *suppression.* Before illustrating these tests I would like to point out that endocrine glands do not operate at a fixed or static level. Hormone release is stimulated or inhibited depending on the need of the moment. For example, if the blood sugar begins to rise, insulin release from the pancreas is stimulated in order to lower it. If the blood glucose falls, insulin release is inhibited. Pancreas and parathyroid glands are regulated directly by the substances they control (glucose, amino acids, fats for the former; calcium for the latter) while the adrenal glands, thyroid and gonads are linked in more complicated fashion with the hypothalamus and pituitary gland. The regulatory system (called *feedback control*) can be illustrated for the thyroid as follows. Suppose for some reason the production of thyroid hormone by the thyroid gland decreases. The hypothalamus recognizes a fall in its plasma concentration and immediately secretes thyroid releasing hormone (*TRH*) which passes to the pituitary and causes release of thyroid stimulating hormone (*TSH*) into the bloodstream. TSH, on reaching the thyroid, then induces the synthesis of additional thyroid hormone. Conversely, if thyroid hormone production increases (or the patient is given thyroid hormone therapeutically), the production of TSH by the pituitary is inhibited, resulting in a fall of hormone production by the thyroid gland. In this way the circulating level of thyroid hormone is maintained within narrow limits. The same type of tight control operates throughout the endocrine system.

Stimulation tests are done when the clinical picture is compatible with deficiency of hormone production; they are designed to localize the site of abnormality to the target organ or the hypothalamic-pituitary control area. For example, deficiency of hydrocortisone (the major adrenal hormone) could be due to primary disease of the adrenal gland or to a central nervous system abnormality that results in impaired production of ACTH, the adrenal stimulating hormone. The two possibilities can be distinguished by injecting ACTH and measuring hydrocortisone response. If plasma hydrocortisone levels fail to rise, the presumption is that the defect is in the adrenal itself; on the other hand, if hydrocortisone concentration increases, it is clear that nothing is wrong with the adrenal and that the problem lies in a failure of stimulating hormone release by the hypothalamus or pituitary. A variety of such stimulation tests are used in endocrinology. *Suppression tests* address the opposite problem. When an endocrine gland becomes overactive, it usually becomes *autonomous* (independent of its normal control mechanisms). This is proved by administering exogenous hormone and showing that the gland does not stop the production of endogenous hormone as it should if the feedback system were working. For example, in Cushing's syndrome the adrenal glands make too much hydrocortisone. Administration of a powerful hydrocortisone analogue (*dexamethasone*) causes the normal adrenal to stop making hydrocortisone but does not suppress the Cushing's gland (or suppresses it only at supranormal doses).

OTHER TESTS

The *CAT scan* and *skull X-rays*, previously mentioned in the section on neurological disease, are extremely helpful in identifying lesions in the pituitary gland. The *radioactive iodine uptake* is a test done to evaluate thyroid function. Iodine is necessary for synthesis of thyroid hormone, and the degree to which radioactive iodine is taken up by the gland indicates whether it is functioning normally or in excess. A *radioactive scan* of the thyroid is done when cancer is suspected.

DIABETES MELLITUS

Diabetes mellitus is by far the most common of the endocrine and metabolic disorders.[3] Overt disease is present in about 2–4 percent of the American population and the incidence appears to be increasing. The *sine qua non* for diagnosis is elevation of the blood sugar (hyperglycemia).[4] Hyperglycemia then causes the symptoms that characterize the disease: *polyuria* (increased urine output), *polydipsia* (increased thirst) and *polyphagia* (increased food intake).[5] The symptoms result from the fact that glucose in the plasma passes through the glomerular apparatus of the kidney into the renal tubule. At high concentrations it cannot be reabsorbed and passes out into the urine. Because

---

[3] *Diabetes mellitus* refers to the spontaneous form of the disease that usually occurs in patients who have a positive family history for the illness: a genetic predisposition is readily discernible. An elevated blood sugar occurring secondary to destructive inflammatory disease in the pancreas, Cushing's syndrome, pheochromocytoma or other diseases is called *secondary diabetes*.

[4] The blood sugar is elevated because the liver makes too much glucose and because both dietary and endogenously produced glucose cannot be metabolized normally by nonhepatic tissues. These changes result because insulin, the glucose-lowering hormone is deficient and because glucagon, the glucose-elevating hormone, is released excessively. While insulin is routinely used in treatment, major efforts are being made to develop a glucagon-blocking drug. *Somatostatin*, a naturally occurring hormone, has this capacity but its biological activity is very short. It is possible that long-acting analogues of the hormone can be developed which will do the job. An antiglucagon agent should markedly simplify the management of diabetes.

[5] In the past diabetes was often diagnosed on the basis of the *oral glucose tolerance test*. In this test 50 to 100 grams of pure glucose is taken orally and the blood sugar response measured. A value at 2 hours of greater than 140 milligrams per 100 milliliters of plasma was once considered to indicate diabetes. It is now recognized that the test results in many false positives: normal persons are often diagnosed as having diabetes. For this reason the National Institutes of Health in 1979 issued new guidelines for the oral glucose tolerance test which reserve the diagnosis of diabetes for a 2-hour value of 200 milligrams per 100 milliliters of plasma or greater, with at least one other value reaching that level in the interval before 2 hours. My view is that glucose tolerance testing should be abandoned and that the diagnosis of diabetes should be made only if there is persistent elevation of plasma glucose after an overnight fast. While most normal persons have fasting values below 100 milligrams per 100 milliliters of plasma, diabetes cannot be definitely diagnosed unless fasting concentrations are above 140 milligrams per 100 milliliters.

water is required to maintain glucose in solution, its reabsorption is also impaired and urine output increases dramatically (there is an osmotic diuresis). The accelerated loss of water makes the patient thirsty while excretion of large amounts of glucose represents a drain of calories from the body, requiring increased food intake.

Patients with diabetes are susceptible to acute metabolic emergencies (the *diabetic comas*) and, over time, to a series of *degenerative complications* affecting the eyes, kidneys, nerves and blood vessels.

Types of Diabetes. Diabetes is not a single homogeneous disease, but a group of distinct illnesses. *Juvenile diabetes* (insulin-dependent diabetes, Type I diabetes), as the name implies, tends to appear in young persons (often before the age of 10) but may develop at any stage of life. Typically the patients are thin, have low or immeasurable plasma insulin levels and require exogenous insulin for treatment. When control is inadequate they are prone to develop the acute complication called *diabetic ketoacidosis.* While the disease clearly has a genetic component, it is now recognized that environmental factors are extremely important. This follows from the observation that when one of a pair of identical twins (whose genetic makeups are precisely the same) has diabetes, the disease develops in the other twin in only about 30 percent of cases. (In a pure genetic disease the concordance rate would be 100 percent.) The environmental factor is widely thought to be one of several viruses; recently a virus (called Coxsackievirus B_4) was isolated from the pancreas of a 10-year-old boy who died in diabetic coma, and it was shown to produce diabetes when inoculated into animals. In some cases autoantibodies that attack the pancreatic islets may be important. *Maturity-onset diabetes* (non-insulin-dependent diabetes, Type II diabetes) usually appears in subjects over the age of 40; most affected individuals are fat. In contrast to the juvenile form, plasma insulin levels are not low (in absolute terms), yet the blood sugar is high. The problem is a resistance to the action of insulin that is induced by obesity: while maturity-onset patients do have a modest decrease in insulin reserve, more than enough insulin is present to maintain plasma glucose levels in the normal range if obesity were not present. Support for this interpretation comes from many studies demonstrating that increased body fat (with or without diabetes) inhibits the action of insulin; moreover, when obese maturity-onset diabetics lose weight, remission of diabetes is often observed. Most patients with this form of the disease respond to oral sulfonylureas (which stimulate endogenous insulin secretion) and do not require insulin injections. Studies in identical twins indicate that the concordance rate is close to 100 percent suggesting that genetic factors are overwhelmingly important for development of the disease. Patients with maturity-onset diabetes do not develop ketoacidosis but may suffer *hyperosmolar, nonketotic coma* as a complication. *Lipoatrophic diabetes,* a very rare condition, is a synonym for the *lipodystrophic states.* These disorders, which may be genetic or acquired, and which may be partial or involve the entire body, are characterized by a total absence of fat in affected areas. Almost always a disease of women, the most common form has normal or excess fat below the waist with a cadaverous appearance to the upper part of the body—every bone is visible through the tightly stretched skin. The diabetes is due to profound insulin resistance rather than insulin deficiency.

Acute Metabolic Complications. Diabetic ketoacidosis is a serious complication of juvenile diabetes which may occur because the patient does not take the prescribed insulin or be a consequence of infection, surgery or emotional stress. The plasma glucose is very high, and there is a severe metabolic acidosis due to the accumulation of acetoacetic and beta-hydroxybutyric acids (the *ketoacids*) in the blood. The syndrome begins with nausea, vomiting and increased urine output; as the patient worsens respiration becomes deep and driven as a consequence of the acidosis (*Kussmaul breathing*). Untreated patients lapse into coma and die in shock but with prompt therapy more than 95 percent survive. *Hyperosmolar, nonketotic coma* occurs in uncontrolled maturity onset disease and differs from ketoacidosis in that overproduction of acetoacetic and beta-hydroxybutyric acids does not occur. The reason is not known. In this syndrome the plasma glucose rises to astronomical levels (as high as 2000 milligrams per 100 milliliters) resulting in profound polyuria and massive depletion of body fluids with shock and kidney failure. Convulsions, coma and widespread clotting in the vessels of the brain complete the picture. The complication usually develops in elderly diabetics who live alone and develop an infection, stroke or other illness that throws them out of control. Mortality rates are greater than 50 percent even with treatment.

Degenerative Complications. A significant percentage of all diabetics develop late degenerative complications that appear on average 15 to 20 years after onset of the disease. These changes involve the eyes, nerves, kidneys and blood vessels. Eye involvement, called *diabetic retinopathy,* is accompanied by retinal hemorrhages, exudates (yellow-white spots reflecting loss of blood supply) and microaneurysms (small, round, red dots representing dilated capillaries). Such changes only rarely impair vision significantly. In some patients a much worse form of retinopathy develops with growth of new blood vessels across the retina, extensive scar formation, retinal detachment and major bleeding into the internal eye (*vitreal hemorrhage*). This complication is called *proliferative diabetic retinopathy.* While only a relatively small percentage of diabetics advance to the proliferative stage, because there are so many diabetics it is now the leading cause of blindness in the United States. *Diabetic neuropathy* is the term used to describe nerve degeneration in diabetics. The usual symptoms are numbness, tingling and pain in the extremities. Impaired perception of pain and position sense may lead to pressure sores and ulcer formation in the feet. Involvement of intestinal nerves causes a persistent form of diarrhea while disease of pelvic nerve branches leads to bladder paralysis (a dread complication requiring chronic catheterization). Rarely sudden cardiac or respiratory arrest results from diseased nerves controlling the heart and lungs. *Diabetic nephropathy* (also called Kimmelstiel-Wilson disease) indicates destructive disease in the kidney due to diabetes. Kidney failure is now the leading cause of death in diabetic patients. Finally, *atherosclerosis* occurs at an accelerated rate in both coronary and peripheral vessels (the latter predisposing to development of gangrene in the lower extremities).

The cause of diabetic complications remains unknown. Many physicians believe that hyperglycemia itself is responsible while others feel that factors other than elevated blood sugar are involved since complications occasionally develop *before* the plasma glucose is ever elevated.

Treatment. All patients with diabetes require careful *dietary therapy* which proscribes sweets and refined sugars. In obese subjects normalization of body weight is of first priority. Juvenile patients are treated with *insulin* (usually one or two injections a day of a long-acting preparation such as NPH or Lente insulin; occasionally a small amount of short-acting regular insulin is added as well).[6] Maturity-onset disease often responds to *sulfonylureas* which can be given by mouth.[7] Diabetic comas are treated with intravenous regular insulin and large amounts of IV fluids. Therapy of diabetic retinopathy has improved dramatically through use of the *laser beam* to prevent hemorrhage and repair retinal detachments. Painful diabetic neuropathy can often be controlled by combination therapy with the drugs *fluphenazine* and *amitriptyline*. Kidney failure requires chronic dialysis or kidney transplantation. Active research continues into the possibility of doing pancreatic transplantation in diabetics, but at present the barriers appear overwhelming.

DISEASES OF THE THYROID

The thyroid gland controls multiple functions in the body but its primary role is regulation of metabolism. When thyroid hormone is released, general tissue metabolism speeds up: the heart rate accelerates, oxygen uptake increases and the generation of heat is enhanced. If thyroid hormone excess is persistent, weight loss occurs because ingested calories are wasted as heat rather than being coupled to useful energy formation.[8]

---

[6] Details of insulin therapy are too complicated to be discussed here. The problem is to administer insulin in sufficient amounts to control symptoms but not so much as to cause hypoglycemia (*insulin reactions*). This is not always easy. A promising approach is the use of small, battery-driven insulin pumps that administer insulin subcutaneously at a constant basal rate with burst injections before meals. Such pumps, which are only a little larger than a pocket calculator, are undergoing widespread clinical trials.

[7] The oral antidiabetic agents are the subject of much controversy among physicians. A famous study (the *UGDP study*) suggested that one of the sulfonylureas (tolbutamide) might increase deaths from heart attacks. Critics have vociferously disputed these conclusions. Those interested in reading about the controversy are referred to an excellent summary in *Science* 203:986–990, 1979. My own bias is that the drugs are safe and useful in a number of patients.

[8] The hormone produced by the thyroid gland is called *thyroxine* (or T_4, indicating that the molecule contains 4 iodine atoms). In order to exert its metabolic effects, thyroxine must be converted to its active form, *triiodothyronine* (T_3), by the splitting off of one specific iodine atom. This conversion takes place in liver and other peripheral tissues. If an alternative iodine is removed, a metabolically inactive product called *reverse triiodothyronine* (rT_3) is produced. It turns out that in acute illness, starvation or other conditions where tissue wasting is expected, T_3 levels fall and rT_3 concentrations rise, presumably to slow metabolism and minimize weight loss.

Conversely, a deficiency of thyroid hormone results in a slow-ing of body metabolism, failure of heat generation and weight gain. Both hyperfunction and diminished activity of the thyroid are frequently seen in clinical medicine. Two other thyroid diseases are common: thyroiditis, in which the gland is infil-trated by inflammatory cells that disrupt its function, and be-nign or malignant nodule formation.

HYPERTHYROIDISM (THYROTOXICOSIS)

Patients with thyrotoxicosis exhibit nervousness, emotional lability, tremors, weight loss (despite increased food intake), sweating, heat intolerance, rapid heart rate and abnormal car-diac rhythms (especially the type called *atrial fibrillation*). True heart failure may occur. Cessation of menses is common in women. Increased frequency of defecation or frank diarrhea is not unusual. The thyroid gland is almost always enlarged. The skin is smooth and velvety; spotty depigmentation (*viti-ligo*) may develop. The hair tends to become very fine, and the nails frequently separate from their underlying beds (*onycho-lysis*). A distressing feature is *exophthalmos,* a condition in which the eyes bulge from their sockets resulting in inflamma-tion, ulceration of the corneas (because lids cannot cover the eyes during sleep) and pain. Older patients may exhibit *apa-thetic hyperthyroidism*, meaning that signs of nervousness and hypermetabolism are missing, and only the weight loss and heart findings are present. An acute exacerbation of symptoms, often produced by infections, surgery or other stress, is called *thyroid storm.* Signs are high fever, heart failure, worsening diarrhea and altered central nervous system function (stupor or coma). This complication is serious and potentially fatal.

Most cases of thyrotoxicosis appear to be due to autoimmune disease: antibodylike molecules appear in the blood that stim-ulate thyroid hormone overproduction. As with all autoimmune phenomena, the cause is unknown. A few cases are due to au-tonomously functioning thyroid nodules (single or multiple). Very rarely pituitary overproduction of thyroid-stimulating hor-mone may be responsible for the disease. Diagnosis is usually clear from the clinical picture but is confirmed by finding an *elevated concentration of thyroid hormone* in the blood, a *high radioactive iodine uptake* and a *low level of TSH* (because of feedback inhibition by the elevated thyroxine levels). The latter is *unresponsive to stimulation by exogenous thyroid-releasing hormone.*

Three forms of treatment are available. If severe symptoms are present, initial therapy is carried out with *propylthiouracil,* a drug that both blocks glandular production of thyroxine and inhibits its peripheral conversion to triiodothyronine. About 25 percent of patients undergo permanent remission following prolonged treatment with propylthiouracil, but definitive therapy by *surgery* or *radioactive iodine administration* usually is required. The former is used in young persons and women during the child-bearing period (because of the outside possibility that radioactive iodine might cause a mutation if given during growth periods or pregnancy). Partial thyroidectomy is a safe procedure although rarely the parathyroid glands are damaged during surgery, requiring treatment for hypoparathyroidism. Even less frequently the recurrent laryngeal nerve is injured resulting in permanent hoarseness. Most patients are now treated with radioactive iodine to destroy the overactive gland. The procedure is quick, painless and very effective. Mild cases can be treated without first controlling the disease with drugs. The only problem is that hypothyroidism frequently results (sometimes years later) requiring therapy with thyroid hormone. Experience with thousands of patients (over many years) clearly indicates that radioactive iodine does not induce thyroid cancer. *Thyroid storm* requires aggressive therapy if the patient is to survive. In addition to large doses of propylthiouracil, *sodium iodide* is infused intravenously to block release of preformed hormone from the gland. *Dexamethasone* and *propranolol* are also given to enhance the inhibition of $T_4 \rightarrow T_3$ conversion and slow the heart rate. There is no specific treatment for exophthalmos, but if the condition progresses to the point where sight is threatened (malignant exophthalmos), a trial of high-dose steroids (prednisone) is given. Success is variable.

HYPOTHYROIDISM

Hypothyroidism results in fatigue, slowed mental and physical activity, cold intolerance (because of inability to increase heat production), hoarseness, constipation, personality change (apathy, irritability) and dry skin. In women menstrual flow may become excessive. Fluid often accumulates in the sac surrounding the heart (*pericardial effusion*) but heart failure does not occur. Extreme cases progress to *myxedema coma,* a state in which body temperature is extremely low, respiration is impaired (such that CO_2 accumulates in the blood) and consciousness is lost. Mortality rates are high. Hypothyroidism occurring in the fetus results in *cretinism.* Affected children are mentally retarded (brain development is impaired), do not grow, have delayed tooth and bone formation and exhibit a characteristic facies with narrow forehead, puffy eyes, pug nose, protruding tongue and thick neck. The abdomen is markedly distended and hernias are frequent.

Hypothyroidism may be primary or secondary. In primary disease the abnormality is in the thyroid gland itself while in secondary forms the pituitary does not release TSH normally, either because it is diseased or because hypothalamic control is impaired. Primary disease may occur *idiopathically* or develop as a late consequence of *Hashimoto's thyroiditis,* an illness caused by autoantibodies directed against the thyroid. Many cases also result from *radioactive iodine* or *surgical treatment of hyperthyroidism.* Rarely *congenital enzyme defects* occur which block thyroxine synthesis.

Diagnosis is based on the finding of low thyroxine levels in blood. Measurement of TSH will usually differentiate primary from secondary forms: if the defect is in the thyroid gland and the pituitary-hypothalamic axis is normal, TSH levels will be high in an attempt to overcome the thyroid deficiency. If TSH and T_4 levels are both low, the problem is likely in the pituitary or hypothalamus. Confirmation that the defect is in central control comes by showing that administration of TSH normalizes radioactive iodine uptake (which is initially low) and thyroxine production.

Treatment of hypothyroidism is extremely simple since purified hormone is available as a pill that can be taken orally.[9]

THYROIDITIS

Several types of thyroiditis are recognized. *Subacute thyroiditis,* which may be virus induced, is associated with fever and pain in the neck, particularly on swallowing. The pain may

---

[9] Thyroid hormone is often administered indiscriminately to "tired" patients who have no evidence of hypothyroidism or to obese subjects in an attempt to induce weight loss. Both practices are to be condemned.

radiate to the ears. On examination the thyroid gland is enlarged and tender. Some patients have symptoms similar to thyrotoxicosis because the inflammatory process causes leakage of excess thyroid hormone into the blood. As a consequence T_4 levels in plasma may be high. In contrast to ordinary thyrotoxicosis, however, the radioactive iodine uptake is low. The disease is self-limited (1 to 3 months) and symptoms can be controlled by aspirin. *Hashimoto's thyroiditis* is a chronic disorder that usually manifests itself only by the presence of an enlarged, slightly irregular thyroid which is not tender to palpation. Progressive damage to the gland results in a high percentage of permanent hypothyroidism. The disease is thought to be autoimmune in nature, and the diagnosis is suggested by the finding of high levels of antithyroid antibodies in the blood. Treatment is unnecessary unless hypothyroidism supervenes. *Acute thyroiditis* with abscess formation secondary to bacterial infection is rare.

SIMPLE GOITER

The term *goiter* means enlargement of the thyroid gland. Most goiters are associated with recognizable thyroid disease (thyrotoxicosis, Hashimoto's thyroiditis, congenital enzyme defects) but thyroid swelling can occur without hormone dysfunction. Such enlargement is called *simple goiter*. It occurs most often in those parts of the world where iodine deficiency is prevalent (in the United States, primarily the Great Lakes area) but may develop sporadically for unknown reason. Simple goiters are common in pregnancy. The glands can usually be reduced in size by giving thyroid hormone, but treatment is necessary only if the goiter is large enough to be cosmetically unattractive. It is presumed that the process begins with an impairment of thyroxine synthesis which is overcome by increased release of TSH from the pituitary (but at the price of increased thyroid size). By providing exogenous thyroid hormone, TSH release is inhibited and the gland shrinks.

THYROID NODULES AND THYROID CANCER

Thyroid nodules (benign tumors or adenomas) develop in about 10 percent of all thyroid glands for reasons that are not yet known. Frequently more than one nodule is present in which case the designation *multinodular goiter* is used. More worrisome is the *single nodule* which can either be benign or represent a *thyroid cancer*. The incidence of thyroid cancer is increased in patients who have had X-ray to the face or neck (done in the past for acne or thymus gland enlargement) but it can also occur spontaneously. All subjects exposed to radiation should have the thyroid examined for nodules at yearly intervals. If a nodule is felt, the first step in workup is to get a radioactive scan of the gland. If the scan shows multiple nodules or if there is a single nodule that takes up radioactivity ("hot" nodule), nothing else need be done. If the isolated nodule does not take up radioactivity ("cold" nodule) cancer has to be considered. The general rule is that single cold nodules should be removed in men of any age and women under 40. In women over 40, a trial of thyroid suppression (like that described for simple goiter) is acceptable. If the nodule shrinks, surgery is not necessary, but failure of suppression or further growth is indication for surgical removal. Even if cancer is found, the vast majority of patients have a benign course. Only a few patients (usually those with anaplastic or undifferentiated lesions) undergo metastases and die from their disease. All patients with carcinoma of the thyroid gland must be treated for life with exogenous thyroid to suppress TSH release since many of the tumors appear to be dependent on TSH for growth. *Medullary carcinoma of the thyroid,* a rare neoplasm associated with the multiple endocrine neoplasia syndrome, is described on page 328.

DISEASES OF THE ADRENAL GLAND

The two adrenal glands are located just above the kidneys. Each gland consists of an outer *cortex* and an inner *medulla*. Hormones produced by the cortex are involved in the maintenance of the blood sugar and blood pressure (*hydrocortisone*), reabsorption of salt and regulation of potassium excretion in the kidney (*aldosterone*) and development of certain secondary sexual characteristics (adrenal *estrogens* and *androgens*). The medulla produces *epinephrine* and *norepinephrine,* powerful hormones that increase the heart rate, raise blood pressure and elevate the blood sugar, particularly during periods of stress. The syndromes of hormone excess and deficiency that characterize disease of the adrenal reflect the actions of these hormones.

ADRENAL INSUFFICIENCY (ADDISON'S DISEASE)

Primary adrenal insufficiency is due to disease in the adrenal glands themselves. By far the most common cause is an idiopathic autoimmune disorder[10] in which antibodies directed against the cortex cause atrophy and scar formation. The adrenals can also be destroyed by tuberculosis (not nearly so common now as in the past), metastatic cancer, hemorrhage and chronic diseases such as sarcoidosis. *Secondary adrenal insufficiency* is due to dysfunction in the pituitary or hypothalamus. Whatever its etiology, adrenal insufficiency causes marked weakness and fatigue, often accompanied by salt craving and intermittent nausea and vomiting. In primary forms patients develop darkening of the skin which resembles a deep suntan except that areas not exposed to sun are also involved. Scars (which ordinarily are lighter than surrounding skin) become pigmented, the nipples are a deep brown color and dark spots are seen in the mouth and gums. The pigmentation is due to the fact that ACTH, the adrenal-stimulating hormone, is released in excessive amounts in an attempt to drive hormone production up in the diseased adrenals. A side effect of ACTH action is dispersal of pigment granules called *melanin* in the skin. Stress of any kind may induce *adrenal crisis*, a potentially fatal state manifested by nausea, repeated vomiting, diarrhea, fever and vascular collapse (shock).

Diagnosis is made by the finding of low levels of plasma hydrocortisone and/or the demonstration that urinary 17-hydroxysteroid levels (metabolic products of adrenal steroid metabolism) are diminished. Separation of primary and secondary forms is accomplished by administering exogenous ACTH. A rise in plasma hydrocortisone concentration after ACTH indicates that the adrenal glands are intact (the problem is in the hypothalamus or pituitary) while failure of response indicates primary disease. Confirmation of ACTH deficiency can be obtained by doing a *metyrapone test*. Metyrapone is a drug that

---

[10] At times antibodies develop against more than one endocrine gland in the same person. The most frequent constellation is autoimmune hypothyroidism and adrenal insufficiency (*Schmidt's syndrome*), but any endocrine gland may be involved, leading to various syndromes of combined endocrine failure (*immune endocrinopathy*).

blocks hydrocortisone synthesis and thereby stimulates ACTH release in normal subjects. Should this response not occur, pituitary or hypothalamic disease is present.

Adrenal crisis is treated by infusion of large amounts of *intravenous fluids* (patients are volume depleted because of vomiting and diarrhea coupled with impairment of salt reabsorption in the kidney) and intravenous *hydrocortisone*. Following recovery hydrocortisone can be given orally; lifelong replacement therapy is necessary. Many subjects also need small amounts of a salt-retaining hormone called *fludrocortisone* (which substitutes for aldosterone). During stressful periods (infections, surgery) extra hydrocortisone must be given. (The adrenals normally increase hormone production threefold to sixfold during stress.)

CUSHING'S SYNDROME

Cushing's syndrome is a term applied to any condition in which there is excess production of hydrocortisone (and other cortical hormones) by the adrenal gland. There are three major causes: overproduction of ACTH by the pituitary gland (which results in enlargement of both adrenals), benign or malignant tumor formation in the adrenal cortex, or abnormal (*ectopic*) ACTH production by cancers elsewhere in the body, especially in the lung.[11] Hyperfunctioning tumors in a single adrenal cause atrophy of the normal gland on the opposite side (because excess hydrocortisone from the tumor inhibits pituitary release of ACTH, causing shrinkage and cessation of function in the ACTH-dependent normal partner).

The clinical picture in full-blown Cushing's syndrome is one of the most striking in all of medicine. The face is rounded with full, flushed cheeks (*moon facies*), the central body is massively obese (the arms and legs are not fat and may even be wasted because of muscle atrophy), there is a humplike mass of fat at the junction of the upper back and lower neck (*buffalo-hump*) and wide, purplish breaks (*striae*) appear in the skin of back,

[11] Another common cause is the therapeutic administration of large doses of prednisone or other adrenal steroid analogues. Readers will surely have been struck by the large number of diseases that now appear to be autoimmune in origin, requiring steroid suppression of antibody formation. When one adds patients undergoing organ transplantation and those treated with steroids for other conditions (e.g., asthma, drug reactions) the number of subjects at risk for *iatrogenic* (physician-induced) Cushing's syndrome is truly formidable.

abdomen and axillary areas. The patients bruise easily, high blood pressure is common and muscle weakness (especially in the legs) is profound. Women often become hirsute and may virilize (with clitoral hypertrophy) due to excess of adrenal androgens. Acne is common. Back pain due to thinning of the bone and collapse of vertebrae is not infrequent (X-ray of bone shows extensive osteoporosis). On laboratory examination the blood sugar tends to be elevated while potassium levels are often low. All symptoms are the consequence of the physiological actions of excess hydrocortisone. These include impairment of protein synthesis and acceleration of protein breakdown (causing muscle atrophy, disruptibility of skin, fragility of blood vessels and thinning of bones), stimulation of fat synthesis, enhancement of glucose production and facilitation of potassium loss in the urine.

The diagnosis of Cushing's syndrome depends on two things. *First,* plasma hydrocortisone or urinary 17-hydroxysteroid concentrations must be elevated. *Second,* the elevated steroid levels must not fall during the dexamethasone suppression test. (Obesity and stress can raise hydrocortisone levels into the Cushing's range but these suppress when dexamethasone is supplied.)[12]

Treatment is complicated. In the past patients with pituitary overproduction of ACTH were treated by *removing the adrenal glands.* The disadvantage of this procedure is that it results in permanent adrenal insufficiency necessitating lifelong hormone replacement. More recently *transsphenoidal pituitary surgery* to remove the microadenomas that secrete ACTH has been carried out. Successful in a number of cases, the long-term efficacy of pituitary surgery remains to be established. The concern is that the primary problem may be in the hypothalamus. Should this prove to be true, recurrence of ACTH overproduction (and new microadenoma formation) might be expected from a continued hypothalamic drive. At the time of this writing, however, pituitary surgery appears to be the treatment of choice. *Drug therapy* utilizing a compound called *o,p'*DDD

[12] Dexamethasone suppression can also give a clue as to the cause of Cushing's syndrome. Normal patients and those with obesity and stress suppress hydrocortisone levels on 1 or 2 milligrams per day of dexamethasone. Patients with pituitary ACTH overproduction do not respond to 2 milligrams a day but will decrease plasma hydrocortisone on 8 milligrams per day. Subjects with adrenal tumors or ectopic ACTH do not suppress at any level.

(*ortho, para*-dichlorodiphenyldichloroethane) has been utilized in a number of cases, usually combined with X-ray treatment to the pituitary. While short-term control of the disease has been reported in something over 50 percent of patients so treated, I am not persuaded that the drug will be satisfactory for most patients over the long run.

Adrenal adenomas (benign tumors) and carcinomas obviously require removal of the involved gland. Most of the time the atrophied adrenal on the other side recovers so that permanent adrenal insufficiency is not a problem. Cancers that produce ACTH ectopically are usually beyond treatment when discovered, but symptoms disappear if the primary malignancy can be removed.

PRIMARY ALDOSTERONISM

In this condition hydrocortisone and adrenal sex hormone production is normal and only aldosterone is overproduced. The cause may be *single* or *multiple adenomas,* or the glands may simply hyperfunction without tumor formation (*adrenal hyperplasia*). Primary aldosteronism should always be suspected in a patient who has high blood pressure associated with a low level of plasma potassium. The hormone causes reabsorption of sodium and loss of potassium in the kidney tubule. Reabsorption of sodium chloride is accompanied by an obligatory retention of water so that plasma volume is expanded; this excess volume causes high blood pressure. The urinary potassium wastage accounts for the hypokalemia. Muscle weakness (due to potassium deficiency) may be profound in long-standing or severe disease.

When aldosteronism is suspected, the first step in screening is measurement of urine potassium. A high urine concentration despite low plasma values is suggestive of the disease (provided the patient is not taking diuretic drugs which cause urinary potassium loss). Diagnosis is confirmed by demonstrating that plasma or urine *aldosterone levels are elevated* and that plasma *renin levels are low.*[13] Renin is the hormone that normally controls aldosterone secretion. It is released whenever there is a deficit in body fluid or salt content. If aldosterone and

---

[13] Licorice contains a chemical (*glycyrrhizic acid*) that can cause high blood pressure, low plasma potassium and suppressed renin levels. Heavy licorice eaters may thus appear to have primary aldosteronism.

renin levels are both high, it is assumed that the aldosterone excess is physiological, a response to a need for salt or fluid. In primary aldosteronism, on the other hand, hormone response is autonomous, plasma volume is high and renin is suppressed. Additional evidence for abnormal aldosterone secretion can be obtained by infusing saline intravenously. Normal subjects respond with a fall in plasma aldosterone concentration, but no fall is produced in the disease state.

Treatment of aldosterone-producing adenomas is surgical removal. Adrenal hyperplasia is usually treated with an aldosterone-inhibiting drug called *spironolactone*.

PHEOCHROMOCYTOMA

Disease of the adrenal medulla is less frequent than that of the cortex. The only significant lesion is the tumor called *pheochromocytoma*, which overproduces one or both of the medullary hormones epinephrine or norepinephrine (the *catecholamines*). The major symptom is *high blood pressure* which may be *constant* (and thus clinically indistinguishable from ordinary essential hypertension) or *paroxysmal* (with normal blood pressure between attacks). Paroxysms are signaled by *headache, sweating, nervousness, rapid or pounding heartbeat* and (sometimes) *chest pain*. These symptoms are due to a burst of catecholamine release at the onset of the episode. (The feeling is not dissimilar to the shaky internal queasiness that one experiences immediately after a serious fright.) Attacks may be precipitated by smoking, changing the position of the body, exercise or overeating; they may occur several times a day or months apart. Other findings include weight loss, elevated blood sugar and (often) the presence of skin tumors called *neurofibromas*. Another skin sign is the presence of one or more irregular pigmented (*café au lait*) spots. Pheochromocytomas may be benign or malignant, single or multiple. They exist in isolation but may be part of the *multiple endocrine neoplasia syndrome*.

Diagnosis is made by the finding of *elevated free catecholamine* levels in the urine or plasma or by demonstrating increased concentrations of the metabolic products *vanillylmandelic acid* (VMA) or *metanephrines* in the urine. All patients with hypertension should be screened with urinary metanephrines to rule out the nonparoxysmal form of pheochromocytoma. Once a pheochromocytoma has been shown to be present, major efforts must be made to localize the lesion. This is done by X-ray, angiograms and selective catheterization of blood vessels to find where the hormone is being overproduced. Treatment is surgical removal. Because surgery can precipitate massive outpouring of catecholamines, patients must be prepared with drugs that block the effects of both epinephrine and norepinephrine. These blocking agents are also helpful in chronic treatment when metastasis makes surgical removal impossible.

DISEASES OF THE HYPOTHALAMUS AND PITUITARY GLAND

The pituitary gland synthesizes a number of hormones. The anterior pituitary releases *adrenocorticotrophic hormone* (ACTH), *thyroid-stimulating hormone* (TSH), *luteinizing and follicle-stimulating hormones* (LH and FSH), *prolactin* (PR) and *growth hormone* (GH). These hormones stimulate the adrenals, thyroid gland, gonads, breasts (milk production) and growth, respectively. All but prolactin appear to be controlled by releasing hormones produced in the hypothalamus, although only thyroid-releasing hormone and gonadotropin-releasing hormone have been isolated and purified. Prolactin is under negative control: a *prolactin inhibitory factor* normally keeps it from being released. Except in pregnancy and lactation, elevation of its concentration in blood means altered function of the hypothalamus or pituitary. The primary hormones of the posterior pituitary are *vasopressin* (antidiuretic hormone), which allows conservation of water by the kidney, and *oxytocin*, a hormone thought to be important in the final stages of pregnancy.

Hypothalamic-pituitary disease may result in overproduction or deficiencies of trophic hormones. The former is essentially always due to tumor formation in the pituitary (although not all pituitary tumors secrete hormones). Prolactin-secreting tumors were considered in chapter 12 and ACTH-producing tumors were discussed under Cushing's syndrome.

GIGANTISM-ACROMEGALY

These two conditions are due to overproduction of growth hormone by a pituitary tumor. If the excess growth hormone appears in childhood before postpubertal closure of the epiphyses (the growth regions of long bones), a pituitary giant is produced. Such patients may have heights up to 9 feet and weights of almost 500 pounds. Gigantism is quite rare. Much more commonly growth hormone excess develops in adult life, causing *acromegaly*. Since long bones of the extremities cannot lengthen in the adult, *bony overgrowth occurs in hands, feet and head*. The first sign may be an increase in glove, shoe or hat size. The lower jaw tends to extend beyond its upper mate (*prognathism*) so that chewing becomes difficult. The teeth may separate (spread apart) as the jaw grows. *Joint stiffness* and *pain, headaches* (due to tumor growth) and *visual difficulties* (from compression of optic nerves by the tumor) are noted in a high percentage of cases. Soft tissues of the face hypertrophy and many organs (heart, thyroid, kidney and liver) are enlarged. Excessive sweating is noted. Elevated blood sugar levels are common because growth hormone antagonizes the effects of insulin.

Diagnosis is suggested by the clinical features and the finding of an *enlarged sella turcica* (the bony seat of the pituitary) on skull X-ray. Definitive confirmation is obtained by demonstrating that *elevated growth hormone levels* are present in plasma and that they do not decrease after administration of an oral glucose load as occurs in normal subjects. Treatment consists of surgical removal of the tumor or irradiation to the pituitary. Both forms of therapy are effective. Attempts to block growth hormone release with drugs remain experimental.

PITUITARY INSUFFICIENCY

Pituitary insufficiency may involve all pituitary hormones (*panhypopituitarism*) or only a single hormone may be deficient. The clinical picture will depend on the combination of hormones involved. *Growth hormone deficiency* in children produces the pituitary dwarf but in the adult causes no symptoms. Secondary adrenal insufficiency and hypothyroidism result from *inadequate release of ACTH* and *TSH* respectively. *Gonadotropin deficits* produce sterility, loss of secondary sexual characteristics and, in women, amenorrhea. Failure of *antidiuretic hormone* leads to the massive urine outputs that characterize the state of diabetes insipidus.

Hypopituitarism may appear in many settings. One of the

most common forms in the past was due to postpartum hemorrhage with shock (*Sheehan's syndrome*). Better obstetrical care has made this rare. *Tumors* (primary or metastatic), *sarcoidosis, trauma to the head, infections* and *hemorrhage* from vascular aneurysms are responsible for a significant number of cases. In many patients the disease appears to be idiopathic: no primary cause can be found. It is suspected that in most of these cases there is a deficiency of hypothalamic-releasing factors (occurring for unknown reason).

Diagnosis is made by showing that deficiency of the target hormone is repaired by administration of the proper pituitary trophic hormone. In some cases failure of pituitary hormone release can be demonstrated directly by administering hypothalamic-releasing factors or by carrying out provocative tests (such as the previously mentioned metyrapone procedure).

Treatment of pituitary insufficiency consists of administering thyroxine, hydrocortisone or sex hormones exactly as in the case of primary deficiency states. The only pituitary hormone used directly in treatment is growth hormone in pituitary dwarfs.

NONFUNCTIONING PITUITARY TUMORS AND THE EMPTY SELLA SYNDROME

Tumors of the pituitary that do not produce hormones (*chromophobe adenomas*) ordinarily manifest themselves by headache or visual field defects, but even large tumors may be totally asymptomatic. The diagnosis is made by finding an enlarged sella turcica on routine X-rays of the skull or by taking specialized films of the sella (*tomograms*). Once an enlarged sella is found, the differential diagnosis lies between an expanding *pituitary tumor* and the *empty sella syndrome*. In the latter condition a defect in the membrane that covers the sella allows cerebrospinal fluid to enter, compressing the normal pituitary. Empty sellas cause no symptoms. The two conditions can be differentiated by CAT scanning or pneumoencephalography (see chapter 5), although the latter procedure is now rarely done. The empty sella usually is found in obese women who have mild hypertension. Treatment of pituitary adenomas is surgical removal.

DISEASES OF THE PARATHYROID GLAND

The parathyroid glands (usually 4 in number but sometimes 5 or 6) are located posterior to the thyroid gland. They secrete parathyroid hormone (PTH) which regulates the level of calcium and phosphorus in the blood. The hormone is normally released when plasma calcium concentration falls and is inhibited when it rises. Parathyroid hormone increases levels of serum calcium by two major mechanisms: *first*, it causes dissolution of calcium from bone; *second*, it enhances the conversion of 25-hydroxycholecalciferol to 1,25-dihydroxycholecalciferol, the most potent form of vitamin D. Active vitamin D then accelerates calcium absorption from the intestine. Parathyroid hormone lowers phosphorus concentrations in plasma at the same time that calcium levels rise. This is due to inhibition of phosphorus reabsorption in the kidney tubule with loss of phosphorus in the urine.

HYPERPARATHYROIDISM

Excess production of parathyroid hormone may be due to a *benign tumor (adenoma), parathyroid cancer,* or *parathyroid hyperplasia,* a general enlargement of all four glands that develops for unknown reasons. Hyperparathyroidism also occurs *secondary to kidney failure.* As the kidney is destroyed, the production of 1,25-dihydroxycholecalciferol is impaired, calcium absorption in the intestine is blunted, serum calcium levels fall and parathyroid hormone is released in large amounts in an attempt to compensate.

In the past hyperparathyroidism was said to be a disease of "stones, bones and abdominal groans." This meant that the disorder was associated with a high incidence of calcium-containing *kidney stones* (which form because urine calcium concentrations are abnormally high), *bone pain* and/or *spontaneous fractures* (reflecting resorption of calcium salts and decreased bone density) and the frequent presence of *duodenal ulcers* (presumably secondary to increased acid production consequent to hypercalcemia). Abdominal pain may also be due to *pancreatitis.* Additional problems include *high blood pressure, weakness, fatigue, increased urine flow* and *constipation.* All the above symptoms are features of advanced hyperparathyroidism. In modern times the disease is usually diagnosed in asymptomatic patients because essentially all patients seen by a physician receive screening tests for blood chemistries that include a plasma calcium determination. An elevated calcium level in the absence of another explanation usually indicates hyperparathyroidism. Other causes of hypercalcemia that have to be ruled out in every case include malignancy,[14] sarcoidosis, hyperthyroidism, vitamin D intoxication, the milk-alkali syndrome (in which patients with ulcer disease ingest large amounts of milk and antacids to prevent abdominal pain), excessive use of diuretic drugs and (rarely) Paget's disease of bone.

Diagnosis requires demonstration of inappropriately elevated concentrations of parathyroid hormone (relative to the serum calcium level)[15] by immunoassay of plasma.

Treatment of hyperparathyroidism is surgical removal of the involved glands. If hyperplasia is present all four glands may be excised with transplantation of one of them in the arm or leg to prevent development of hypoparathyroidism. The idea is that if hyperparathyroidism recurs in the transplanted gland it can be easily removed.

HYPOPARATHYROIDISM

Hypoparathyroidism is much less frequent than overactivity of the glands. The most common cause is *surgery in the neck,* especially on the thyroid. The parathyroid glands are quite fragile and easily damaged when the thyroid is dissected out. The disease may also develop spontaneously, either in isolation or as part of the previously described *immune endocrinopathy syndrome* in which antibodies form against endocrine glands. An acquired form of hypoparathyroidism, very common in alcoholics, is due to *depletion of plasma magnesium.*

The symptoms of hypoparathyroidism are due to low levels of calcium in the blood. They include *weakness, fatigue, mus-*

[14] Cancers cause hypercalcemia by several mechanisms. They may produce parathyroid hormone (*ectopic PTH production*), dissolve bone by direct metastasis or secrete the calcium-mobilizing substances prostaglandin E_2 or osteoclast-activating factor (*OAF*).

[15] As in most of endocrinology, hormone levels have to be interpreted in relation to the substances that they regulate. For example, a high plasma PTH is normal when the calcium level is low while even a "normal" level may indicate hyperparathyroidism if the plasma calcium is high (since PTH secretion ordinarily ceases when calcium concentrations rise).

cle cramps, numbness and *tingling* in the extremities and around the mouth, *spasm of the fingers, tetany* [16] and, in extreme cases, *convulsions. Cataracts* are frequently present. In the autoimmune form a defect in cellular defense against infection predisposes to *fungus infestations* in the fingernails and elsewhere in the body.

Diagnosis is made by demonstrating low parathyroid hormone levels in the blood in the face of low calcium and high phosphorus concentrations. Confirmation is obtained by administering exogenous parathyroid hormone and showing a rise in plasma calcium. Unfortunately PTH cannot be given chronically. Long-term therapy thus requires administration of *vitamin D* or *dihydrotachysterol* (a chemical with powerful vitamin D-like effects) together with oral *calcium supplements*. If the phosphorus concentration in plasma remains elevated a *phosphorus-binding antacid* can be given.

PSEUDOHYPOPARATHYROIDISM

Patients with pseudohypoparathyroidism have the same clinical symptoms as subjects with hypoparathyroidism. In contrast to the latter disease, however, circulating levels of parathyroid hormone are elevated. The condition is due to failure of kidney and bone to respond to the hormone rather than to its deficient production by the parathyroid glands. Patients with pseudohypoparathyroidism are short, often mentally retarded and may have an impaired sense of taste and smell. Another extremely characteristic finding is shortening of the 4th and 5th metacarpal and metatarsal bones (the bones of the wide portions of the hands and feet that connect to the fingers and toes). When affected subjects make a fist, the protruding knuckle normally seen is absent (replaced by a dimple) in the 4th and 5 positions.

MULTIPLE ENDOCRINE NEOPLASIA (MEN) SYNDROMES

It has already been mentioned that benign or malignant tumors of endocrine glands can secrete hormones. While these

---

[16] Spasm of the fingers (*carpopedal spasm*) and tetany usually appear together. In the former the fingers, fully extended, are painfully drawn together such that the hand resembles a teepee. *Tetany* refers to cramplike involuntary spasms of muscles throughout the body.

tumors may exist in isolation, it is now recognized that multiple tumors can be present in the same patient. When more than one tumor is present, the patient is said to have a *multiple endocrine neoplasia syndrome*.[17] The diseases run in families and are inherited in dominant fashion. The tumors segregate into two major categories called *MEN type I* and *MEN type II*. *Multiple endocrine neoplasia type I* is associated with neoplasms of the pituitary gland, parathyroids, pancreas, thyroid and adrenal cortex. Fatty tumors of the skin (*lipomas*) are also often present. *Multiple endocrine neoplasia type II* has pheochromocytoma and medullary carcinoma of the thyroid as primary tumors, although parathyroid adenomas may also develop. Bumpy nodules (*neuromas*) of lips, tongue and mucosal membranes are sometimes present. (Some physicians subdivide MEN II into *a* and *b* groups with *IIb* containing those patients with mucosal neuromas.)

The importance of these diseases is that the appearance of any functioning adenoma requires search for other tumors. Once the diagnosis has been made in a patient, all family members must be screened for hormonal abnormalities, even if they are asymptomatic. This is particularly important in MEN II because medullary carcinoma is a malignant lesion. Since the tumor makes the hormone *calcitonin*, measurement of its concentration in plasma is an effective screening procedure.

HYPOGLYCEMIA

Hypoglycemia means the presence of blood sugar levels sufficiently low to cause symptoms. It is a diagnosis made with incredible frequency in the United States, erroneously in the majority of cases. The physiologic background is as follows. Glucose is the most important body fuel because it is ordinarily the sole source of energy for the brain. Elaborate defense systems exist to prevent its concentrations from falling to levels that would cause altered central nervous system function or death. If one undergoes a fast, glucose production by the liver increases to replace sugar ordinarily taken in through diet. For the first 12 to 16 hours, plasma glucose is maintained by breakdown of glycogen, the storage form of sugar in the liver (*glyco-*

---

[17] MEN and multiple endocrine adenomatosis (MEA) are synonymous terms.

genolysis). Beyond this time (when glycogen is depleted) the liver must make glucose from other molecules, primarily amino acids delivered from muscle (*gluconeogenesis*). At the same time that hepatic glucose production accelerates, fat stores in adipose tissue begin to break down and long-chain fatty acids become a major energy source for almost every organ in the body except the central nervous system (which cannot burn fat). The switch to fat energy by these tissues spares glucose for use by the brain. Finally, after about 24 hours of fasting, the liver is able to convert significant amounts of fatty acids to ketoacids; the importance of the ketoacids is that they can be metabolized by the brain, substituting for glucose. Impairment of any of these adaptive responses may result in hypoglycemia when food is unavailable (even during as short a period as the normal overnight fast). Hypoglycemia can also supervene even when compensatory mechanisms are functioning normally if glucose utilization is markedly accelerated as in the case of insulin-producing tumors.

The symptoms of hypoglycemia fall into two categories: those caused by *epinephrine release* and those caused by *central nervous system dysfunction*. When the blood sugar begins to fall, the body signals the liver to start glycogen breakdown and adipose tissue to mobilize fat by releasing epinephrine from the adrenal medulla. The sudden release of epinephrine causes *nervousness, sweating, tremulousness* and *hunger sensations,* a constellation of symptoms that usually first suggests the diagnosis of hypoglycemia. If for any reason the plasma glucose continues to fall, epinephrine symptoms are joined by signs of central nervous system dysfunction: *headache, mental fuzziness, irrational behavior, loss of consciousness* or *convulsions.*

Two types of hypoglycemia are recognized. *Fasting hypoglycemia* usually indicates the presence of disease and is diagnosed by demonstrating a fall of the plasma glucose to below 40 milligrams per 100 milliliters when food is withheld. Diagnostic fasts are continued until symptoms develop or for a maximum of 72 hours (if hypoglycemia has not occurred in 3 days it can be assumed to be absent). Fasting hypoglycemia may be due to insulin-producing tumors, congenital absence of the enzymes necessary for glycogen breakdown or gluconeogenesis, deficiency of the hormones that regulate these processes, severe liver disease, alcohol ingestion in the fasting state (which blocks gluconeogenesis), certain large tumors of the chest and abdomen or overdosage with insulin or sulfonylureas. *Reactive hypoglycemia* refers to the appearance of hypoglycemia 2–4 hours after eating a meal. It is only rarely a sign of disease. True reactive hypoglycemia is almost always found in patients who have had part of the stomach removed surgically. Rapid passage of food into the intestine causes excess insulin release and thus results in hypoglycemia.

A word needs to be said about the epidemic of "reactive hypoglycemia" now sweeping the country. There is an organized group of doctors and laymen who believe that hypoglycemia is extraordinarily common and that it is responsible for everything from fatigue and weakness to crime in the streets. (Proponents have claimed South American headhunters behave as they do because of hypoglycemia and that the Vietnam war was lost because South Vietnamese troops had persistently low blood sugars.) The usual patient has symptoms of nervousness, sweating and weakness several hours after eating, particularly if a high-carbohydrate meal is ingested. A "hypoglycemia specialist" is then consulted and a 5-hour glucose tolerance test is performed. In this test a pure glucose load is administered by mouth and sequential plasma glucose levels are measured. If the glucose value falls below the starting level at any time within the 5 hours, a diagnosis of hypoglycemia is made. The patient is then treated with a high-protein diet (given as frequent feedings), massive amounts of vitamins, a variety of minerals and (often) injections of extracts from adrenal glands.

This is a nondisease. The confusion comes from the fact that essentially everyone has at least a small fall in plasma glucose when given a 5-hour glucose tolerance test (many perfectly normal persons get very low levels without any symptoms whatever). However, since the test is done only in persons who complain of epinephrine symptoms (which in reality are due to anxiety and stress, not hypoglycemia), the diagnosis of hypoglycemia will be made in everyone who is tested. Interestingly, when patients presumed to have this form of "hypoglycemia" have blood glucose levels measured during spontaneous attacks (not after the very artificial circumstance of drinking pure glucose) their values are not low but in the upper normal range or even high! (This is because a normal consequence of stress-induced epinephrine release is elevation of the blood sugar.) If true reactive hypoglycemia is present, plasma glucose values are low during spontaneous attacks. Patients treated by the "hypoglycemia doctors" almost always get better (for a while) because the new diet and medications act as a placebo, relieving their anxiety. The dietary therapy is not harmful and can be used without objection if it helps. Drug therapy should be avoided because it does nothing, because it may not be entirely safe and because it is very expensive.

If true fasting hypoglycemia is demonstrated, the cause must be discerned by sophisticated tests, description of which would probably be of little interest to the reader. Insulin-secreting tumors are treated by surgical removal while other forms of recurrent hypoglycemia are managed by dietary manipulation and drugs. True reactive hypoglycemia (due to rapid intestinal transit) usually responds to a multiple small-meal feeding schedule.

HYPERCHOLESTEROLEMIA AND HYPERTRIGLYCERIDEMIA (THE HYPERLIPOPROTEINEMIAS)

Cholesterol and triglyceride are normal constituents of plasma and subserve important functions in the body. Triglyceride (fat) is a major energy source while cholesterol is necessary for the formation of all cell membranes and is the precursor for sex and adrenal hormones. However, if the concentrations of these molecules become abnormally elevated, disease results.

HYPERCHOLESTEROLEMIA

Cholesterol elevation may occur as a consequence of genetic disease or be secondary to another disorder. The genetic form is called *familial hypercholesterolemia.* In *homozygous familial hypercholesterolemia* (where the patient receives an abnormal gene from each parent) cholesterol levels are around 1000 milligrams per 100 milliliters of plasma (normal upper limits about 250 mg per 100 ml). Affected subjects develop coronary artery disease in childhood and often die of heart attacks before the age of 15.[18] *Heterozygous familial hypercholesterolemia* (one abnormal and one normal gene) results in plasma cholesterol levels of 400–500 milligrams per 100 milliliters of plasma, and heart attacks appear between ages 30 to 50. Cholesterol is transported in blood bound to a carrier lipoprotein (*low density lipoprotein* or *LDL*) that allows it to be solubilized in plasma. Transfer into cells is made possible by a specialized receptor on cell surfaces (the LDL receptor) which binds circulating LDL and internalizes its cargo of cholesterol. The LDL receptor is absent in familial hypercholesterolemia, accounting for the high plasma levels of cholesterol. LDL cholesterol then enters arteries by what is called a salvage pathway, causing atherosclerosis.

Secondary forms of hypercholesterolemia are seen in *hypothyroidism, biliary cirrhosis* and the *nephrotic syndrome.*

HYPERTRIGLYCERIDEMIA

Hypertriglyceridemia may also appear as a familial disorder or be secondary to other disease. While not as dangerous as elevation of cholesterol, hypertriglyceridemia may cause pancreatitis or, in some forms, lead to premature heart disease. Triglyceride is carried in two different lipoprotein particles: dietary fat travels as *chylomicrons* while fat produced in the liver is transported as *very low density lipoprotein* (VLDL).[19] Familial disorders which exhibit elevation of each are known. A separate genetic disorder is *familial combined hyperlipoproteinemia* in which both cholesterol and triglycerides may be elevated in the same family.

The most common causes of secondary hypertriglyceridemia are *diabetes mellitus* and *alcohol ingestion.*

TREATMENT

Hypercholesterolemia is treated by a low cholesterol, high polyunsaturated fat diet combined with bile-acid-binding res-

---

[18] It has been shown that fetuses with this disease have elevated cholesterol levels in plasma even before birth.

[19] The various lipoprotein particles can be separated and identified by electrophoresis of plasma (a technique in which molecules migrate in an electrical field according to their inherent electrical charge) or by a procedure called density centrifugation. Each lipoprotein has a characteristic density (weight per unit of volume); when spun at high speeds in the ultracentrifuge, individual lipoproteins separate on the basis of density and can thus be identified. Hence the names *low density lipoprotein, very low density lipoprotein, high density lipoprotein.*

ins (cholestyramine, colestipol) and nicotinic acid. Hypertri-glyceridemia requires a low total fat diet (for chylomicronemia) or a high-polyunsaturated-fat diet (for VLDL excess). Clofibrate is the initial therapeutic agent used by most physicians, but nicotinic acid is also effective.

16

Infectious Diseases

Before the antibiotic era, infections were the leading cause of death in the world. While advances in sanitary engineering, widespread programs of immunization and the continuing development of powerful antibiotics have markedly diminished the number of deaths attributable to infectious agents, the battle continues. Three factors have prevented the complete eradication of the infectious diseases. *First,* for a whole series of organisms (notably the viruses) no effective antibiotic has been developed.[1] *Second,* bacteria have a remarkable capacity to develop resistance to anti-infectious agents.[2] *Third,* the increasing use of chemotherapeutic drugs (which paralyze the immune defenses of the recipient) has rendered significant numbers of patients susceptible to infection not only by organisms which are capable of attacking normal persons but, importantly, also to agents that cannot infect a well host (*opportunistic organ-*

[1] While effective antibiotics are available for most bacteria, antifungal agents are only moderately effective and no useful antiviral drug has been discovered. Following infections with viruses, human and animal cells make a protein called *interferon* which attaches to noninfected cells and converts them to an "antiviral" state. In a sense it is a naturally occurring antibiotic for viruses, although it really acts by preventing the deleterious biological effects of the virus rather than by killing it. Major efforts are being made to develop drugs that can induce interferon production; hopefully, such drugs would function as viral antibiotics.

[2] Resistance can develop by many mechanisms. For example, a high proportion of staphylococci have developed the capacity to break down penicillin by an enzyme called penicillinase and thus are not killed in its presence. Fortunately penicillinase-resistant penicillin analogues have been developed which have shifted the edge back to the physician (at least temporarily).

335

isms). Patients with cancer, autoimmune disease and organ transplants make up the bulk of those at risk for opportunistic infection.

The body has several defenses against disease. *First,* there are physical barriers to infection such as the skin and the cilia lining the bronchial tree (which continually sweep inhaled bacteria out of the lung). *Second,* circulating white blood cells (particularly those classified as neutrophilic polymorphonuclear leukocytes) have the capacity to sense, trap, engulf and destroy invading agents (a process called *phagocytosis*). *Third,* immune mechanisms exist that assist in the elimination of acute infections and protect against future (return) invasion by similar organisms. The immune defense system is mediated by that class of white blood cells called lymphocytes. There are two major types: *B lymphocytes* and *T lymphocytes. B cells* function by producing antibodies to infectious agents (or any foreign protein). These antibodies circulate in plasma, bind to invading organisms, neutralize their pathologic effects and enhance their destruction by neutrophilic leukocytes. Their continued presence in plasma accounts for the immunity that develops following infection. Antibody formation by B lymphocytes is also the basis of all immunization procedures. Instead of naturally acquired infection, the inducing antigen is either a live organism treated in such a way that it produces only mild disease (*attenuated strains*) or an inactivated (killed) preparation still capable of inducing an immune response. *T cells* do not make antibodies but release protein molecules called *lymphokines* that attract phagocytic cells into tissues and enhance their killing properties. T cells also have the capacity to interact synergistically with B cells, facilitating their capacity to make antibody, a process called the *helper function.*[3]

When host defense mechanisms break down, infection results. The vast majority of infections are eventually thrown off without outside help; however, a particularly virulent organism

---

[3] T cell activity is quite complicated. There are at least three (probably more) cell types. *Effector T cells* carry out functions such as surveillance and killing of cancer cells as they develop in the body. *Helper T cells,* as mentioned, enhance antibody formation by B lymphocytes. *Suppressor T cells* have the capacity to act in the opposite way—blocking antibody formation by B cells and inhibiting effector T cell activity. How these various cells develop and interact is only now being unraveled. It has been speculated that underactivity of suppressors for B cells might allow excessive autoantibody formation and cause autoimmune disease. Conversely, overactivity of suppressors for T effector cells might dampen the effectiveness of the tumor surveillance system and predispose to cancer.

or a weakened host (or both) may result in serious disability or death. In these circumstances antibiotics are required. Antibiotics are of two types. *Bacteriocidal* agents kill organisms directly while *bacteriostatic* drugs simply inhibit bacterial growth and multiplication such that the host's white cells can more easily engulf and destroy them. It is important to recognize that antibiotics are selective in their actions: a drug effective against one group of bacteria will be totally ineffective against other species. Selection of the proper antibiotic thus becomes a major issue in the management of infectious diseases.

Many of the common infectious disorders have been discussed earlier under diseases of organ systems. In this chapter those infections which cause systemic problems will be discussed. Illnesses such as malaria and cholera, which have major world impact but do not occur in the United States (except in foreign travelers), will not be covered.

DIAGNOSTIC PROCEDURES

Microscopic Examination. The first step in identifying an infective organism is to make a smear of the indicated specimen (pus, cerebrospinal fluid, urine, sputum, etc.). The smear is then stained with one of several dyes and examined for the presence of bacteria. The *gram stain* is universally used and divides bacteria into two classes: *gram-positive* (blue-staining) and *gram-negative* (red-staining). Simple identification of gram-staining characteristics markedly narrows the diagnostic possibilities and suggests the type of antibiotic that might work against the agent (some antibiotics are effective against gram-positive organisms, others against gram-negative). Many other stains are available to bring out special characteristics. For example, the *acid-fast stain* identifies the bacteria that cause tuberculosis. In addition to staining characteristics, the smear reveals the anatomy of bacteria: round organisms are called *cocci* (singular, *coccus*) while rod-shaped bacteria are termed *bacilli* (singular, *bacillus*). Also important are association patterns that tend to be characteristic of different species; staphylococci appear in clumps, streptococci in chains, pneumococci and gonococci in pairs and intestinal bacilli as single organisms.

Culture and Sensitivity. While a clue to the cause of infection comes from microscopic examination of smears, precise identification demands isolation of the organism by *culture techniques*. Different bacteria require different nutrients to grow, so in screening procedures culture media of different types are used. Proof of identity comes from growth characteristics and chemical tests. If a culture is positive, the organism's susceptibility to killing or inhibition by antibiotics is then tested (*sensitivity tests*). This is done by adding antibiotic discs to the surface of culture plates or by growing the organism in tubes containing liquid culture media to which are added varying concentrations of the different antibiotics. Determination of antibiotic sensitivity is critically important to patient care since an organism that is generally sensitive to a given antibiotic may be resistant in the patient under study. Since completion of culture and sensitivity tests takes 48–72 hours, ill patients must be started on antibiotics in the absence of specific knowledge of the agent present or its sensitivity. Choice of initial antibiotic is based on past experience with the infection that seems most likely to be causing symptoms.

Serologic Tests. A number of diseases are caused by organisms that cannot be cultured easily. In these cases identification is based on finding antibodies to the organism in serum. (Serum is the fluid remaining after blood has been allowed to clot.) If antibody concentration to a specific organism rises in the second of two blood samples taken several weeks apart, it can be assumed that recent infection has occurred. Serologic tests are required for diagnosis of almost all viral diseases (since viruses do not grow on ordinary culture media), many fungi and some bacteria (e.g., the organism causing Legionnaire's disease). A variety of procedures are available for demonstrating the presence of antibody, details of which are unimportant. They are usually descriptively named according to the basic technique used; e.g., complement-fixation tests, precipitin tests, agglutinin determinations.

Skin Tests. Antigens isolated from infecting organisms can be injected into the skin and the allergic response of the patient tested. Positive tests indicate previous exposure to the infectious agent but do not imply active (current) infection. Negative tests are useful in eliminating diseases that might account for a clinical syndrome. Skin tests are most often used for tuberculosis, mumps, the various fungal diseases and leprosy.

BACTERIAL DISEASES

SEPTICEMIA

Septicemia is a general term referring to invasion of the bloodstream by bacterial organisms. The bacteria may arise from a site of local infection (an abscess, pneumonia, kidney infection), from dental work or tooth extractions (there are many bacteria in the gums around the teeth) or from damaged or devitalized tissues such as ischemic bowel. Septicemia is also a common consequence of the intravenous use of contaminated illicit drugs. The initial symptoms are *chills* and *fever*. Serious complications include *bacterial endocarditis, lung* and *brain abscesses, meningitis* and *infectious arthritis*. Gram-negative organisms cause a special syndrome of high fever and collapse of the blood pressure called *endotoxic shock* (the causal agent is *endotoxin,* a potent toxin released when the bacteria are killed by host defense mechanisms). Gram-negative septicemia may occur spontaneously or result from mechanical manipulation of the urinary tract (catheterization, cystoscopy or transurethral prostatectomy). Uncomplicated septicemia is treated by intravenous antibiotics given for a period of 10 days. Endocarditis requires 4 to 6 weeks of intravenous therapy.

TUBERCULOSIS

Tuberculosis is caused by *Mycobacterium tuberculosis,* an "acid-fast" bacillus that almost always gains entrance to the body through the lungs.[4] The majority of persons exposed to the organism develop *primary tuberculosis:* the infection is effectively contained at the regional lymph nodes without progression to active lung disease. The skin test for tuberculosis turns positive after primary exposure. While full-blown infection may rarely occur following primary contact, usually the organisms lie dormant in a regional lymph node until some later event allows them to break out and cause *active tubercu-*

[4] Before pasteurization of milk tuberculosis was often spread from infected cattle. Bovine tuberculosis causes *scrofula,* a disease characterized by development of a matted mass of infected lymph nodes in the neck with draining sinuses extending through the overlying skin. It has now been essentially eradicated in the United States. Occasionally a tuberculosislike picture is produced by so-called *atypical mycobacteria,* organisms related to *M. tuberculosis* that apparently only attack previously damaged lungs. They are not contagious and do not spread from person to person.

losis. The nature of the precipitating event is usually not identified but presumably represents an acquired deficit in tissue resistance. Many active cases are picked up by routine screening X-rays of the chest. The typical lesion is a *hazy infiltrate* or *cavity* in the upper portion (*apex*) of one or both lungs. If the disease is not detected early, *weight loss, cough* (with purulent or bloody sputum) and *shortness of breath* supervene. Occasionally the only manifestation is a *pleural effusion.* (Fluid in the pleural spaces without apparent underlying lung disease turns out to be tuberculosis about 50 percent of the time.) Tuberculosis may also cause *infection of the kidneys* (with blood or pus in the urine), *meningitis, pericarditis, peritonitis, destruction of the adrenal glands* and *infection of bone,* particularly of the spine (*Pott's disease*). The diagnosis is suggested by finding acid-fast bacilli on smear of sputum, pus, urine, spinal fluid or gastric contents and confirmed by culture of the organism. Fortunately good antibiotics are now available for treatment and cure is almost always obtained. The major drugs are *isoniazid (INH), rifampin, ethambutal* and *streptomycin.* Two or three drugs are used in combination in all active cases. INH and rifampin are often the initial choice. Most patients can now be treated without hospitalization. Persons with close exposure to an active case and those with recent conversion of the tuberculin skin test are usually treated prophylactically for a year with INH alone.

TETANUS

Tetanus is due to infection with *Clostridium tetani,* an organism that grows only in the presence of low oxygen concentrations (such bacteria are called *anaerobes*). It exists in an inactive form (spore) that is transformed to an active (multiplying) bacillus. Tetanus spores are essentially ubiquitous in dirt, dust and manure. As a consequence every wound must be considered potentially contaminated with the organism. Clinical disease is relatively rare in advanced societies only because the bulk of the population has been immunized during childhood; even so, the number of nonimmune persons is not insignificant. Tetanus of the newborn (*tetanus neonatorum*) is a significant problem in primitive or developing countries because of nonsterile obstetrical techniques. A subpopulation of adults at unusual risk is the narcotics culture; this is because illicit drugs frequently contain tetanus spores.

Proliferation of organisms occurs in those wounds that have oxygen tension lowered by foreign debris, dead tissue or simultaneous infection with other bacteria. Clean wounds are much less susceptible. The incubation period between receipt of the wound and onset of clinical symptoms varies from 2 days to 2 months but most of the time is around 2 weeks. The organism does not leave the site of injury (it is noninvasive) but produces a toxin that passes up nerve trunks to reach the central nervous system. The clinical picture is that of intense muscle contraction with repetitive *painful involuntary spasms* superimposed on *a generalized rigidity of the body.* Involvement of the face muscles gives rise to the familiar picture of "lockjaw" (*trismus*) in which there is difficulty in opening the mouth. Spasm of the facial muscles pulls the lips into a grimacing smile (*risus sardonicus*). *Pneumonia* is common because difficulty in swallowing leads to aspiration. Death results from pneumonia or from spasm of the muscles of the larynx and chest causing *asphyxia.*

Once symptoms develop admission to an intensive care unit is mandatory. *Human tetanus immune globulin* (an antibody against tetanus toxin) is administered and the patient is *sedated with barbiturates.* Muscle spasm is treated with *diazepam. Tracheostomy* is often necessary to allow support of the respiration in the face of intense contraction of laryngeal muscles that blocks airflow from the throat. Advanced disease may require administration of a derivative of *curare* to paralyze all muscles (and thus relieve spasm). Under these circumstances respiration must be supported with a respirator. Mortality rates in established tetanus are in the range of 50 percent or higher.[5] It cannot be stated too strongly that every individual should be immunized against tetanus; prevention is still the best form of treatment.

DIPHTHERIA

Diphtheria, caused by *Corynebacterium diphtheriae,*[6] is a completely preventable disease. Unfortunately laxness in see-

[5] It is an interesting fact that survivors of active disease are not immunized by their experience. Active immunization by vaccination must be carried out on recovery.

[6] It is now known that bacteria as well as humans can be infected by viruses. Bacterial viruses are called *bacteriophages.* They penetrate through the bacterial cell wall, become attached to the chromosomes and act like acquired genes, inducing the bacteria to make viral proteins. (Like genes, they are also passed down from generation to generation.) Toxin production in *C. diphtheriae* is due to phage infection: in the absence of the virus the bacterium is innocent (nonvirulent).

ing that children are immunized, particularly in lower socio-
economic populations, has resulted in several recent mini-
epidemics. The diphtheria bacillus initially invades the throat
and upper airways producing *fever* and a *thick, leathery membrane* over the mouth and throat. The latter, consisting of dead
tissue, bacteria and white cells, is so tightly attached that bleeding occurs when it is scraped off. The membrane obstructs airflow producing *stridor* (noisy respiration), *hoarseness* and
swelling of the neck ("bull neck"). Toxin produced by the organism causes inflammatory changes in the heart muscle (*myocarditis*) and frequently leads to dangerous cardiac arrhythmias
or heart failure. The toxin also causes an extensive *peripheral
neuritis* that results in widespread paralysis of muscles. Death
occurs from respiratory failure, abnormal heart rhythms or secondary infection. The only form of treatment is administration
of *diphtheria antitoxin.* The antitoxin is available only as a
horse serum preparation; allergy to horse serum (which is common) requires desensitization before treatment can be given.

TYPHOID FEVER

Typhoid fever is now a relatively rare disease in the United
States although it remains common in underdeveloped countries with poor sanitary systems. It is due to ingestion of water,
food or milk contaminated with *Salmonella typhi.* Once ingested the organisms enter the bloodstream from the small intestine and come to lodge in cells of the reticulo-endothelial
system (the early septicemia is transient). There they multiply
and eventually reenter the blood to initiate symptomatic disease. The period from exposure to symptoms varies from 3 days
to 2 months. Onset is signaled by the appearance of *severe
headache, fever* and *chilliness* (sometimes frank chills). Fever
may last 2–4 weeks in untreated cases. A *dry cough* is prominent. *Constipation* is usual in the early stages but changes to
diarrhea in some patients. Round, red spots (*rose spots*) appear
on the abdomen during the second week of the disease and are
highly suggestive of the diagnosis. The *liver and spleen are
enlarged* but jaundice is only rarely present. *Weakness* is severe. Two serious, potentially fatal complications may result
from proliferation of bacteria in the intestinal wall: *perforation
with peritonitis* and *gastrointestinal hemorrhage.* Other problems, less common, include *acute renal failure, osteomyelitis,*

meningitis and *peripheral neuritis*. Diagnosis is made by culturing the organism from blood or feces. *S. typhi* usually responds well to treatment with chloramphenicol or ampicillin.

It is possible to be a chronic carrier of the typhoid organism without being sick. Carriers spread the organism through the stool. In a significant proportion of cases the reservoir is the gallbladder. Carriers must be treated for 6 weeks with antibiotics; if gallstones are present or the gallbladder is abnormal, surgical removal is required.

BRUCELLOSIS

Brucellosis (*undulant fever*) is an occupational disease of farmers, ranchers, veterinarians and packinghouse workers. Goats, hogs and cattle are natural hosts for Brucella species. (Brucellosis in cattle is called *Bang's disease.*) Infection results from ingestion of milk or contact with infected tissues. The most common clinical presentation is that of *fever* without other specific signs. *Headache, weakness* and *generalized muscular aching* are nondiagnostic accompaniments. Brucellosis thus usually falls into the category of "fever of unknown origin." A clue to diagnosis is the presence of an *enlarged tender spleen* in a person known to have been exposed to domestic animals or their carcasses. Untreated, the disease may run a course of up to six months. Complications include *painful swelling of the testes, arthritis* and *bacterial endocarditis*. Diagnosis may be obtained by culture of the blood or bone marrow but usually is based on serologic tests showing antibodies to the Brucella organism. Tetracycline is effective treatment.

TULAREMIA

Tularemia (*rabbit fever*) is due to *Pasteurella tularensis* and is transmitted to man through contact with infected flesh of rabbits, squirrels, foxes, opossums, woodchucks, skunks, coyotes and some birds. It is thus a disease of hunters. However, transmission can also occur via bites of insect vectors such as ticks and the deer fly. Classically the first sign is a *reddened bump* on the exposed extremity; the lesion subsequently *ulcerates* and regional *lymph nodes become enlarged, red* and *tender*, occasionally draining spontaneously through the skin. *Fever, chills* and *prostration* are common and *pneumonia* is not unusual. *Ocular infection* produces redness, pain and swelling in the eyes. *Enlargement of the spleen* is frequent. Diagnosis requires culture of an affected lymph node or demonstration of a rising antibody titer to *Pasteurella*. Streptomycin, tetracycline and chloramphenicol have all been used successfully in treatment.

BOTULISM

Botulism is caused by ingestion of a toxin produced by *Clostridium botulinum,* an anaerobic, gram-positive soil bacillus that contaminates canned and processed foods. Most cases result from inadequate home canning procedures, but outbreaks from commercial sources still occasionally occur. The bacterium exists in soil as a spore which becomes activated and toxin-producing under conditions of low oxygen tension and heat (as occur during canning). Both bacteria and their elaborated toxin are destroyed provided heating is adequate. Botulinum toxin is probably the most powerful of all naturally occurring poisons. It paralyzes nerves throughout the body. Initial symptoms (which occur a few hours to a few days after ingestion of toxin-containing foods) include *double vision, difficulty in swallowing* and *impaired speech. Paralysis* then spreads throughout the body. The *bladder may become nonfunctional* and *constipation* is almost invariable. *Nausea* and *vomiting* afflict about half the patients. Some 25–30 percent of patients die, generally from *respiratory paralysis* or *pneumonia*. Diagnosis ordinarily requires injection of suspected material into mice with demonstration of paralysis and death within 24 hours. Suspected foods, containers and feces from the patient should be tested. In some cases the organism can be identified directly, utilizing anaerobic culture techniques. Treatment consists of support of respiration and administration of *botulinum antitoxin*. This material is also carried in a horse serum vehicle, requiring testing for allergy before use.

PLAGUE

Bubonic plague, which in its epidemic form has been responsible on three occasions in history for wiping out large populations (the dread *black death*), occurs sporadically in the United States. The plague bacillus (*Yersinia pestis*) is transmitted to man from infected rodents by bite of the rat flea. The disease is characterized by *high fever, chills, headache, vomiting, en-*

larged regional lymph nodes (bubos), severe bleeding tendency, delirium and shock. (Extensive hemorrhage into the skin gave rise to the appellation "black death.") The disease may also take the form of a *fulminating pneumonia* which can be transmitted between humans (through droplet spread during coughing) without necessity of a flea vector. In the absence of therapy, the pneumonic form is universally fatal. Diagnosis is made by culture of infected material or guinea pig inoculation. Treatment must be initiated immediately with streptomycin, tetracycline or chloramphenicol if a fatal outcome is to be prevented.

GONORRHEA

Gonorrhea, the most common of the venereal diseases, is due to *Neisseria gonorrhoeae* (the gonococcus). It is spread by direct sexual contact. In the male a *pus-containing urethral discharge* ("clap") develops 2 to 6 days following exposure. *Frequent, painful urination* is usual. Homosexuals may have *anorectal infection* with burning, itching, painful defecation and a mucus or pus-containing rectal discharge. If oral sex has been performed *infection of the throat* may result. Women may have *frequency of urination, dysuria* and a *vaginal discharge*, but many are completely asymptomatic.[7] If the disease is contracted around or during the menstrual period, extension of the infection to the fallopian tubes may result. This complication, called *acute salpingitis* (or *pelvic inflammatory disease*, PID), results in excruciating lower abdominal pain. Vaginal (pelvic) examination shows marked tenderness in the area of the tubes and ovaries. Untreated the disease progresses to abscess formation with high fever. The infection may spread upward to the liver, causing right upper quadrant abdominal pain. Sterility is a late complication.

In both sexes gonococci may invade the bloodstream and spread throughout the body. The most common manifestation is *septic arthritis*, but occasionally *bacterial endocarditis* and *meningitis* may result.

[7] While men generally seek treatment because the urethral discharge points to the presence of venereal disease, this is not necessarily the case for women, a higher percentage of whom are asymptomatic. (The prevalence of asymptomatic men appears to be increasing but is still much less than in women.) Untreated patients are a major reservoir for continuing infection in the community. Efforts to develop a vaccine for gonorrhea persist but so far have not been successful.

Diagnosis is made by culture of the organism in urethral or cervical discharges, joint fluid or blood. Most strains of gonococci are killed by penicillin, but resistant organisms are now appearing with increasing frequency. Ampicillin, tetracycline and spectinomycin are also effective. The latter two drugs are recommended in penicillin-resistant cases.

LYMPHOGRANULOMA VENEREUM

Lymphogranuloma venereum, one of the venereal diseases, is due to infection with *Chlamydia trachomatis*.[8] The disease begins with a *painless blister, ulcer* or *bump* on the penis or female genitalia which heals without scarring. Subsequently (2 to 6 weeks after exposure) *lymph nodes in the groin enlarge* and become *painful (lymphadenitis)*. Untreated they break down into *draining fistulas. Fever, chills* and *muscle aches* accompany the lymphadenitis. Women and homosexual men may develop *disease in the rectal area* with formation of abscesses or fistulas between the rectum and bladder or vagina (a terrible complication which results in drainage of feces into the urine or vaginal secretions). Diagnosis may be made by culture of pus from an infected lymph node but usually is based on a positive complement-fixation test showing antibodies to the organism. Treatment with tetracycline is curative.

PSITTACOSIS

Psittacosis (also called *ornithosis* and *parrot fever*) is a disease of birds that is easily transmitted to humans. Exposure can occur from the environment without the actual handling of the infected fowl. The causative organism is *Chlamydia psittaci,* a close relative of the species causing lymphogranuloma venereum. Symptoms include *fever, chills, severe headache, muscle pains* and a *skin rash* not dissimilar to that seen in typhoid fever. Other findings include *nosebleeds, enlargement of lymph nodes* (especially in the neck) and *cough*. Chest X-ray shows a patchy *bronchopneumonia*. Diagnosis is suspected from a history of exposure to birds and is confirmed by demon-

---

[8] This organism is almost identical to that which causes *trachoma*, an infection of the eyes that is the leading cause of blindness throughout the world. The disease is usually transmitted by direct contact with secretions from infected eyes. Large numbers of persons are affected in Africa, the Middle East and India. A few cases result from transfer of infection from genitalia to the eye.

stration of a rise in complement-fixing antibody to *Chlamydia* during recovery. The disease responds promptly to treatment with tetracycline.

VIRAL DISEASES

Most viruses cause annoying but insignificant illnesses such as colds or gastroenteritis. Only the major (serious) viral illnesses will be considered in this chapter.

INFLUENZA

Influenza can be produced by three distinct viruses (A, B and C); epidemic disease is due to the A type. The various strains of the A group (Asian, Hong Kong, swine) are identified by differences in proteins contained in the viral coat. Onset of influenza is usually abrupt with *fever, headache, chilliness* and, outstandingly, *muscle aches (myalgias)*. The latter are so characteristic that their presence during a nonspecific febrile illness suggests the presence of "flu" while their absence casts doubt on the diagnosis. *Cough* is usually present early, but manifestations suggesting a *cold* (runny nose, sneezing and redness of the eyes) may not appear until a day or two later. The chief complication is *pneumonia* which may be due to the influenza virus itself or a superimposed bacterial infection (often staphylococcal). Either type is extremely serious and mortality rates are high despite the use of antibiotics. The diagnosis of influenza is based on serologic tests, but the virus can be isolated if desired by injection of throat washings into chick embryos or cells in tissue culture.

There is no specific treatment but prophylaxis is reasonably effective. Immunization is recommended for all patients with heart disease, chronic pulmonary dysfunction, diabetes and adrenal insufficiency. Persons over 65 should also be routinely vaccinated. While influenza vaccine is not entirely without danger, it is felt that the risk of the disease in the above segments of the population is greater than the risk of immunization.[9]

---

[9] Side effects of influenza vaccine include fever and allergic reactions. Recently a number of persons receiving swine vaccine developed the Guillain-Barré syndrome (see page 116). As a consequence the national immunization program was temporarily suspended. Some authorities still question a direct causal link between vaccine and paralysis.

POLIOMYELITIS

Poliomyelitis should have been eliminated from the world because of one of the great triumphs of modern medicine, the development of the polio vaccine. Unfortunately, because of failure to vaccinate, the disease has reappeared in the United States, a situation that is truly tragic. Polio virus is spread in the feces of asymptomatic carriers and is ingested in contaminated food or water. Most exposed persons develop no symptoms. Symptomatic disease usually occurs in three phases: the *minor illness, nonparalytic* and *paralytic polio*. A given patient may stop at any level or progress through the entire spectrum. The *minor illness* manifests itself as a cold with sore throat, a flulike syndrome or gastroenteritis with nausea and vomiting. *Nonparalytic polio* consists of the minor illness plus headache, stiff neck and cerebrospinal fluid, findings of viral (aseptic) meningitis. *Paralytic polio* may follow phases one and two or appear with no premonitory symptoms save pain or spasm in the muscles to be involved. Paralysis, which may be partial or complete, usually supervenes within a short period of the onset of pain. Any part of the body (including the face) may be involved. Death ordinarily results from *failure of the respiratory muscles* or *aspiration pneumonia* secondary to weak or nonfunctioning throat musculature. Many patients with paralytic symptoms recover, but for some paralysis is permanent.[10] For this reason it is mandatory that immunization against polio be provided all children and adults. (With rare exception oral "live" vaccine should be used rather than the injectable inactivated virus.)

RABIES

The rabies virus is usually transmitted by a bite from diseased animals but rarely may enter the host via the respiratory tract or by ingestion of virus-infested tissue. Traditionally the dog has been the important vehicle of transmission, but in the United States (because of the effectiveness of pet immunization) skunks and other wild species (squirrels, raccoons, bats) are now the primary source. Following exposure infected indi-

---

[10] My medical career extends far enough back to have participated in the yearly polio epidemics. The sympathy evoked for patients in the iron lungs with paralyzed limbs, bladders and bowels was matched by the fear that one would, caring for them, contract the disease oneself.

viduals pass through a period of nonspecific symptoms—*mild
fever, malaise, nausea, cough, sore throat* and *numbness* or
tingling at the site of the bite. After several days the toxin
(which like tetanus toxin travels by nerve trunks) reaches the
central nervous system and produces the dysfunction that char-
acterizes fully developed disease. Basically the picture is that
of an *encephalitis* with involvement of the brain stem. *Hyper-
activity* is accompanied by intermittent periods of *confusion* or
hallucinations. Muscle spasms, stiff neck and *high fever* appear
as the disease progresses; *convulsions* are not unusual. Spasm
and weakness of throat muscles *makes swallowing difficult.*
Because of this patients who are alert refuse to drink water,
recognizing that they will choke (accounting for the synonym
for rabies, *hydrophobia*—fear of water). *Excessive salivation*
gives the impression that patients "foam at the mouth." These
signs are rapidly followed by *coma* and *death* due to cessation
of activity of the respiratory centers in the brain stem.

When a person has been bitten by a known or presumed
rabid animal, the wound is cleaned, dead tissue is removed and
active immunization is started with *duck embryo vaccine*
(which is much safer than previous vaccines). In addition,
human antirabies antiserum is injected into the wound area
and also intramuscularly to provide passive antibody protection
until the body can make its own antibody in response to the
vaccine.[11] Immediate treatment is imperative since rabies, once
developed, is essentially uniformly fatal.

SMALLPOX

Smallpox has been essentially eliminated as a public health
problem because of a worldwide program of immunization and
an international cooperative program for early identification
and isolation of persons contracting the disease. Eradication
was possible because the virus is not maintained in nonhuman
species and because asymptomatic carriers do not exist. The
last reported natural case of smallpox appeared in Somalia in

[11] The difficult decision comes when the rabidity of the animal is not known. Wild
animals attacking without provocation must be presumed rabid. If the animal is killed
at the time of the attack, its carcass is sent to the state public health laboratory for
examination. Vaccination is started pending evidence the animal is free of rabies. If
domestic animals are captured following a bite and appear well, vaccination need not
be given unless the animal becomes ill; the holding (observation) period should be 10
days.

1977 (although a fatal laboratory-acquired infection occurred in England in 1978). For this reason routine immunization is no longer recommended either for children or adults. Clinically smallpox is a *febrile illness* (102° to 106°F) associated with *headache, nausea, vomiting, muscle pains* and a *skin rash* which begins as blisters (vesicles) that become pus filled and finally rupture, leaving a scar. The lesion initially resembles chicken pox. A *fulminant variant* manifests itself by *bone marrow depression, hemorrhage throughout the body* and *death in shock* before the rash has time to develop. No specific treatment is available.

INFECTIOUS MONONUCLEOSIS

This disease of adolescents and young adults is due to infection by the Epstein-Barr virus.[12] Symptoms include *fever, sore throat* and *prominent enlargement of lymph nodes* in the neck and elsewhere in the body. *Weakness* and *fatigue* are marked. Additional findings include *small hemorrhages in the hard and soft palate* and *enlargement of the spleen.* Occasionally a *rash* and *liver enlargement* are seen. Symptoms may persist for several weeks but recovery is usually complete. Serious complications include *aseptic meningitis* and the *Guillain-Barré syndrome.* The diagnosis is suggested by finding a high percentage of large, atypical-appearing lymphocytes on smear of the blood and confirmed by a serological test called the *heterophile antibody reaction.* There is no treatment, but bed rest is usually required during the acute phase.

HERPES

The *herpes simplex* virus[13] consists of two types. *Type 1 virus* causes *fever blisters* on the lips; in a few patients it also results in the picture of *aseptic meningitis* or *encephalitis.* A serious complication is involvement of the eye (*herpes keratitis*) which

[12] In Africa Epstein-Barr virus causes lymphoma in young persons (*Burkitt's lymphoma*). Why the virus is associated with neoplastic disease in that continent and with a benign illness like infectious mononucleosis in the West is not completely clear, although genetic explanations have been put forth.

[13] *Herpes zoster* ("shingles"), a disease causing extreme pain and overlying blister formation in the distribution of thoracic, lumbar, cervical and (occasionally) cranial nerves, is due to the chicken pox virus. The disease usually occurs in adults who have had chicken pox as children; it is thought to be due to reactivation of virus that has remained dormant in the nerve ganglia since the childhood episode. Presumably an acquired depression in the immune suppressive response allows it to break out.

may lead to corneal scarring and blindness. *Type 2 virus* causes *venereal disease*. The primary manifestation is development of *small blisters on the genitalia* which ultimately ulcerate to form open sores. At the outset *fever, malaise* and *localized lymph node enlargement* result. If infection is present during pregnancy, the virus may be transmitted to the newborn infant on passage through the vagina. *Neonatal herpes* is a serious disease which may kill the child; it causes widespread vesicle formation, liver disease, adrenal insufficiency and encephalitis. Herpes keratitis can be treated with *idoxuridine* added topically. No treatment is available for other forms of type 1 disease or the type 2 virus.

DISEASES DUE TO SPIROCHETES

SYPHILIS

Syphilis is due to infection with *Treponema pallidum*. It causes disease in three stages. *Primary syphilis* usually appears about 3 weeks after exposure and consists of a painless bump or nodule (*chancre*) at the contact site (genitalia, mouth, throat). *Secondary syphilis* follows about 6 weeks after healing of the chancre and manifests itself by fever and an extensive skin rash (occasionally with symptoms due to involvement of liver, kidney, joints and eyes). The patient is highly contagious in this stage. The disease then enters a latent (asymptomatic) phase which may last for years before appearance of the signs of *tertiary syphilis*. The cardiovascular and nervous systems are preeminently involved in the tertiary stage. *Cardiovascular syphilis* causes aortic valve incompetency and heart failure. It may also produce aneurysms of the aorta. *Neurosyphilis* is of three types: meningovascular syphilis, general paresis and tabes dorsalis. *Meningovascular syphilis* usually manifests itself as a syndrome of small or large strokes while *paresis* results in mental dysfunction ranging from delusions and hallucinations to loss of memory and frank psychosis. *Tabes dorsalis* causes loss of equilibrium and position sense coupled with episodes of lightninglike pain in the extremities, abdomen or chest (*tabetic crisis*). An additional feature is blindness due to atrophy of the optic nerves. Both tabes and paresis are associated with a characteristic physical sign, the *Argyll Robertson pupil.* Such pupils do not constrict when exposed to light as is expected in normal eyes. The ability to contract during accommodation (the act of focusing on objects approaching the eye) is preserved.

Diagnosis of syphilis is based on positive serologic tests in the blood and cerebrospinal fluid.[14] Treatment is penicillin, with large doses required if neurosyphilis is present (diagnosed by finding a positive serologic test for syphilis in the cerebrospinal fluid).

LEPTOSPIROSIS

Leptospirosis, a disease that primarily affects farmers, veterinarians and slaughterhouse workers, is transmitted to humans from a variety of domestic and wild animals. The organism is passed in the urine, thus contaminating the environment. The clinical picture consists of the *acute onset of chills* and *fever* with *headache* and *severe muscle pain. Nausea, vomiting* and *loss of appetite* are prominent. A clinical clue to diagnosis is the appearance on the third or fourth day of a severe *conjunctivitis* with redness of the eyes and excessive tear formation. With severe disease many organ systems are involved. Outstanding are *aseptic meningitis, liver disease with jaundice* and *inflammation of the kidney* with cells and protein in the urine. Diagnosis is based on recovery of the organism by culture or positive serologic tests. A variety of antibiotics are effective in treatment, but penicillin and tetracycline are preferred by most authorities.

DISEASES CAUSED BY FUNGI

Fungi, which differ in morphologic and chemical characteristics from bacteria, produce diseases that are similar to bacterial infections; pneumonia and meningitis are the outstanding manifestations. The organisms are found in soil and generally cause disease following inhalation of infected dust. One fungus (*Candida albicans*) and a funguslike bacterium (*Actinomyces*

---

[14] The most common screening test for syphilis is the *VDRL exam;* however, this test may be falsely positive in the collagen-vascular diseases and other autoimmune disorders. The *fluorescent treponema antibody absorption test* (FTA) or *treponema pallidum immobilization test* (TPI), which are specific for syphilis, must be ordered if a false positive reaction is suspected.

israelii) are found normally in the intestinal tract of man. The fungi are identified by culture of infected material on special media or serologic tests showing a rise in antibody to the responsible organism.

CRYPTOCOCCOSIS

Cryptococcus neoformans causes *pneumonia* and also commonly *invades the central nervous system.* Symptoms of CNS infection include *headache, double vision, loss of balance, vomiting* and *convulsions.* A wide variety of other neurologic deficits may appear. Treatment requires long-term intravenous administration of a toxic antifungal drug called *amphotericin B.* The antibiotic may have to be added directly to spinal fluid as well. It may cause anemia, hypokalemia and damage to the kidney, but with cryptococcal meningitis its use is absolutely required.

COCCIDIOIDOMYCOSIS

This disease, caused by *Coccidioides immitis,* produces *pneumonia* (with pleural effusions), *joint pains,* an *itchy skin rash* and a nodular reddish lesion of the skin of the lower extremities called *erythema nodosum.* If the disease becomes *generalized,* the patient may develop ulcerating lesions of the skin, lymph node enlargement and invasion of bone. *Meningitis* results in headache, nerve palsies and hydrocephalus (increased fluid content of brain). Coccidioidomycosis is also treated with amphotericin B, but the outlook with meningitis is grim.

HISTOPLASMOSIS

Like the two previous diseases, histoplasmosis (caused by *Histoplasma capsulatum*) results most often in *pneumonia* but can produce *disseminated disease* with involvement of many organ systems including the brain and meninges. A special feature not seen in the other fungal infections is the presence of *ulcer formation in the mucous membranes of the mouth, throat, genitalia* and *bladder.* Again, amphotericin B is the only available treatment.

OTHER FORMS OF FUNGAL DISEASE

Sporotrichosis develops following penetration of the skin by thorns of the fungus-laden plant (such as a rosebush). A red or purple nodule develops at the puncture site, and lymph nodes in the drainage tract enlarge with red streaks connecting them to the primary lesion. Generalized disease may occur but is unusual. *Moniliasis* (*Candida albicans* infection) is usually localized to the oral cavity where it produces a white, patchy membrane (*thrush*), or the vagina where it causes a vaginal discharge with itching.[15] Skin infections, especially around the nails, are not unusual. In debilitated patients the organism may get in the bloodstream and invade many organs. A dangerous complication is *Candida endocarditis* where the fungus lodges on and damages the heart valves. *Actinomycosis* is a condition manifested by an abscesslike swelling of the jaw ("lumpy jaw"), enlarged lymph nodes in the neck and draining sinuses. *Blastomycosis*, relatively rare in the United States, causes pulmonary disease that may be confused with pneumonia, cancer of the lung or other fungal diseases. It also produces a nodular skin lesion. *Nocardiosis*, caused by a funguslike bacteria similar to that causing actinomycosis, usually produces the picture of lung abscess but can also cause abscess formation in the brain and elsewhere.

RICKETTSIAL DISEASES

Rickettsiae are parasites about the size of bacteria that are transmitted between infected animals and from animals to man by arthropod vectors such as ticks, fleas and lice. *Rocky Mountain spotted fever*, conveyed by tick bite, begins with high fever and chills. Two to six days after onset, round red spots appear in the skin; bleeding into the spots occurs with time, leading to large bruiselike or hemorrhagic areas. With severe disease shock supervenes. Treatment is with chloramphenicol or tetracycline. *Murine typhus* follows bite by an infected flea. It is a febrile illness with a skin rash that may mimic Rocky Mountain spotted fever. Typhus can be differentiated because it tends to occur in city dwellers rather than in rural areas (where ticks abound) and because the rash occurs predomi-

---

[15] Vaginal moniliasis is very common in diabetic women because the sugar content of vaginal secretions is high, promoting growth of the fungus. However, normal women may also become infected with *Candida*. The treatment is nystatin vaginal tablets or (in resistant cases) a dye called gentian violet.

nantly over the trunk rather than over extremities, palms, soles and face as is the case with spotted fever. Antibiotic therapy is identical in the two diseases. *Epidemic typhus*, as the name indicates, occurs in vast waves in susceptible populations, spread by the body louse. The last epidemic in the United States occurred in the 19th century. The disease resembles murine typhus but is more severe. *Q fever* is a rickettsial pneumonia occurring primarily in Australia, although the agent has been found in North America.

IMMUNODEFICIENCY SYNDROMES

A number of diseases are known in which the immune defense systems of the body are incompetent. Defects in both B and T cell function have been identified, occurring singly and in combination. Deficiency states may be either congenital or acquired. Current classifications are quite complicated and will not be discussed here. Treatment is difficult. If circulating gamma globulin (the plasma protein fraction that contains the bulk of antibodies) levels are low, intermittent transfusion of pooled gamma globulin from normal subjects may be helpful. Some patients have had restoration of immune competence by transplantation of bone marrow, thymus glands or liver from a normal donor, but these are research procedures not yet available for general application. Once infection has developed, treatment with antibiotics is carried out as in normal persons. Some children with extreme forms of deficiency have been kept isolated in sterile environments for years.

17

Eating Disorders:
Obesity and Anorexia Nervosa

In this chapter two disorders at the extremes of the eating spectrum will be considered: obesity and anorexia nervosa. In the former caloric intake is inappropriately high resulting in abnormal accumulation of body fat; in the latter it is so low that affected subjects may die of voluntary starvation.

OBESITY

The treatment of obesity is a major industry in the United States with millions of dollars spent yearly in the quest for weight reduction. Overweight persons are willing to try almost anything to lose a few pounds, and money freely flows to any entrepreneur with a diet or mechanical aid that promises "weight loss without dieting or hunger." The truth is that apart from surgical treatment and a drug therapy that constitutes poisoning, weight loss cannot be achieved without restricting caloric intake or experiencing the discomfort of hunger.

DEFINITION, INCIDENCE AND TYPES OF OBESITY
Since body weights span a continuous spectrum from thin to fat, the diagnosis of obesity is somewhat arbitrary. In the medical literature tables of *ideal body weight* are often used. These

tables are based on actuarial figures compiled by insurance companies and indicate the range of weight (for a given height) that is associated with a normal life expectancy. Most studies suggest that a weight 20 percent above the ideal imparts some degree of health risk. However, it must be pointed out that some large-framed individuals with heavy musculature may have body weights above the ideal and still not be obese; another way of saying this is that obesity should be defined as excess weight due to accumulation of adipose tissue.[1] Nevertheless, if obesity is considered to be a weight greater than 20 percent above the ideal, about 20–30 percent of men and 30–40 percent of women in the United States are obese. For those who do not have access to tables of ideal body weight, calculation of the *body mass index* (BMI) is useful. The formula is weight (W) in kilograms divided by the square of the height (H) in meters (W/H^2).[2] Excess mortality begins to appear at values above 25.

There are a number of forms of obesity. The most common is the modest *obesity of middle age* in which persons gain 15 or 20 pounds over their ideal weight as they enter the middle years. The mechanism is a modest decrease in physical activity that is unmatched by a decrease in caloric intake. *Social obesity* refers to the fact that in some segments of human society, moderate obesity is considered a sign of health and beauty. Such patients have no desire to lose weight and often refuse to do so even when a specific health indication exists. *Massive obesity* is usually defined as a weight 100 percent above ideal. The mechanisms underlying massive obesity are probably quite different from the first two types. Ordinarily such obesity begins in childhood and continues throughout life. Health risks are maximal in these patients. *Secondary obesity* is a state of excess adiposity due to the presence of an underlying disease process. The major causes are Cushing's syndrome, hypothyroidism, some forms of hypogonadism and congenital disorders affecting the hypothalamus. The latter include the *Prader-Willi syndrome,* in which children have major obesity, sexual infantil-

---

[1] Total body fat can be accurately assessed by several methods, but these are not routinely available to physicians. An estimate of adiposity that is reasonably precise can be obtained by measuring the thickness of the fat pad in the triceps area (the back part of the upper arm) using specialized calipers that are commercially available.

[2] The weight in pounds divided by 2.2 yields the equivalent value in kilograms. The height in inches can be converted to meters by dividing by 39.4.

ism, abnormally small hands and feet and a peculiar flaccidity of muscles, and the *Laurence-Moon-Biedl* syndrome wherein major obesity is associated with polydactyly (increased numbers of fingers and toes), mental retardation, pigmented changes in the retina, nystagmus, hypogonadism and abnormalities of the urinary tract. The latter disease usually results from marriage between relatives.

DETRIMENTAL EFFECTS OF OBESITY

Most affected persons are concerned about obesity for cosmetic and not health reasons. The physician, on the other hand, worries about effects on health. Minor (but annoying problems) include *shortness of breath, decreased exercise tolerance* and *fatigue. Degenerative arthritis* of the spine, hips and knees occurs much earlier than in normal persons because of increased pressure loads on the joint cartilages. More serious is the fact that obesity is associated with a greatly increased incidence of *high blood pressure, diabetes* and *hypertriglyceridemia.*[3] All three are risk factors for development of *coronary artery disease* and *heart attacks.* Massive obesity can also cause *congestive heart failure* in the absence of underlying primary heart disease. *Ventilatory failure* (low oxygen concentrations and retention of carbon dioxide in blood) and *pulmonary embolism* occur with increased frequency. Finally, the heavy chest wall and high diaphragms that predispose to ventilatory failure make anesthesia and surgery high risk propositions in obese subjects.

WHAT CAUSES OBESITY?

The answer is that in many cases we don't know. The mild obesity of middle age seems straightforward, as indicated above, but massive obesity is a different matter. It likely is polyfactorial in origin, meaning that there is no one causal mechanism. A number of interesting facts are known from studies in both animals and humans. These will be briefly reviewed.

[3] In some patients obesity itself appears to cause high blood pressure; others have hypertension which exists independent of obesity but is made worse by its presence. As pointed out in chapter 15, obesity causes maturity-onset diabetes to become clinically manifest by producing tissue resistance to the action of insulin. Hypertriglyceridemia is due to obesity-induced overproduction of very low density lipoproteins in the liver. All three conditions improve or disappear if weight loss can be achieved.

Hypothalamic Centers. Central nervous system control of eating is largely vested in two centers located in the hypothalamus.[4] The *feeding center* is located in the lateral hypothalamus; if this center is stimulated chronically through an implanted electrode, animals overeat and become obese. Conversely, destruction of the center causes animals to cease eating and lose weight. The *satiety center* is found in the ventromedial hypothalamus. Stimulation in this area causes weight loss while destruction causes massive obesity. The satiety center is the only area of the brain that is sensitive to insulin. It has been speculated that obesity in some persons might be the consequence of satiety center dysfunction (perhaps a resistance to insulin), but no direct evidence is available to support the hypothesis.

Absence of a Humoral Satiety Factor. Parabiosis is a technique in which the circulatory system of one animal is connected to that of another such that there is complete exchange of blood between the two. If an electrode is placed in the feeding center of one parabiotic partner and chronically stimulated, that animal becomes fat. The normal partner, in contrast, ceases to eat (in the face of abundant food) and will eventually die of starvation. This strongly suggests that a factor enters the blood of normal animals following eating and signals cessation of food intake by suppressing appetite (the *humoral satiety factor*).[5] In a similar type of study, genetically obese mice (*ob/ob* strain) have been parabiosed to normal weight animals. Under this circumstance the obese animals lose weight (despite free access to food). The interpretation is that the *ob/ob* mouse may be unable to produce the putative satiety factor and thus overeats. Satiety factor arising in the normal partner replaces the deficit and reverses the obesity. Preliminary studies suggest that a satiety factor may normally be made in the pancreatic islets of Langerhans. This follows from the observation that transplantation of islets from normal animals into obese recipients cures their disease. Islets from obese animals do not work. Two possible candidates for the pancreatic satiety factor are the islet

---

[4] These centers are doubtless controlled by a variety of signals, but some circulating nutrient (such as plasma glucose) probably plays the primary role. Overriding signals from higher up in the central nervous system clearly operate. For example, anxiety may cause signals to pass from the cerebral cortex to the feeding center and result in "nervous eating" even though the satiety center is receiving input that no food is needed.

[5] *Humoral* means circulating in blood.

hormones *pancreatic polypeptide* and *somatostatin*. While much work remains to be done, both hormones have been reported to cause weight loss in experimental animals. Despite these intriguing results, there is at present no evidence for satiety factor deficiency in man.

Abnormal Metabolism. Almost all fat people believe they have something wrong with their metabolism. They commonly state that they gain weight on amounts of food that do not make lean persons add pounds. As will be seen later, essentially all obese patients overeat. Nevertheless, the question of abnormal metabolism is legitimate. Some recent studies are of interest in this regard.

Ingested calories have three possible fates. They may be oxidized in biochemical reactions that convert food energy into useful work, they may be stored in tissues as potential or reserve energy (primarily as fat in adipose tissue) or they may be metabolized in such a way that energy is released as heat (i.e., the energy is uncoupled from useful work). The latter reactions are usually carried out by what biochemists call *futile cycles*.[6] Such futile cycles are important for generating extra body heat on exposure to cold environments. Theoretically, activation of futile cycles could also be useful in protecting against fat formation when excess calories are ingested: insofar as calories could be utilized for heat production, they would be shunted away from fat formation. An exciting recent discovery is the observation that rats and mice genetically destined to become obese lack the ability to generate heat on exposure to cold (they die of hypothermia with temperature exposures that do not affect normal animals). These animals appear to be deficient in an enzyme called *sodium-potassium ATPase* whose biochemical characteristics allow it to function as a futile cycle. The implication is that their obesity might be due to an impaired ability to dispose of ingested calories as heat. In other words, it is assumed that normally a portion of ingested food is oxidized

[6] In a futile cycle one chemical compound is converted to a second in a reaction requiring the input of energy from ATP, the primary high-energy chemical of the body. This product is then immediately broken back down to the first compound by an opposing enzyme, releasing the energy contributed by ATP as heat. The net result is that tissue content of both chemicals remains constant but the energy of ATP is converted to heat. Regeneration of ATP requires the continual oxidation of ingested food or tissue fat thus "wasting" calories. Since such a cycle is biochemically meaningless (in the sense that no net chemical transformation has been produced), it is designated "futile."

in futile cycles or equivalent energy-wasteful pathways. In the absence of one or more of these pathways, food utilization would become more efficient and weight gain would be greater (for the same number of ingested calories) than in a genetically normal animal with an intact energy-wasting system.

Does an analogous defect exist in obese humans? The answer is unknown, but three lines of evidence suggest that it might (at least in some cases). *First,* when normal lean individuals are overfed for several months, the actual weight gain is less (by about 15–20 percent) than that predicted.[7] Moreover, it has been shown that body heat production after a meal (tested during a standard exercise) rises as caloric content of the meal increases, suggesting the operation of a compensatory mechanism for handling excess calories. *Second,* in a famous study in which massively obese subjects were compared with volunteers who were overfed to the same approximate weight, it was observed that there were marked differences in the number of calories required to maintain the obese state. Thus the normal volunteers eating a mixed diet needed 1,800 calories per square meter of body surface per day to keep weight constant before the experiment and 2,700 calories per M^2 once they had become obese. The spontaneously obese subjects, on the other hand, required only about 1,400 calories per M^2. Interestingly, volunteers made obese with a high-fat diet could be maintained by 1,800 calories per M^2, emphasizing the fact that high-fat diets tend to cause more weight gain than mixed or high-carbohydrate diets. Exercise levels were equivalent in spontaneously obese subjects and volunteers. The conclusion was that lean volunteers, even when they overate sufficiently to become massively obese, converted far fewer calories to fat (and thus, necessarily, more to heat) than obese subjects. *Third,* deficient heat production during exposure to cool environmental temperatures has been demonstrated in certain aboriginal tribes living in the Australian desert. They thus resemble the temperature-sensitive obese rodents described above. It has been pointed out that when primitive tribes move to areas of abundant food they tend to become fat. A heat-generating defect is conceiv-

---

[7] Provided calories were given as carbohydrates or a mixed diet (carbohydrate, protein, fat). If a high-fat diet was given weight gain was exactly as predicted: wastage of calories as heat was not apparent. This is important since many of the fad diets are high-fat regimens.

ably partially responsible. On balance it seems possible that more efficient metabolism may play a role in some human obesity.[8]

Fat Cell Size and Fat Cell Number. If rats are overfed in the first 3 weeks of life (to weaning), they become permanently obese compared to their normally fed litter mates. This brief period of overfeeding causes a significant increase in the total number of fat cells in the body, each of which is also larger than normal adipose tissue cells (contains more fat). In contrast, if rodents are overfed as adults, there is no increase in fat cell number, only an increase in fat cell size. Subsequently it was found that humans who had been obese since childhood also had an increased number of fat cells compared to persons becoming obese as adults. On the basis of such studies, the concept arose that obesity might be related, in part, to overfeeding in infancy. The anatomical consequence of that overfeeding, an increased fat cell number, would significantly increase the potential for total body adiposity in the future (since a single fat cell can hold only a given amount of fat).[9] Support for the concept that food intake during infancy may at least partially determine weight in later life comes from observations made of the offspring of parents living under famine and nonfamine conditions during World War II. The prevalence of adult obesity was significantly higher in children who had adequate food during infancy than in the group who were malnourished.

Eating Cues. Experimental studies have shown that laboratory animals can be made to overeat simply by making food

[8] The prevalence of obesity is increasing throughout the world. Some scientists have postulated that the increase is the consequence of an evolutionary adaptation—a so-called "thrifty" mutation. They suggest that in times or environments where food was scarce or only intermittently available, persons with the most efficient fuel utilization systems had survival advantage. When these persons ate they stored almost every calorie as fat and thus could survive during prolonged periods of food shortage. Lean persons, in contrast, would die during famine because of limited fat stores. In this way the species might have become enriched with efficient utilizers of calories. In modern times, where food for the most part is continually available, such persons would become fat. There is an analogy in the *desert sand rat.* Living in the desert under conditions of intermittent food supply, these rodents are lean and healthy. Transported to a laboratory where food is freely available, they not only become fat, they develop diabetes. A human counterpart may exist in the Pima Indians of Arizona, a desert tribe that exhibits a remarkable prevalence of obesity and diabetes in the setting of reservation life.

[9] Obesity acquired during adult life usually results in a pot-bellied picture with relative sparing of the arms and legs because there are limited numbers of fat cells in the extremities in persons not overfed early in life, and these cells are limited in their expansile capacity by surrounding muscle. Fat cells in the abdominal cavity, on the other hand, can expand to their maximal limit.

more attractive (adding sugar or fat). It is therefore no surprise that food intake in humans is influenced by its look, taste and smell. Thus a dual system of stimuli determines eating patterns: *internal signals* of hunger or satiety and *external cues* of physical attractiveness. In normal-weight persons, the former signals dominate. On the other hand, a number of studies suggest that obese persons respond more to external cues than they do to physiologic signals; if they are exposed to food that looks or smells good, the tendency will be to eat regardless of whether they are hungry. Some psychoanalysts believe this type of reliance on external cues is produced early in life by overfeeding (e.g., if the mother puts a bottle of milk in the baby's mouth every time the baby cries, the infant learns to eat whenever food is available). Whether this is in fact the case is not known.

Exercise. Many studies show that obese children and adults exercise less than their normal-weight compatriots. For example, if one places a pedometer on normal weight and obese housewives, it can be shown that the lean subjects walk many more miles during a day than those who are obese. Obese subjects tend, therefore, to accentuate the weight-producing effect of excess food because they do not burn calories normally through exercise. It is not known whether decreased exercise is always secondary to obesity (it is hard to exercise when one is fat), or whether low levels of physical activity (genetically determined?) might predate the onset of weight gain and contribute to its development.

Ponderostat. There is increasing evidence that the total amount of fat in the body somehow controls eating. Such regulation has been called the *ponderostat*. The concept is still incompletely developed but is based on evidence like the following. If one destroys the satiety center in a rat, the animal becomes obese but eventually reaches a steady weight. If one now further overfeeds that rat by some means (such as tube feeding), additional weight gain is produced. Once a new plateau has been obtained, the animal is then allowed to eat what it wishes. Invariably, food intake ceases until weight falls to the previous (still obese) level. Then food intake is resumed to maintain that weight. Human volunteers who are made massively obese for experimental reasons rapidly return to their preexperimental weight (spontaneously) once the study is completed. Similarly, obese persons brought to normal weight during prolonged hospitalization almost always rapidly regain to prehospitalization values on discharge. There thus appears to be some sort of "set" weight perceived as normal by the individual's central nervous system. Psychological studies in obese subjects show emotional deterioration when major weight loss has occurred and lend additional support to the concept that a powerful drive emanates from the fat cell mass to sustain itself.[10] How these signals arise and exert their effect is totally unknown.

Summary. While no final answers can be given, it is attractive to assume (tentatively) that massive obesity is both genetically and environmentally determined. It may well turn out that many obese patients have extraefficient metabolism due to a genetically acquired impairment of some futile cycle activity or perhaps a deficiency of or resistance to a humoral satiety factor that signals the sense of fullness. From the environmental standpoint, overfeeding in infancy may have two major effects —the foundation structure of adipose tissue (cell number) is expanded, setting the ponderostat high, and eating patterns become externally cued rather than physiological. Finally, decreased exercise removes the compensating effect of caloric expenditure. The end result is increased food intake, frugal metabolism of ingested calories and diminished utilization of calories for mechanical (muscular) work. A person in this situation is destined for a lifelong fight if obesity is to be controlled or reversed. Unfortunately, statistics show that the battle is almost always lost.

TREATMENT

Regardless of the underlying mechanisms that predispose to development of obesity, weight loss can be achieved only if

---

[10] In a famous study done at Rockefeller University, massively obese persons were brought to normal weight by fasting. Psychologic testing revealed severe emotional distress during weight loss. The investigators carrying out the study rigged up an adjustable lens system that could distort photographic images (like sideshow mirrors that make a person look thin or fat). If a current photograph of nurses or doctors was distorted by the lens, obese patients were able to adjust the image to the way the person actually looked (exactly as did control subjects). However, they dialed themselves fat (even though at the time of the test their weight was normal). It is almost as if obese persons have implanted in their central nervous system an image of fatness. Presumably if weight loss were maintained for a long enough period, body image perception might normalize, but to my knowledge such a study has not been carried out.

caloric intake is restricted or if caloric expenditure is increased; usually both are required. While short-term weight loss is fairly easily achieved, long-term success in normalizing weight in moderately or massively obese persons is minuscule—about 5 percent. What usually happens is that obese persons embrace every new diet that comes along and, because it is new, are motivated to lose weight for several weeks. As the novelty wears off they rapidly regain. Many obese persons lose literally hundreds of pounds over a lifetime. The only problem is that they also regain hundreds. This cycle, dismal from the patient's point of view, is an economic godsend for the weight-loss entrepreneurs. The first step in dealing with the problem is to acknowledge that achievement of weight loss and its maintenance will be difficult (every serious experimental study yet reported indicates this to be the case). This means that widely advertised popular schemes, despite their glowing claims and pseudoscience, should be avoided (unless there is an underlying desire to redistribute one's financial resources). A review of acceptable and unacceptable approaches to treatment follows.

Diet. The ideal weight reduction diet should be nutritionally balanced, differing from a normal diet only in that total calories are limited. Caloric restriction need not be rigid for weight loss to occur. From chapter 2 it will be recalled that a normal person utilizes about half the daily caloric intake to sustain the basal metabolic rate while the other half is expended in physical activity. Most adults take in 2,400 to 3,000 calories a day. (Studies have shown that the massively obese may ingest up to 5,000 calories in 24 hours.) It follows that a diet of less than 2,400 calories will cause weight loss in most people. Physicians usually prescribe more severely restricted diets (in the range of 1,000 to 1,500 calories per day) in order to speed weight loss. If one cuts the intake from 2,400 calories to 1,000 calories per day, weight loss over the long range will average a pound every 2½ days. (Recall that a deficit of 3,500 calories is roughly equal to 1 pound.)[11] *High-fat diets* (the "ketogenic" diets recommended in many popular books) should be avoided for two reasons. First, they tend to promote elevation of cholesterol and triglyceride levels in the blood (which is bad from the standpoint of

---

[11] Weight loss in the first day or two of dieting consists of considerable amounts of fluid. The fact that the rate of weight loss rapidly slows after the initial few days of dieting discourages many people, even though it is totally predictable.

accelerating atherosclerosis and coronary artery disease). Second, as previously noted, fat appears to be used more efficiently than carbohydrate or protein. *High-protein diets* are also frequently recommended. They have two real advantages. First, the specific dynamic action (the calories required to get food absorbed) is higher for protein than for carbohydrate and fat; thus net calories absorbed per calories ingested is lower. Second, it is harder to eat large amounts of protein calories than it is a mixed meal (proteins tend to satiate earlier). For these reasons increasing the protein content of the diet is probably helpful. Since animal proteins contain high concentrations of saturated fat, it is preferable to use fish and fowl (chicken and turkey) as the protein source. The recently popularized *liquid-protein diets* should never be used. Sudden and unpredictable death has occurred on these diets even with patients under medical supervision. The cause of death is cardiac arrhythmia, but the mechanism of induction is not known.

Fasting. Maximal rates of weight loss are achieved by total fasting. Massively obese patients have been kept without food (given only fluids and vitamins) for many months with no difficulty. However, the procedure is expensive (because hospitalization is required) and not a practical solution for the vast majority of patients. Short-term fasts (1 day per week) are useful as an aid in speeding weight loss, providing the patient does not compensate by eating much more on the day after the fast. Four fasting days a month (assuming a basic therapeutic diet of 1,500 calories per day) would lead to a net extra deficit of 6,000 calories (about 1.75 pounds) per month.

Behavior Modification. Behavior modification techniques are important as an adjunct to diet. Such programs may be formal (under direction of a therapist), but the principles are simple and can be learned with the help of the primary physician. A careful history of eating habits is obtained (Does one eat only at meals? Does one snack continuously while watching TV? Does one eat in the middle of the night? etc.) to pinpoint areas of difficulty. New rules for eating are then adopted. For example, all obese persons are taught to eat only at meals and to eat the meals in one place away from distracting influences such as TV (it is amazing how much one can eat absentmindedly while attention is directed at the small screen). Emphasis is placed on eating slowly with small bites which are thoroughly chewed so that the taste of the food can be enjoyed. Along the same lines patients are instructed to put eating utensils down on the table between bites (many obese persons gulp food down, thus eating more calories per unit time than does a subject of normal weight). If hunger returns between meals, low-calorie foods (such as celery) are prescribed to fill the stomach. It is repeatedly drummed home as of preeminent importance that a change in life-style is required—not fad diets or other short-term measures.[12]

Drugs. Several types of drugs are used by those physicians who specialize in the treatment of obesity.[13] These include: *appetite suppressants, thyroid hormone* and *human chorionic gonadotropin.* Appetite suppressants are related to the amphetamine class of drugs (central nervous system stimulants or "uppers"). They cause loss of small amounts of weight for 2 to 3 weeks but afterward simply become habituating (because of the stimulant effect). Thyroid hormone can only cause weight loss if the patient is given enough hormone to produce thyrotoxicosis: by producing one illness to combat another, a very unwise maneuver. Human chorionic gonadotropin has been shown to be worthless in carefully controlled studies; it acts as a placebo. (The placebo effect is enhanced because the drug must be injected.) Reputable authorities on obesity do not recommend the use of any of these drugs. I wholeheartedly concur.

Exercise. Exercise is an important feature of weight reduction, but it must be realized that a good bit of exercise is required to overcome excess calories. For an average-size person, approximate caloric expenditures (calories per minute) for four common activities are: walking, 5.2; bicycling, 8.2; swimming, 11.2; running, 19.4. Thus a bowl of ice cream containing 193

[12] In this regard patients need to learn that a single meal off diet is not harmful. Most patients on reducing diets eat little when out in public and cheat at home (usually on junk foods). Exactly the opposite behavior should be followed: observe the diet at home and break over (if one has to) on special occasions when the food is good. It is far better to eat a large meal when entertaining (or being entertained) at a nice restaurant than to waste calories on chips and soft drinks at home.

[13] Some physicians who treat obesity exclusively are legitimate. Be suspicious, however, of any doctor who has a high patient turnover per day, who prescribes multiple drugs (especially if drugs are dispersed in the office) without taking a history or doing a careful physical examination, and who indicates that weight loss will be achieved without dieting. This mode of operation usually indicates a money-generating (and very lucrative) business which is on the very fringe of legitimate medicine (if not outside its bounds).

calories (⅙ of a quart) would require (for neutralization) 37 minutes of walking, 24 minutes of cycling, 17 minutes of swimming or 10 minutes of running. Still, a net increased expenditure of only 100 calories a day by exercise (say a 20-minute walk) would lead to a weight loss of 10 pounds in a year. Coupled with a decrease in intake of only 100 calories a day (1 serving of potato chips or a soft drink), weight loss of 20 pounds would be produced. It seems incredibly simple (and it is), yet even these minimal adjustments appear to be beyond the capability of most obese subjects.

Surgery. Because of the aforementioned difficulties in achieving weight loss in the massively obese, surgery has come to play an increasingly important role in its management. In general any patient under 50 who is at least 100 pounds overweight and has no complication that would be expected to shorten normal life expectancy (e.g., heart failure, severe pulmonary disease, cancer) would now be considered eligible for surgical treatment. The 50-year cutoff point is not absolute, but older patients have a substantially higher surgically related mortality and lesser overall weight loss than younger subjects. Two procedures are used. The first is called *jejunoileal bypass* and until recently was the most widely performed operation. In this technique the jejunum (the second portion of the small intestine) is transected at a point 35 centimeters below its origin at the junction with the duodenum, and this 35 cm segment is anastomosed to the terminal 10 cm of the ileum (the third portion of the small intestine) just before it joins the cecum. This effectively excludes (bypasses) a very large segment of jejunum and ileum which is left in the peritoneal cavity as a blind loop with the jejunal end closed by suturing. Since the bypassed segment contains most of the absorptive area of the small intestine, absorption of calories is markedly diminished and weight loss ensues. Food intake also tends to decrease (for reasons that are uncertain), contributing to the weight loss. Mortality rates during surgery or from postoperative complications are about 2–4 percent (because of the previously mentioned risks imposed by obesity). While most patients who have the procedure consider it successful, an inevitable consequence is persistent diarrhea (3–4 stools per day). The most serious late complication is development of liver disease that may be very severe. Other problems stemming from malabsorption include vitamin deficiencies, electrolyte abnormalities, kidney stones, joint pains, gallbladder disease and gout. Although reanastomosis of the bypassed intestine usually reverses the complications, I do not recommend the operation to any patient. A far preferable procedure in my experience (and one that has gained wide acceptance over the last 2–3 years) is the *gastric bypass*. In this operation the stomach chamber is drastically reduced in size (to a volume of about 60 ml), either by surgically transecting the upper stomach and anastomosing the pouch to the jejunum (bypassing the lower stomach and duodenum) or by simply closing off the bulk of the gastric cavity with surgical staples without anastomosing the upper portion to the jejunum. Weight loss is not produced by interfering with absorption of food but as a consequence of the fact that capacity of the newly created pouch is so small that the patient cannot get much food in even with constant eating. Results are equivalent to those obtained with the jejunoileal bypass procedure but without serious complications. Nausea and vomiting occur early but rapidly disappear as the patients learn to eat small volumes at frequent intervals rather than larger meals three times a day. In my opinion this is the operation that should be carried out in massively obese patients who fail dietary management.

It is extremely interesting that the psychological disintegration seen in patients who lose weight by dieting is not seen with surgically induced weight loss. The reasons are not known, but it may have something to do with the fact that they are not forced to limit food intake.[14]

ANOREXIA NERVOSA

Anorexia nervosa is a relatively rare disease that seems to be increasing in frequency.[15] It occurs almost exclusively in adolescent girls and young women in the twenties (the disease is

[14] One unique psychological change was observed in a selected group of obese subjects who underwent jejunoileal bypass. With weight loss, libido and sexual activity markedly increased, introducing major stress in previously stable marriages. The non-operated partner was the one who became distressed. It turns out that for complicated reasons most had married the massively obese subjects precisely because sex was not commonly demanded (or even possible). A significant number of the partners appeared to be overt or latent homosexuals. Appearance of the sexual drive following surgery made the marriage threatening or unacceptable and divorce followed.

[15] The diagnosis of anorexia nervosa is restricted to patients who have no underlying mental illness. Schizophrenic or depressed patients may refuse to eat and lose weight, but this is called *secondary anorexia* and is unrelated to the illness under discussion.

rare in men and almost never occurs in black women). These young women voluntarily cease to eat and may lose so much weight that they die from starvation. They are absolutely obsessed with food and have a desperate fear of becoming fat.[16] If forced to eat by social convention (e.g., attending a banquet), they excuse themselves, retreat to the restroom and induce vomiting. Most patients carry out extensive exercise, usually in ritualized fashion (doing calisthenics or running at set times throughout the day). Affected subjects exhibit a characteristic triad of denials: (1) they deny hunger (2) they deny that they are wasted and (3) they deny fatigue. When fully clothed the degree of malnutrition is often not appreciated. This is because protein deficiency lowers the plasma albumin concentration, causing marked edema. Thus the legs may not appear wasted because they are swollen with fluid. The face looks full because of edema and because salivary glands are enlarged (a common consequence of starvation or malnutrition). When undressed, however, the patients look like one of the skeletal victims of the concentration camps at Dachau or Auschwitz. No body fat can be seen and every bone is visible. Blood pressure is low and the pulse is slow. A fine covering of hair (*lanugo*) covers the body. Menstruation stops early in the syndrome because gonadotropin release from the pituitary is impaired (luteinizing and follicle-stimulating hormone levels resemble those of prepubertal girls). An interesting oddity is that breast tissue is usually relatively preserved in anorexia nervosa in contrast to imposed starvation where breast atrophy is universal. The reason for this difference is not known.

The cause of anorexia nervosa is obscure. Since the girls are often obese early in life, one theory is that it is a psychological reaction to being fat in childhood, but this remains speculative. Almost always there is excessive conflict between the patient and her family; often the parents are overweight themselves and have overfed the children in early life. Treatment is ineffective, although psychiatric therapy is generally prescribed. If body weight reaches 65 percent of normal, where danger of sudden death is real, forced feeding by stomach tube is required.

[16] Occasionally they lose control and go on giant eating binges. This indicates that the disease is somehow connected with a hatred (and fear of) being fat but that an underlying drive to eat is present—just oversuppressed.

18

Living and Dying

Having come to the end of this book, which has been about the diseases that afflict humankind, I want to say a word about the anxieties that arise when one faces serious illness and death. There are, it seems to me, five common fears regularly induced by the diagnosis of a fatal or potentially fatal disease. These are: (1) fear of the unknown, (2) fear of suffering, (3) fear of incapacitation, (4) fear that life will be fruitlessly prolonged by artificial means and (5) fear of dying.[1] Not every person experiences all of these fears and some seem to experience none. Nevertheless, they are very real and need to be dealt with.

FEAR OF THE UNKNOWN

This fear often surfaces first with the initial development of symptoms. It peaks when an ominous diagnosis is made and continues throughout the course of the disease. The first-stage question (What is wrong with me?) is usually the easiest to answer since most of the time the physician is able to come up with the correct diagnosis. The second set of questions, prompted by the identification of a prognostically grave illness, is more difficult: Is there treatment? How does the disease manifest itself? How long do I have to live? Despite their difficulty they should be asked directly and not be allowed to race cease-

[1] In this discussion I have omitted the fear of economic disaster. As noted in chapter 1, this is currently a real problem that needs to be solved, probably by some form of universal insurance against catastrophic illness.

lessly but silently through the mind. If they are not asked, the physician may be hesitant to discuss the situation in detail fearing that the absence of questions indicates a psychologic protective mechanism (denial) that should not be breached until the patient is ready. While precise answers cannot always be given ("You have 6 weeks to live"), experience with the illness usually allows a rough projection of the expected course. The wise physician attempts to be realistic but not dogmatic, especially about predicting demise. All of us have seen patients with cancer or heart disease who live far beyond the statistically predicted point of death. The aim of the discussion (which needs to be continuing) is threefold: to convey the reality of approaching death,[2] to remove (insofar as possible) the mystery about what lies ahead and to preserve the element of hope.

Once the diagnosis is made and its implications explored, the final set of questions surfaces: Can I go through with what I have to go through? Do I have courage? Will I be able to finish the course with dignity? Answers cannot be given prospectively; they are only provided in the experience itself. Yet, to anyone asking such questions I would say: Almost certainly yes. I never cease to be amazed at the quiet bravery of ordinary men and women facing serious illness and death. That courage can be manifest in human beings is not surprising; what is astonishing is its common presence (sometimes in the most unlikely candidates). The physician's role (priestly function) in the experience is not inconsequential. I find it very helpful in activating strength and courage to say: "Whatever you have to face, I'll accompany you down the way."[3] One needs a medical companion.

FEAR OF SUFFERING

Usually the fear of suffering focuses on pain. It is most often present in patients given a diagnosis of cancer but also is seen

[2] Apart from everything else, the patient, particularly if the breadwinner in the home, needs to prepare or update a will and get financial affairs in order.

[3] It is important for family and friends of the critically or fatally ill to be open, concerned and *present*. If one is unsure that the patient wants to talk about his condition, doubts and fears (but thinks he might), a good approach is to say something like "How are your spirits facing this thing?" (If the question is simply "How are you?" the response will usually be in terms of physical, not emotional feelings.) On the other hand, if one is nervous about initiating such a conversation, nothing specific need be said. The visit itself bespeaks concern without verbalization. Some theologians, in a phrase I like, speak of such visits as a "ministry of presence."

in pain-producing illnesses other than cancer such as crippling rheumatoid arthritis, severe neuropathies and coronary artery disease with recurrent angina. It is not clear why the public associates neoplastic disease with extreme pain. There is no question that certain cancers do cause pain, particularly if there is metastasis to bone. However, there is almost no situation in which the physician cannot either remove the pain or attenuate it to the point where it is only a discomfort that is easily bearable. In advanced malignancy there is no hesitation to use powerful narcotic drugs that would not be prescribed with ordinary pain syndromes because of the fear of addiction. Fear of pain should not be an overwhelming worry. One way or the other it can usually be handled.

FEAR OF INCAPACITATION

The fear of incapacitation (the loss of the ability to maintain oneself as an intact, self-determining unit) usually occurs in those diseases that are potentially or actually paralytic, cause loss of intellectual capacity, result in blindness or lead to the inability to swallow. Classic examples would be spinal cord injuries, crippling arthritis, brain tumors (requiring extensive surgical extirpation of cerebral tissue) and strokes. In these situations imminent death usually is not the problem; rather it is the fear that one will live so depleted of one or more critical functions that mere survival is dependent on the actions of others.[4] Such injuries and illnesses occur every day, and they are extraordinarily difficult to deal with (provided brain function is intact, allowing recognition of one's state). The important issue is to sustain hope.[5] A caring family unit often makes this possible. They must be taught to meet the patient's needs without crushing the spirit through pity and overconcern. Emotional support is much more difficult for the person who is alone in the world although society will provide physical sustenance. Fortunately volunteer agencies and medical personnel (nurses,

[4] A disability that allows one to function independently or semi-independently is not nearly so hard to bear. For example, a quadriplegic bound to a wheelchair may live a full and happy life because he can do many things for himself.

[5] Psychiatrists have distinguished between the states of *helplessness* and *hopelessness*. The latter is far more devastating. A totally paralyzed (thus helpless) young person may be hopeful about life if surrounded by a loving cadre of significant others (family and friends) while a physically normal person with deep depression (thus hopeless) may kill himself in despair.

social workers, physical therapists) take up some of the gap. Many of the latter truly care even though they are paid to do their work. It should be noted that significant advances have been made by specialists in physical and rehabilitative medicine, and these also are a source of hope. Increasing numbers of patients who only a decade or so ago would have been abandoned to their fate can now be restored to a useful existence.

FEAR THAT LIFE WILL BE FRUITLESSLY PROLONGED

The tremendous technical advances in life-support systems now available to the physician have made it possible to sustain life for prolonged periods in the absence of spontaneous respiration or adequate circulation. Such techniques are absolutely marvelous in an acute illness or injury from which recovery is expected provided the patient can only be kept alive through the crisis period. Examples would be the patient with myocardial infarction who goes into shock or the young person comatose from meningitis. Yet these same support systems can also be used to maintain vegetative life in subjects who are irretrievably ill. It is here that the problem comes. Increasingly I find patients broaching this issue directly. I do not want you, they say, to keep me alive by extraordinary means. (Most often the issue arises in persons with cancer or those facing serious surgery, particularly on the heart and brain.) Their concern is not only for themselves; it is for the financial and emotional protection of the loved ones who watch. I think it healthy to discuss such issues openly. I usually respond by saying that this is one fear they need not have; that I will do everything in my power to preserve life as long as the issue is in doubt, but that I will not sustain life artificially once a clearly nonredeemable state is reached.[6] I find that such assurance almost always allows a

[6] I recognize that the physician cannot always tell when death has become inevitable. If the EEG shows no electrical activity in the brain, there is no problem; however, an irreversible state may precede brain death by a considerable period. One can only go on experience and one's best judgment. As a consequence most physicians tend to continue support systems for a reasonable period (say 24 hours) beyond the time of apparent irreversibility. Withholding or withdrawal of extraordinary support measures should be sharply differentiated from *euthanasia* (mercy killing). The latter refers to a positive act by which a pain-ridden, hopelessly ill patient is put to death (e.g., by the injection of a chemical to paralyze respiration). I strongly oppose such acts not because I do not understand that death sometimes appears to be the only mercy but because I do not wish to see the arbitrary power of life and death placed in any human hands. It might be that no physician would ever abuse that power or make a wrong decision; however, since humans are humans I want no one put to such a test.

lightening of the burden of possible death in the patient. The contract also seems to draw patient and physician into a closer relationship than existed before, one which quite often is special for both.

FEAR OF DEATH

The final fear is death. From antiquity, it seems men have been afraid to die. There are two components to that fear. The first is fear of the act of dying. We somehow seem to think it will be painful or traumatic. In fact it is usually very quiet and peaceful.[7] In recent years there has been a great deal of study directed to the remembrances of those who have approached death (e.g., had a cardiac arrest) and then revived. These "near-death" experiences strongly suggest that the act of dying is not frightening.[8] Dr. Lewis Thomas, famous for his books on biological science for lay persons and his column "Notes of a Biology Watcher," comments on this as follows:

"Here's a thing we need to learn more about, if we are to go on living here. What about this dying? Is it really true that such a universal process, in a living system that in so many other respects can strike us dumb with its harmony and beauty, can turn vicious at the end with all its creatures? Or have we got it wrong?

"I think we have, maybe. There are some odd things about human dying, anyway, that don't fit at all with the notion of agony at the end. People who almost die but don't, and then recover to describe the experience, never mention anguish or pain or even despair; to the contrary they recall a strange, unfamiliar feeling of tranquility and peace. The act of dying seems to be associated with some other event,

---

[7] I have seen death many times. The experience is always quite remarkable. One moment there is life, the next it is gone. Most things still work—one can take out the heart or kidney and transplant it for long years of additional function in another living person or isolate a hundred enzymes and show they function perfectly in the test tube, but life is gone. It always reminds me of the sparse recapitulation of creation by some ancient Hebrew scribe: "Then the Lord God formed man of dust from the ground, and breathed into his nostrils the breath of life; and man became a living being" (Genesis 2:7). With death one watches the breath of life vanish.

[8] I am not prepared, as some are, to equate "near-death" with actual death. The visions reported are interesting but for the present, in my opinion, should be considered simply that—visions. A common experience seems to be that the patient floats in the air and watches his own resuscitation. Details are very clear in his memory. There is a sense of great calm and often a luminosity or religious figure fills the room bringing a sense of love and beauty. Frequently past events of the life are visualized. The experience ends with a return of consciousness.

perhaps pharmacologic, that transforms it into something quite different from what most of us are brought up to anticipate. We might be
learning more about this, especially if we were to discover (as might
be the case) that there is a similar event in all sentient creatures. It
might be mediated by the release of peptides of the endorphin class,[9]
which could have the simultaneous effect of suppressing pain and
switching on a level of consciousness previously unknown to most of
us, or all of us. This is wishful guessing, of course, but you can see
what I'm getting at. Something is probably going on that we don't yet
know about."[10]

Whether Dr. Thomas's interpretation of a pharmacologic
event at the end is correct or not, I am convinced that the act of
dying (in itself) should not be feared.

The second component extends beyond fear of the transition
event between life and death. It might be called the fear of
nonbeing or the awareness of finitude. All of us know intui-
tively (for we have observed the endless cycle of death in the
world) that we must die. But in ordinary life we submerge that
knowledge and never think of it. Others die but we live. Then
comes illness (in ourselves or a significant other) and suddenly
we are (frighteningly) aware of our transitoriness. That recognition produces anxiety. Why this should be so cannot be answered in biological terms. As far as one knows nonhuman life
does not consciously fear death. The deer may, by instinct, flee
the danger that comes with the hunter, but I doubt that it con-
templates the possibility of death even when it is imminent.
Theologians would say that the anxiety about finitude derives
from an instinctual awareness that somehow there is a principle
of judgment inherent in the Universe, outside of and transcen-
dent to biological life. Further, that in that judgment we fear
we will be found wanting.[11] Since this is a book about medicine

[9] Endorphins are the recently discovered morphinelike chemicals that exist in the
brain of humans and animals.
[10] Thomas, L. *New England Journal of Medicine* 296:1462–1464, 1977.
[11] Perhaps nowhere in literature is this better expressed than in the words of Job:

"*Now I have had a secret revelation,*
  a whisper has come to my ears.
At the hour when dreams master the mind,
  and slumber lies heavy on man,
A shiver of horror ran through me,
  and my bones quaked with fear.

and not theology, I will not explore this issue further except to recall the statement of the late great philospher-theologian, Professor Paul Tillich:

"If anxiety is defined as the awareness of being finite, God must be called the infinite ground of courage."

LIVING

It is quite paradoxical that life seems most beautiful to those who are about to die. It has been my repeated experience that this is so.[12] To one who has received an announcement of impending death (whether weeks or months ahead), the sun is no longer just there, trees and flowers do not just exist, the rains are not just to be endured; rather every aspect of nature seems rich and precious. Relationships change and become of ultimate importance; friends and family (despite their annoying habits and irritating features) are somehow poignantly loved.[13] Leave-taking and greetings become more than casual events. Things (particularly luxuries) become totally uninteresting. Almost always sensitivity to the plights and needs of others increases.[14] Everything is more intense. In short it is almost as though the awareness of approaching death causes a radical

---

A breath slid over my face,
   the hairs of my body bristled.
Someone stood there—I could not see his face,
   but the form remained before me
Silence—then I heard a Voice,
   'Was ever any man found blameless in the presence of God,
   or faultless in the presence of his Maker?"
            Job 4:12–17 *The Jerusalem Bible*

[12] It is much harder to have a tranquil end if one is poor and alone in society. As a physician who has spent a great many years working in a large metropolitan hospital that cares for the poor, what seems to me a wonder is that despite all the barriers it still occurs.

[13] Some seriously ill people react by becoming embittered, angry and withdrawn, activating personal traits that separate rather than unite. Faced with such a person, the physician and family should not adopt a posture of rejection but seek to break down the wall of fear and hostility (sometimes you can; sometimes you can't).

[14] It always moves me to see a patient I know to be terminally ill caring for others. Not too long ago (about a month before she died), one of my patients with widespread metastatic breast cancer drove (as a Red Cross volunteer) another patient with some degenerative arthritis to the Parkland Memorial Hospital clinic. Throughout the ride the arthritic patient complained of her aches and pains. On arrival she concluded by saying, "But I guess you wouldn't know anything about pain, would you, dearie?" My patient (with cancer in every bone of her body) responded, "Perhaps I don't. I'm sorry you are hurting."

reorientation of all one's priorities; the superficial fun and games and inane trivialities that so clutter up most of our lives are discarded easily and without regret. In place of a future-oriented, goal-driven existence ("Someday, when I make it, I'm really going to enjoy life") is substituted the desire to live in the "now," extracting from it and giving to it everything there is. Perhaps the message to the rest of us (who differ from the ill only in that the signs of our inevitable approaching death are still hidden) is simply this: The only way to live is as if one is about to die.

Appendix

TRADE NAMES OF SOME COMMON DRUGS MENTIONED IN THE TEXT

Only a fraction of the multitudinous drugs available to the physician were mentioned in this book. Many excellent preparations were omitted simply because it was not my purpose to get into details of therapeutics. Generic (general) names were used for all. In this table the registered trade names available in the United States are given. No attempt has been made to list every brand when multiple alternatives are available. Some drugs described in the text will not be found either because they are too new to have been assigned a name or because they are so widely used that they are generally prescribed by their generic nomenclature. Compactin is an example of the former and penicillin the prototype of the latter. An excellent reference for all prescription drugs, their generic and brand names, therapeutic indications and potential hazards is the *Physicians' Desk Reference*, published yearly by the Medical Economics Company. It is readily available in public libraries.

GENERIC NAME—REGISTERED TRADE NAME

acetaminophen—Datril, Tempra, Tylenol
actinomycin D—Cosmegen

GENERIC NAME—REGISTERED TRADE NAME *(cont.)*

adrenocorticotrophic hormone (ACTH)—ACTHar, ACTHar gel,
    Cortrosyn
allopurinol—Zyloprim
amitriptyline—Amitril, Elavil, Endep
amphotericin B—Fungizone
ampicillin—Amcill, Omnipen, Pen A, Penbritin, Pensyn, Polycillin,
    Principen
androgens—Delatestryl, Depo-Testosterone Cypionate, Dianabol,
    Halotestin
azathioprine—Imuran
beclomethasone—Vanceril
benzathine penicillin—Bicillin
bis-hydroxycoumarin—Dicumarol
bromocriptine—Parlodel
calcitonin—Calcimar
carbamazepine—Tegretol
chloramphenicol—Chloromycetin
chloroquine—Aralen, Plaquenil
chlorothiazide—Diuril
chlorpromazine—Thorazine
cholestyramine—Questran
cimetidine—Tagamet
clindamycin—Cleocin
clofibrate—Atromid-S
clomiphene—Clomid
clonidine—Catapres
colestipol—Colestid
coumarin derivatives—Coumadin, Dicumarol, Panwarfin
cromolyn sodium—Intal
curare—Tubocurarine
cyclophosphamide—Cytoxan
dexamethasone—Decadron, Deronil, Dexone, Hexadrol
diazepam—Valium
digitalis—Crystodigin, Digitoxin, Digoxin, Lanoxin
dihydrotachysterol—Hytakerol
dipyridamole—Persantine
L-dopa (levodopa)—Larodopa
dopamine—Intropin
doxorubicin—Adriamycin
edrophonium chloride—Tensilon
estrogen—Estrace, Evex, Hormonin, Menest, Ogen, Premarin
ethambutol—Myambutol

GENERIC NAME—REGISTERED TRADE NAME (*cont.*)

ferrous gluconate—Fergon, Ferralet
ferrous sulfate—Feosol, Fer-In-Sol
fludrocortisone—Florinef
fluphenazine—Permitil, Prolixin
furosemide—Lasix
gentamicin—Garamycin
gentian violet—HYVA vaginal tablets
gold thiomalate—Myochrysine
gonadotropins—Pergonal
guanethidine—Ismelin
halothane—Fluothane
human chorionic gonadotropin—A.P.L., Follutein, Profasi HP
hydralazine—Apresoline
ibuprofen—Motrin
idoxuridine—Stoxil
indomethacin—Indocin
isoniazid—INH, Nydrazid
isoproterenol—Isuprel, Proternol
lactulose—Cephulac, Duphalac
lidocaine—Xylocaine
lincomycin—Lincocin
medroxyprogesterone—Amen, Depo-Provera, Provera
melphalan—Alkeran
meperidine—Demerol
methimazole—Tapazole
methyldopa—Aldomet
methyltestosterone—Android, Metandren, Oreton, Testred, Virilon
methysergide—Sansert
metyrapone—Metopirone
neomycin—Mycifradin, Neobiotic
neostigmine—Prostigmin
nicotinic acid—Nicalex, Nicolar, Nico-Span
nystatin—Mycostatin, Nilstat
pancreatic enzymes—Cotazym, Ilozyme, Pancrease, Viokase
D-penicillamine—Cuprimine
pentagastrin—Peptavlon
phenylbutazone—Azolid, Butazolidin
phenytoin sodium—Dilantin
prednisolone—Delta-Cortef, Sterane
prednisone—Deltasone, Meticorten, Orasone
probenecid—Benemid
procainamide—Pronestyl

GENERIC NAME—REGISTERED TRADE NAME (cont.)

propranolol—Inderal
pyridostigmine—Mestinon, Regonol
quinidine—Cardioquin, Quinaglute, Quinidex, Quinora
rifampin—Rifadin, Rimactane
spectinomycin—Trobicin
spironolactone—Aldactone
streptokinase—Streptase
sulfasalazine—Azulfidine
sulfinpyrazone—Anturane
sulfonylureas—Diabinese, Dymelor, Orinase, Tolinase
terbutaline—Brethine, Bricanyl
tetracycline—Achromycin, Panmycin, Sumycin
thiazide diuretics—Diuril, Dyazide, Esidrix, Exna, Metahydrin,
     Naqua, Oretic, Renese
thyroid—Proloid
L-thyroxine—Levothroid, Synthroid
tolbutamide—Orinase
urokinase—Abbokinase
vasopressin—Pitressin
vincristine—Oncovin
warfarin—Panwarfin

INDEX

ABOUT THE AUTHOR

DR. DANIEL W. FOSTER'S face and reputation are extremely well known to all those people who enjoyed and were intrigued by his very popular weekly television program, "Daniel Foster, M.D.," which was aired nationally by the Public Broadcasting System until Dr. Foster's resignation in 1978. It can still be seen on reruns. In informal style Dr. Foster explained the whole of medicine for the layman and answered barrages of questions. In this book he offers the reader the same perceptive and sound knowledge that he brought to the program.

Born in Marlin, Texas, he has made that state his essential base for many years. He received his M.D. degree in 1955 from the University of Texas Southwestern Medical School, where his academic record was the highest in his class. He served his internship and residency in Dallas and then accepted postdoctoral fellowship appointments in biochemistry, first at the same medical school and then at the National Institutes of Health, Bethesda, Maryland.

He is Professor of Internal Medicine at the University of Texas Health Science Center, and serves as Senior Attending Physician at Parkland Memorial Hospital, Dallas, as well as Consulting Physician at other local hospitals. He is currently Editor of *Diabetes* and has served as Associate Editor of *Metabolism Clinical and Experimental* and *The Journal of Clinical Investigation*.

Dr. Foster has served in government advisory positions, particularly in the area of metabolism study, and is considered a world authority in that subject and the abnormalities of diabetes. He has published many papers in the scientific literature and has been a contributing author to Harrison's *Principles of Internal Medicine* and other books and monographs.

Dr. Foster has been elected to numerous professional societies, including the prestigious American Society of Clinical Investigation and the Association of American Physicians. He and his wife, the former Dorothy Skinner, have three sons and make their home in Dallas.